Noninvasive Imaging of Cerebrovascular Disease

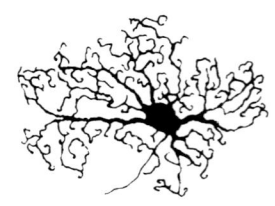

Frontiers of Clinical Neuroscience

Series Editors

Ivan Bodis-Wollner, M.D.
Mt. Sinai School of Medicine
New York

Earl A. Zimmerman, M.D.
Oregon Health Sciences University
Portland

VOLUME 1	**Neurobiology of Mood Disorders** Robert M. Post, M.D., and James C. Ballenger, M.D., *Editors*
VOLUME 2	**Norepinephrine** Michael G. Ziegler, M.D., and C. Raymond Lake, M.D., Ph.D., *Editors*
VOLUME 3	**Evoked Potentials** Roger Q. Cracco, M.D., and Ivan Bodis-Wollner, M.D., *Editors*
VOLUME 4	**Clinical Neuroimaging** William H. Theodore, M.D., *Editor*
VOLUME 5	**Noninvasive Imaging of Cerebrovascular Disease** Jesse Weinberger, M.D., *Editor*

Frontiers of Clinical Neuroscience
VOLUME 5

NONINVASIVE IMAGING OF CEREBROVASCULAR DISEASE

Edited by
JESSE WEINBERGER, M.D.
Department of Neurology
The Mount Sinai School of Medicine
New York, New York

ALAN R. LISS, INC.
New York

Address all Inquiries to the Publisher
Alan R. Liss, Inc., 41 East 11th Street, New York, NY 10003

Copyright © 1989 Alan R. Liss, Inc.

Printed in the United States of America

Under the conditions stated below the owner of copyright for this book hereby grants permission to users to make photocopy reproductions of any part or all of its contents for personal or internal organizational use, or for personal or internal use of specific clients. This consent is given on the condition that the copier pay the stated per-copy fee through the Copyright Clearance Center, Incorporated, 27 Congress Street, Salem, MA 01970, as listed in the most current issue of "Permissions to Photocopy" (Publisher's Fee List, distributed by CCC, Inc.), for copying beyond that permitted by sections 107 or 108 of the US Copyright Law. This consent does not extend to other kinds of copying, such as copying for general distribution, for advertising or promotional purposes, for creating new collective works, or for resale.

While the authors, editors, and publisher believe that drug selection and dosage and the specifications and usage of equipment and devices, as set forth in this book, are in accord with current recommendations and practice at the time of publication, they accept no legal responsibility for any errors or omissions, and make no warranty, express or implied, with respect to material contained herein. In view of ongoing research, equipment modifications, changes in governmental regulations and the constant flow of information relating to drug therapy, drug reactions and the use of equipment and devices, the reader is urged to review and evaluate the information provided in the package insert or instructions for each drug, piece of equipment or device for, among other things, any changes in the instructions or indications of dosage or usage and for added warnings and precautions.

Library of Congress Cataloging-in-Publication Data

Noninvasive imaging of cerebrovascular disease / edited by Jesse Weinberger.
    p.   cm. — (Frontiers of clinical neuroscience ; v. 5)
  Includes bibliographies and index.
  ISBN 0-8451-4504-5
  1. Cerebrovascular disease—Diagnosis. 2. Brain—Blood-vessels—Imaging. 3. Diagnosis, Noninvasive. 4. Cerebral circulation—Measurement. I. Weinberger, Jesse. II. Series.
  [DNLM: 1. Cerebrovascular Disorders—diagnosis. 2. Diagnostic Imaging. W1 FR946DM v. 5 / WL 355 N813]
RC388.5.N65   1988
616.8'1—dc19
DNLM/DLC
for Library of Congress   88-8293
                                            CIP

Contents

Contributors vii

Preface
JESSE WEINBERGER, M.D. ix

1. **Cardiac Ultrasound in Cerebrovascular Disease**
   MARTIN E. GOLDMAN, M.D. 1

2. **Noninvasive Carotid Artery Testing in Cerebrovascular Disease**
   JESSE WEINBERGER, M.D., AND VICTORIA BISCARRA, R.N. 17

3. **Continuous-Wave Doppler Sonography of the Extracranial Brain-Supplying Arteries**
   ERICH BERND RINGELSTEIN, M.D. 27

4. **Duplex Scanning of the Carotid Arteries**
   STEPHEN C. NICHOLLS, M.D., R. EUGENE ZIERLER, M.D., AND D.E. STRANDNESS, JR., M.D. 49

Color Figure Section 67

5. **A Practical Guide to Transcranial Doppler Sonography**
   ERICH BERND RINGELSTEIN, M.D. 75

6. **Magnetic Resonance Imaging (MRI) and Computerized Tomography (CT) in Cerebrovascular Disease**
   GARY GERARD, M.D., DEBRA SHABAS, M.D., AND VIDIA MALHOTRA, M.D. 123

7. **SPECT Perfusion Imaging in Cerebrovascular Disease**
   B. LEONARD HOLMAN, M.D., JEAN-LUC MORETTI, M.D., PH.D., AND THOMAS C. HILL, M.D. 147

8. **Functional Imaging of Brain Ischemia**
   MICHAEL KUSHNER, M.D., AND MARTIN REIVICH, M.D. 163

9. **Cerebral Blood Flow Measurements During Carotid Endarterectomy**
   THORALF M. SUNDT, JR., M.D. 175

Index 187

Contributors

Victoria Biscarra, R.N., Vascular Laboratory, Department of Surgery, The Mount Sinai School of Medicine, New York, NY 10029 **[17]**

Gary Gerard, M.D., Department of Neurology, Winthrop-University Hospital, Mineola, NY 11501 **[123]**

Martin E. Goldman, M.D., Non-Invasive Cardiology, Division of Cardiology, Mount Sinai Medical Center, New York, NY 10029 **[1]**

Thomas C. Hill, M.D., Department of Radiology, Harvard Medical School, Brigham and Women's Hospital and New England Deaconess Hospital, Boston, MA 02115 **[147]**

B. Leonard Holman, M.D., Department of Radiology, Harvard Medical School, Brigham and Women's Hospital and New England Deaconess Hospital, Boston, MA 02115 **[147]**

Michael Kushner, M.D., Cerebrovascular Research Center, Department of Neurology, University of Pennsylvania School of Medicine, Philadelphia, PA 19104-6063 **[163]**

Vidia Malhotra, M.D., Department of Neuroradiology, Beth Israel Medical Center, New York, NY 10003 **[123]**

Jean-Luc Moretti, M.D., Ph.D., Department de Biophysique et Medecine Nucleaire, Bobigny, Paris 13-93, France **[147]**

Stephen C. Nicholls, M.D., Department of Surgery, School of Medicine, University of Washington, Seattle, WA 98195 **[49]**

Martin Reivich, M.D., Cerebrovascular Research Center, Department of Neurology, University of Pennsylvania School of Medicine, Philadelphia, PA 19104-6063 **[163]**

Erich Bernd Ringelstein, M.D., Department of Neurology, Technische Hochschule, 5100 Aachen, Federal Republic of Germany **[27,75]**

Debra Shabas, M.D., Department of Neurology, Beth Israel Medical Center, New York, NY 10003 **[123]**

D.E. Strandness, Jr., M.D., Department of Surgery, School of Medicine, University of Washington, Seattle, WA 98195 **[49]**

Thoralf M. Sundt, Jr., M.D., Department of Neurosurgery, Mayo Clinic, Rochester, MN 55904 **[175]**

Jesse Weinberger, M.D., Department of Neurology, The Mount Sinai School of Medicine, New York, NY 10029 **[17]**

R. Eugene Zierler, M.D., Department of Surgery, School of Medicine, University of Washington, Seattle, WA 98195; present address: Vascular Surgery Section, Seattle VA Medical Center, Seattle, WA 98108 **[49]**

The number in brackets is the opening page number of the contributor's article.

Preface

The last decade has produced significant advances in the understanding and management of ischemic cerebrovascular disease. Laboratory studies of the mechanisms of cerebral ischemic damage and clinical studies of new treatment modalities promise still greater progress in the next decade. However, ischemic stroke has a variety of causes. Atherosclerotic occlusive disease of the extracranial vessels, proliferative vasculopathy of intracranial vessels associated with hypertension, and cardioembolic phenomena account for the majority of cerebral infarctions. Both to treat patients with stroke appropriately and to interpret the potential benefit of experimental therapeutic regimens, modern imaging techniques are necessary to define the source of cerebral ischemia.

The purpose of this volume is to provide the clinician caring for stroke patients with a working knowledge of current noninvasive techniques employed to visualize the pathophysiology of cerebral ischemia without exposing the patient to risk. Information about the etiology and mechanisms of stroke derived from such studies can be invaluable in determining the optimal therapy and prevention of stroke in individual patients.

The first four chapters in this volume concentrate on imaging the extracranial sources of cerebral ischemia. The first chapter provides a summary of cardiac imaging techniques that define cardioembolic sources of stroke. The next three chapters delineate noninvasive tests now available to determine the extent of extracranial atherosclerotic vascular disease and how to apply this information to the clinical management of patients with transient ischemic attacks and stroke.

The second half of the volume is devoted to imaging studies of the intracranial vessels by transcranial Doppler techniques and magnetic resonance imaging (MRI) and imaging of the pathophysiology of cerebral ischemic damage by MRI, single photon emission tomography (SPECT), and positron emission tomography (PET). The last chapter describes cerebrovascular imaging techniques employed during artificial occlusion of a carotid artery during endarterectomy. While carotid artery surgery is certainly not noninvasive, the information obtained about cerebral circulatory and physiologic function during iatrogenic carotid artery occlusion is invaluable to further understanding of the mechanisms of ischemic stroke.

The contributors trust that this volume will provide new insight for the clinician caring for stroke patients. We also hope that it will stimulate new interest in the field of cerebrovascular disease that could lead to new advances.

JESSE WEINBERGER, M.D.

Cardiac Ultrasound in Cerebrovascular Disease

Martin E. Goldman, MD

Non-Invasive Cardiology, Division of Cardiology, Mount Sinai Medical Center, New York, New York 10029

CARDIAC ULTRASOUND FOR THE NEUROLOGIST

Cardiac ultrasound is a totally noninvasive technique utilizing high frequency sound waves to evaluate motion and functioning of the heart muscle and valves. First efforts to use reflected sound waves to evaluate cardiac function were obtained with a commercial ultrasonoscope. The first clinical application of echocardiography was a single beam for the detection of mitral stenosis [1]. Since then, significant strides have been made in ultrasound equipment, which can now image the heart in real-time and evaluate blood flow parameters. Specifically, the development of Doppler echocardiography and color flow Doppler mapping facilitates simultaneous evaluation of anatomic and blood flow information.

M-MODE AND 2-D ECHOCARDIOGRAPHY

The initial echocardiographic equipment utilized a single, thin sound wave beam to interrogate the cardiac chambers, termed an m-mode view of the heart. Subsequently, multiple beams were coalesced to image the heart simultaneously, yielding a wide sector or wide beam through the heart called two-dimensional echocardiography (Fig. 1-1).

M-mode echocardiography provides information about a single perpendicular line through the heart over time: an easily quantifiable hard copy printout of linear information obtained over several seconds.

Two-dimensional echocardiography (2-D echo) images a wide sector of the heart with multiple beams (while being recorded on video cassette recorder) to provide rapid, on-line qualitative information. Currently, both m-mode and 2-D echoes are performed simultaneously, with accurate alignment of the m-mode beam by 2-D echo guidance. Therefore, a routine ultrasound exam today incorporates both 2-D and m-mode information.

There are several routine echocardiographic views obtainable by two-dimensional echocardiography. The transducer placed in the third left intercostal space provides the long axis view of the heart, which demonstrates the left atrium, aorta, mitral valve, aortic valve, and the basal half of the left ventricle (Fig. 1-2). By rotating the transducer 90°, the short axis view of the left ventricle is seen (Fig. 1-3). This view is similar to putting the ventricle through a slicer and seeing sequential round slices of the heart from base to apex. This view is extremely important to evaluate regional ventricular function. By placing the transducer on the apex of the heart, all four chambers can be visualized (Fig. 1-4). From the apical four-chamber view, the relative sizes of the atria and ventricles can be determined. The transducer can also be placed subxyphoid to obtain a four-chamber view or over the suprasternal notch to evaluate the great vessels. Obtaining multiple views facilitates a stereoscopic anatomic approach. Similarly, multiple views are often required, to obtain maximum blood flow velocities by Doppler.

Noninvasive Imaging of Cerebrovascular Disease, pages 1–15
© 1989 Alan R. Liss, Inc.

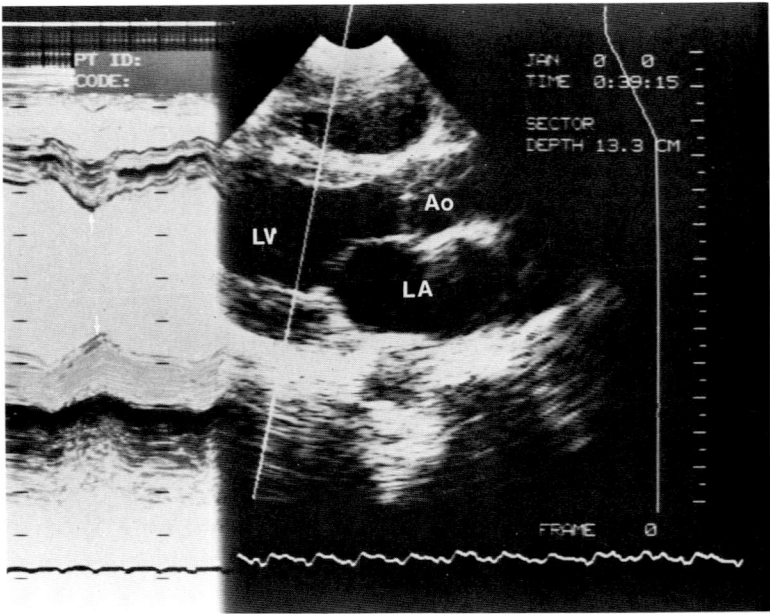

Figure 1-1. Simultaneous m-mode and 2-D echo. Right side image is of long axis left ventricle (LV). A perpendicular, "ice pick" beam is isolated to obtain the m-mode (left side). Note the 2-D is a single frozen frame of a wide sector, while the m-mode is an isolated view of the LV muscle over a longer period of time, showing thickening (systole) and relaxing (diastole). Ao, aorta; LA, left atrium.

DOPPLER ECHOCARDIOGRAPHY

The Doppler principle was first formulated by Christian Doppler in 1842 [2]. Since then, the principle has been utilized to evaluate blood flow in large blood vessels as well as inside the cardiac chambers.

The Doppler shift defines a change of a sound wave frequency as a function of the velocity of an observed moving object. A practical example of the use of Doppler is the evaluation by a radar gun of the speed of a car in motion. A sound wave directed parallel to the vehicle is emitted at a given frequency to assess the speed of the car. As the sound wave is reflected back off the car to the emitting source, its frequency is shifted as a function of the speed of the car. This Doppler shift can be calculated to determine the precise velocity of the moving vehicle. Doppler can also determine flow direction: flow towards the transducer is positive, flow away is negative. Additionally, in biological systems, blood flow is either laminar, with all of the fluid flowing with a similar velocity, or turbulent, as seen with stenotic or regurgitant lesions in which blood flow velocities are varied and much higher than normal. These two types of flows can be detected both by their display on the video screen as well as by their distinctive auditory pattern. Doppler is displayed as a time interval histogram of different velocities so that blood flow moving in a uniform velocity is an envelope edge rising and falling coinciding with blood flow, whereas turbulent blood flow is a grayish, filled-in, higher envelope incorporating multiple velocities (Fig. 1-5).

Types of Doppler

PULSED MODE

This mode utilizes a single beam directed through the heart that can localize information along any point of that beam. Sound wave is sent to a specific location along that beam and returns to the emitting source, providing precise localizing information about blood flow velocity only at the sampled site (Fig. 1-5).

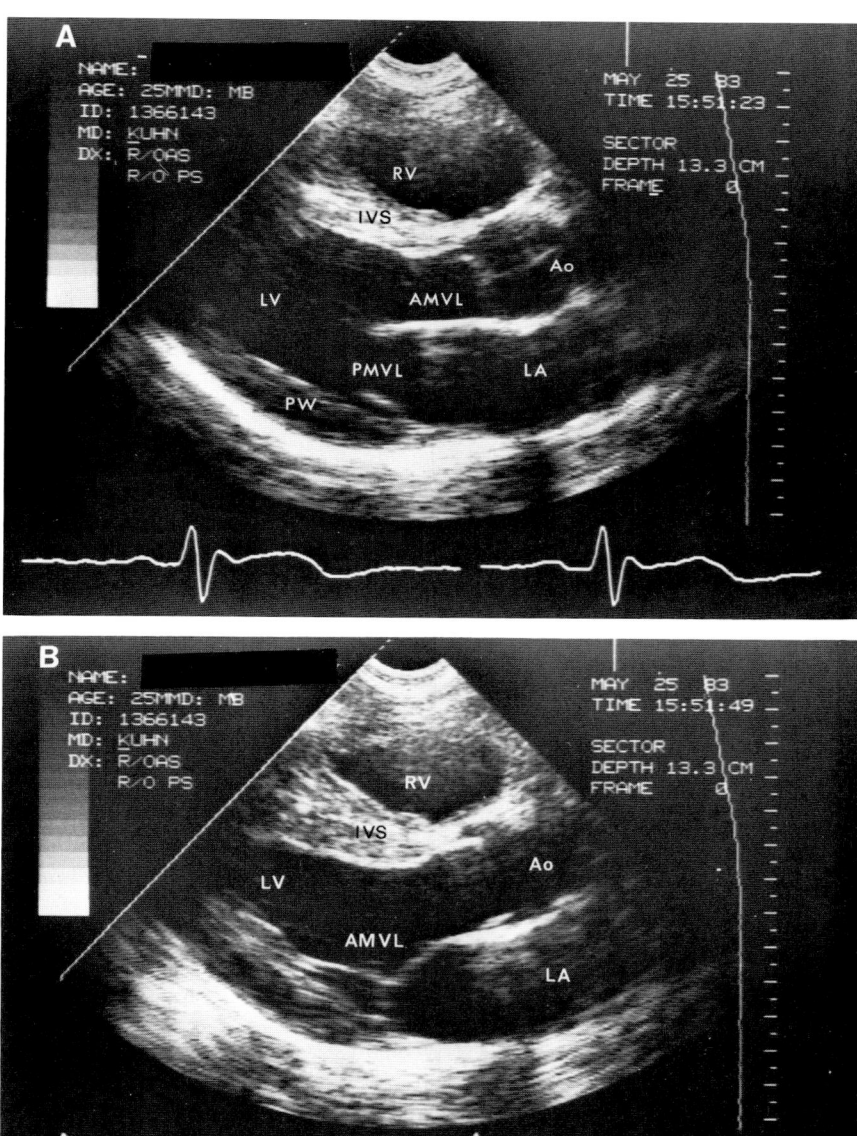

Figure 1–2. A: Long axis view. Diastole: the mitral valve is open, the aortic valve closed. **B:** Long axis view. Systole: the ventricle contracts, forcing blood out the aortic valve. AMVL, anterior mitral valve leaflet; A, aorta; IVS, interventricular septum; LA, left atrium; LV, left ventricle; PMVL, posterior mitral valve leaflet; PW, posterior wall of LV.

4   Goldman

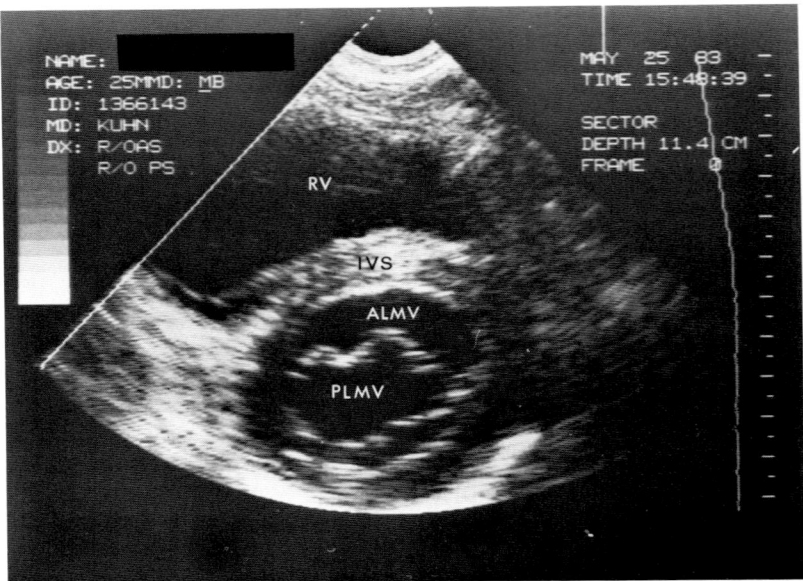

Figure 1–3. Short axis. Mitral valve level, diastole. ALMV, anterior leaflet mitral valve; IVS, interventricular septum; PLMV, posterior leaflet mitral valve; RV, right ventricle.

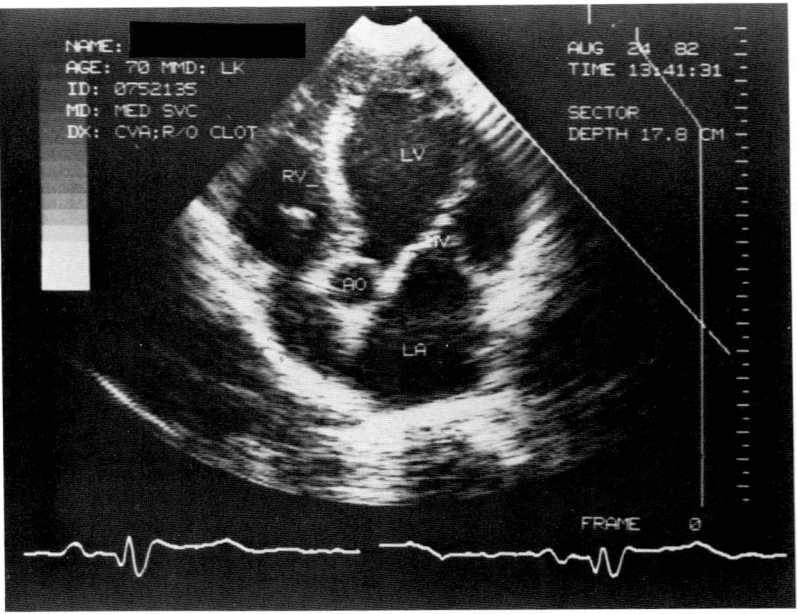

Figure 1–4. Apical view. AO, aorta; LA, left atrium; LV, left ventricle; MV, mitral valve; RV, right ventricle.

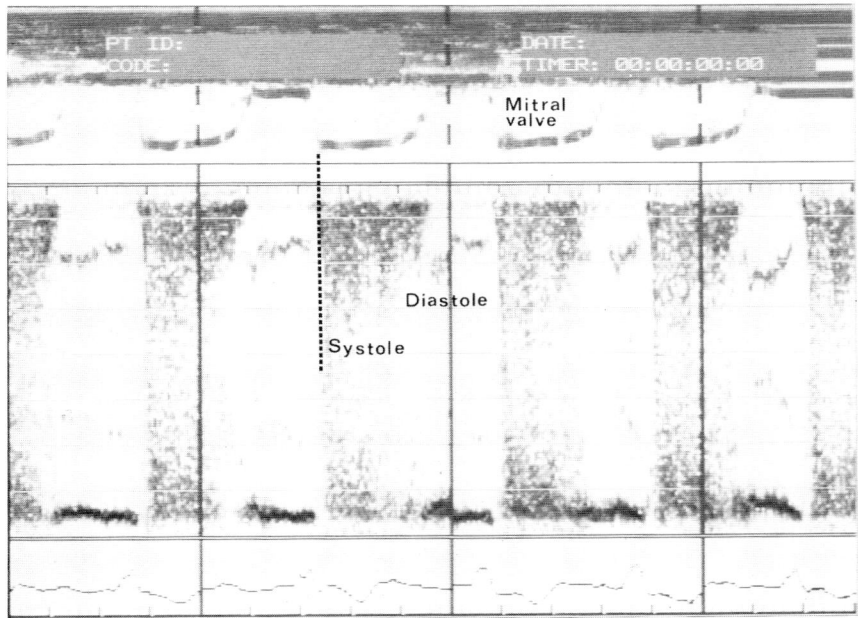

Figure 1–5. Pulsed doppler. Patient with mitral regurgitation. The m-mode of mitral valve on top, Doppler below. Simultaneously with mitral valve closure (dotted line), the Doppler demonstrated turbulent flow consistent with mitral regurgitation.

However, because of the necessary time for the sound wave to be emitted and to return, higher velocity events such as stenotic lesions cannot be accurately assessed by the pulsed technique.

CONTINUOUS-WAVE

This mode assesses the ultrasound shift along a continuous line, emitting and sampling simultaneously. Because there is no time delay in waiting for a return of a given packet of sound wave, there can be continuous sampling and even high velocities can be assessed (Fig. 1-6). Therefore, continuous-wave Doppler is valuable for the assessment of stenotic lesions, while pulsed Doppler provides specific localization of murmurs such as mitral or aortic regurgitation or ventricular septal defects. However, quantification of regurgitant lesions is difficult by the single-beam technique.

COLOR-FLOW

Color-flow or real-time Doppler imaging allows visualization of blood flow information

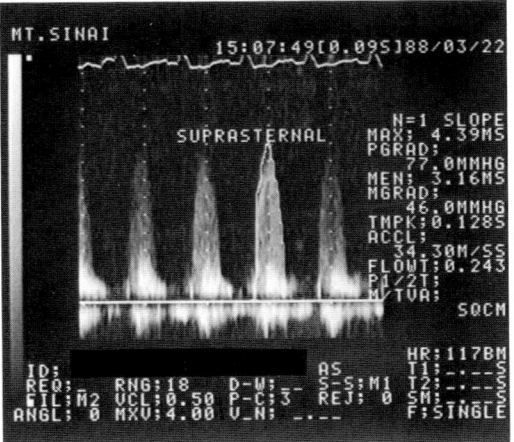

Figure 1–6. Continuous-wave Doppler. Suprasternal notch Doppler of patient with aortic stenosis. The peak gradient was 77 mmHg, the mean 46 mmHg, consistant with severe aortic stenosis.

6 Goldman

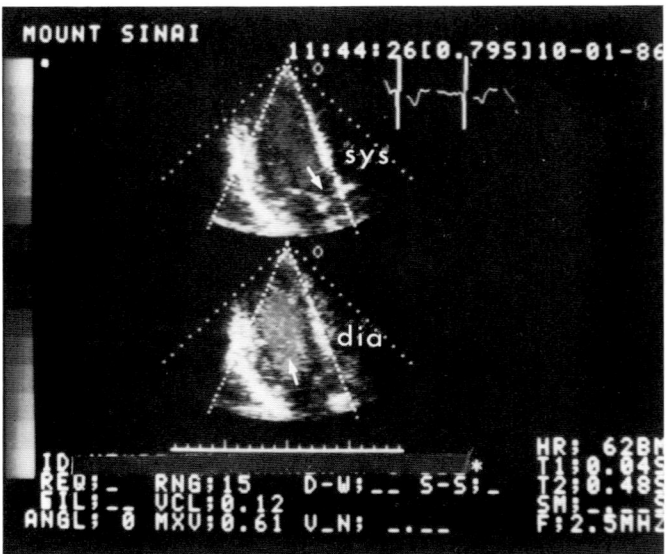

Figure 1–7. Color Doppler. During diastole (**lower**), blood moving into the ventricle (and toward transducer) is depicted in orange, while during systole (**upper**), blood moving out the aorta is depicted in blue. (Reproduced in color on page 68.)

over a wide sector. The following analogy can be applied: single beam imaging is to wide beam imaging as m-mode is to 2-D echocardiography or as pulsed Doppler is to color-flow Doppler. Color-flow samples Doppler frequency shifts over a wide sector simultaneously. The Doppler shift is represented in color-coded information: blood flow moving towards the transducer in shades of red or orange, blood flow moving away from the transducer in shades of blue (Fig. 1-7). The higher velocities are in lighter colors. Because color-flow Doppler is a pulsed system, blood flow movement exceeding the assigned frequencies cause "aliasing" and is presented in a mosaic or multicolored pattern. Therefore, stenotic lesions cannot be assessed easily. However, the major advantage of color flow mapping is the ability to localize abnormal (regurgitant or congenital defect) flow patterns and to potentially quantify their severity [3].

CLINICAL APPLICATION

Mitral Stenosis

The first cardiac disease to be described by echocardiography was mitral stenosis. Rheumatic disease causes fibrosis with subsequent calcification and fusion of the mitral commissures and thickening of the leaflets and gradual narrowing of the valve orifice. The cardiac sequelae are dilation of left atrium, atrial arrhythmias, particularly atrial fibrillation and the development of atrial thrombi. The left ventricle is usually not involved in the disease process unless there is concomitant rheumatic myopathy. M-mode echocardiography will show thickening of the anterior and posterior leaflets. The posterior leaflet, which normally moves separately from the anterior leaflet, moves anteriorly in an abnormal fashion, and a large left atrium is also seen. By two-dimensional echocardiography, doming of the valve and the actual valve orifice itself can be planimetered to obtain the actual valve area (Fig. 1-8). Doppler pressure half-time calculation can also accurately determine the mitral valve area [4]. Color-flow Doppler facilitates identification and quantification of potential mitral regurgitation.

Mitral Regurgitation

Mitral regurgitation can be caused by multiple disease entities: endocarditis, mitral valve prolapse, ruptured chordae, ruptured papillary muscle, inferior wall myocardial infarction, or ventricular dilation in cardiomyopathies. Spe-

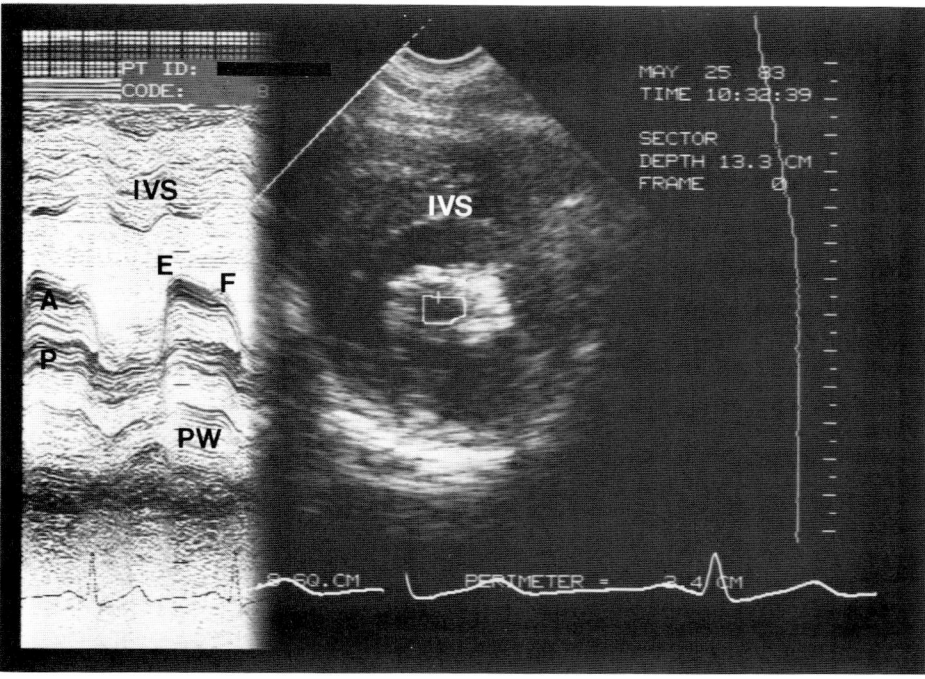

Figure 1–8. Mitral stenosis. M-mode echo (**left**) demonstrated the thickened anterior (A) and posterior (P) leaflets of the mitral valve, and decreased E-F slope, consistent with delayed LV filling 2-D echo (**right**), shows a thickened mitral valve that can be planimetered to obtain an accurate valve area (2.4 cm^2).

cific valvular pathology can be determined with echocardiography, and the extent and severity of regurgitation can be assessed by color-flow Doppler (Fig. 1-9). Mitral valve prolapse, which is probably the most common cardiac abnormality, is caused by myxomatous degeneration and thickening of the mitral valve leaflets and their support apparatus. During systole, either the anterior, posterior, or both mitral valve leaflets prolapse backwards into the left atrium (Fig. 1-10). The left atrium may be enlarged depending upon the severity of mitral regurgitation. Mitral valve prolapse has been associated with cerebral vascular events including microemboli to the ophthalmic or retinal arteries, whose source may be platelet aggregates on the ruffled and redundant mitral leaflets. An m-mode echocardiographic study reported that those mitral valve prolapse patients with the most redundant, thickest valves were at greatest risk for subsequent complications. Dental prophylaxis is recommended by the American Heart Association only for those patients with mitral valve prolapse who also have mitral regurgitation.

Aortic Stenosis

Aortic stenosis can be due to rheumatic heart disease, aortic sclerosis (progressive degeneration and calcification of the valve with aging), or a congenital, bicuspid aortic valve. The etiology of the stenosis will usually dictate when symptoms will develop (bicuspid in the fifth decade, sclerosis by the sixth or seventh). The major presenting symptoms are syncope, shortness of breath, congestive heart failure, angina, and sudden death. The extent of aortic valve stenosis can be assessed directly by two-dimensional echocardiography (Fig. 1-11), and the exact valve area can be measured by Doppler echocardiography (Fig. 1-6) [5].

Tumors of the Heart

Left atrial myxomas are the most common primary malignancies of the heart. They can

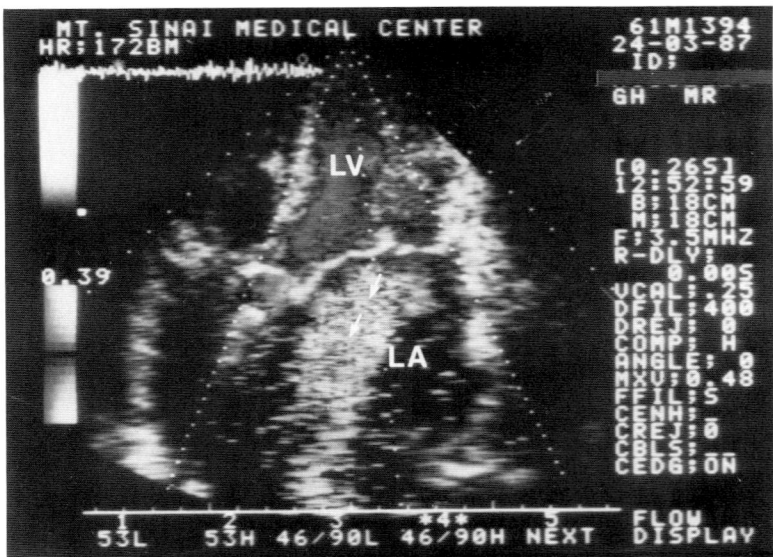

Figure 1–9. Color Doppler. Mitral regurgitation. During systole, blood moving out the left ventricle into the aorta is in deep blue, while mitral regurgitation (arrows) into a large left atrium is a turbulent mosaic pattern of turquoise and yellow. LA, left atrium; LV, left ventricle. (Reproduced in color on page 69.)

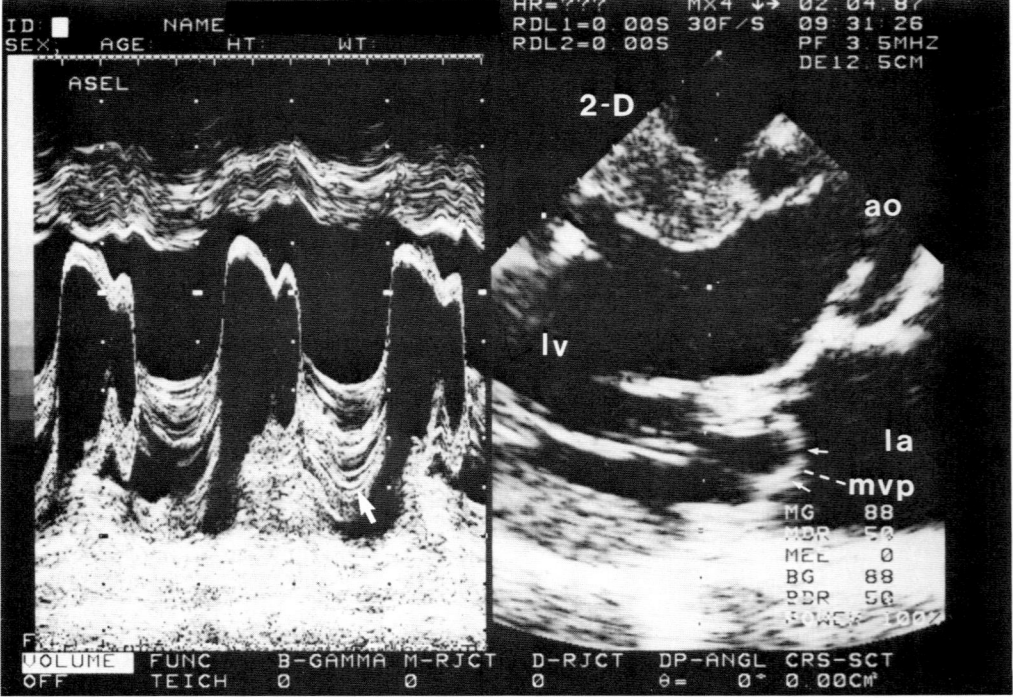

Figure 1–10. Mitral valve prolapse (mvp). 2-D echo (**right**) demonstrates hammocking posteriorly (small arrows) of the mitral valve. The m-mode image (**left**) also shows systolic hammocking (large arrow).

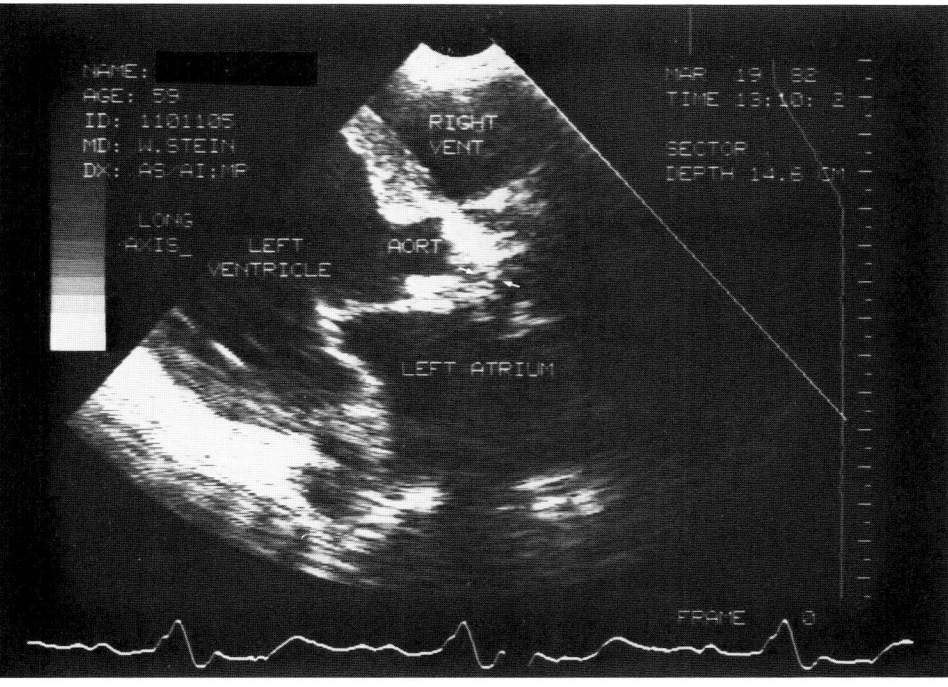

Figure 1–11. Aortic stenosis. Long axis view demonstrating heavily calcified aortic valve (AORT) with very stenotic orifice (arrow).

present as arrhythmias, syncope, congestive heart failure, or with systemic symptoms. By echocardiography, the myxomas are easily imaged as large masses attached to the interatrial septum flopping into the left ventricle in diastole from its left atrial attachment and prolapsing back in the left atrium during systole (Fig. 1-12). They are usually benign and can be excised from their base quite easily. Other tumors of the heart include myxomas in other cardiac chambers, leiomyosarcomas, or metastatic lesions such as melanomas and lymphomas.

Pericardial Diseases

The pericardium is a membrane surrounding the heart that contains a small amount of serous fluid for lubrication of the contracting heart. In certain diseases such as renal failure, congestive heart failure, viral illnesses, thyroid disease, or malignant metastatic disease, large pericardial effusions can develop that can cause hemodynamic compromise (cardiac tamponade). Two-dimensional echocardiography can clearly delineate the extent and location of the pericardial effusion. Echo can also help differentiate the potential etiology by determining the nodularity and extent of pericardial thickening.

Myocardial Function

One of the most important applications of echocardiography is in the evaluation of myocardial contractility. Two-dimensional echocardiography is the only technique that allows direct assessment of ventricular muscle thickening. Other techniques such as gated blood pool scanning or even cardiac catheterization show motion of the endocardium indirectly and myocardial function is inferred. Two-dimensional echocardiography directly evaluates muscle thickening. Areas of abnormal function related to myocardial infarction, ischemia, or cardiomyopathy may be located and their extend quantified [6]. Therefore, 2-D echo is extremely valuable in the differential diagnosis of congestive heart failure and identifying ventricular aneurysms, frequently the

10 Goldman

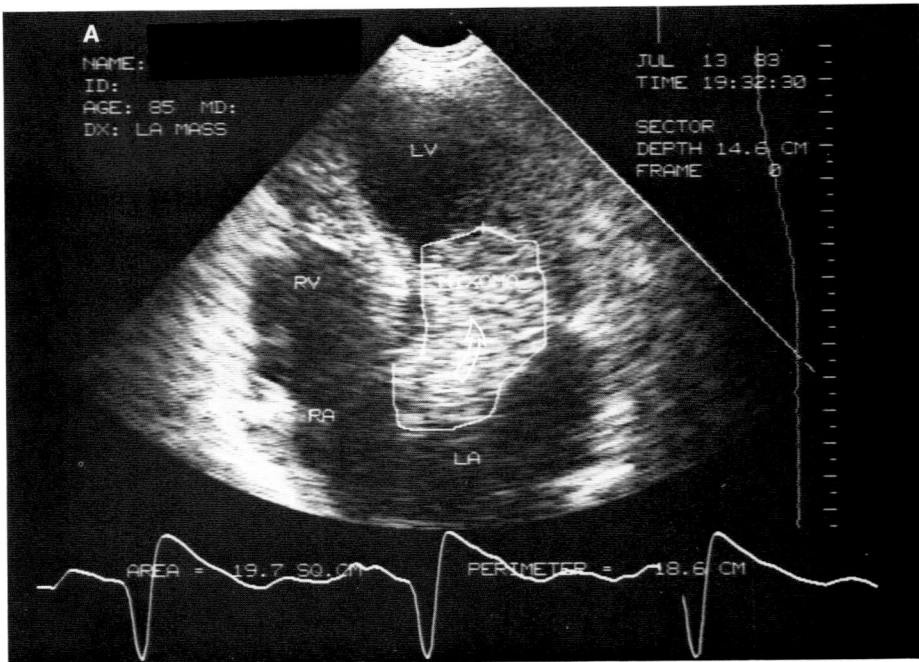

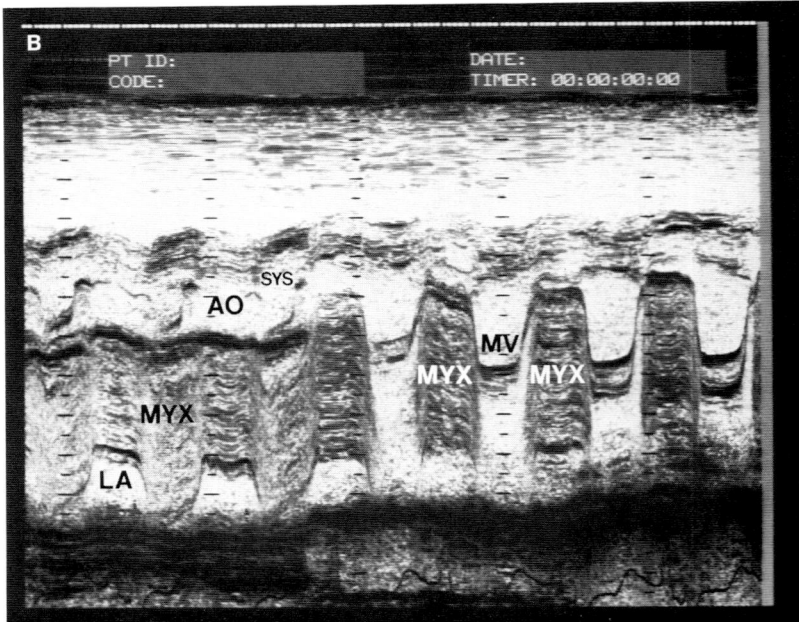

Figure 1–12. Left atrial myxoma. **A:** 2-D echo apical view demonstrating large myxoma (19.6 cm^2) prolapsing into the left ventricle during diastole (arrow). **B:** Classic m-mode echo demonstrating the diastolic motion of the myxoma through the mitral valve (right side) and returning on its stalk to the atrium (left side).

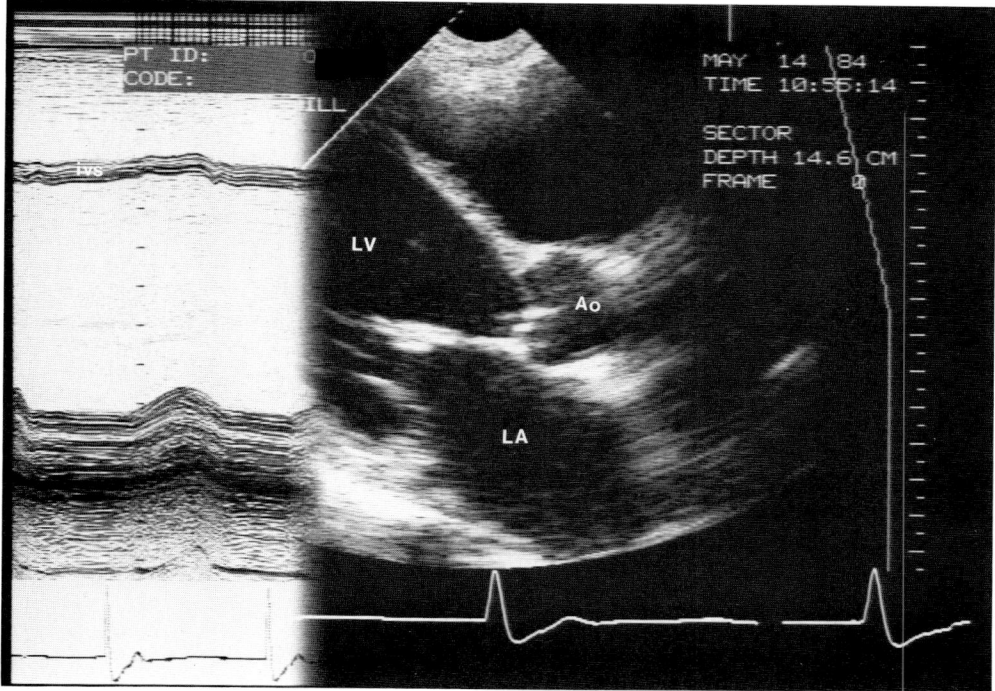

Figure 1–13. Dilated cardiomyopathy. 2-D echo (**right**) demonstrated a dilated cavity and thin walls. The m-mode (**left**) also showed an enlarged cavity with thinned septum (ivs) and minimal systolic thickening.

source of thrombi, In dilated cardiomyopathy, the left ventricular cavity is dilated and the walls are hypocontractile (Fig. 1-13).

In Hypertrophic cardiomyopathy, a segment of the ventricular muscle (usually the septum) is asymetrically thickened, causing LV outflow tract obstruction during systole, mimicking aortic stenosis (Fig. 1-14). Restrictive myopathy is due to infiltration of the myocardium causing initially diastolic dysfunction and subsequent systolic dysfunction. Heart failure, arrhythmias and ventricular thrombi can be complications of any of the cardiomyopathies.

Embolic Events

Potential sources of emboli from the heart include left atrial masses (myxomas, thrombi; Fig. 1-15), left ventricular masses (thrombi, Fig. 1-16; tumors), vegetations (endocarditis, Fig. 1-17), calcification (aortic, Fig. 1-11, or mitral stenosis, Fig. 1-8), platelet emboli (mitral valve prolapse, Fig. 1-10), parodoxical emboli (via a right to left shunt at the atrial or ventricular level, or via patent foramen ovale, Fig. 1-18), or thrombus on a prosthetic valve. Echocardiography can clearly identify each of these abnormalites.

Evaluating the Stroke Patient

Evaluation of a patient with a cerebrovascular event should include a two-dimensional echocardiogram under certain circumstances. The highest yield will be obtained in those patients having a positive cardiac history (a myocardial infarction on electrocardiogram, atrial, arrhythmias (particularly atrial fibrillation), physical evidence of heart failure, the presence of a heart murmur or known valvular disease, or possible endocarditis), therefore increasing the likelihood of a cardiac source. Younger people may have mitral valve prolapse, other valvular disease, or intracardiac shunts previously undetected may also be worthwhile candidates for an echocardiographic evaluation.

SUMMARY

Two-dimensional echocardiography with Doppler can provide rapid noninvasive infor-

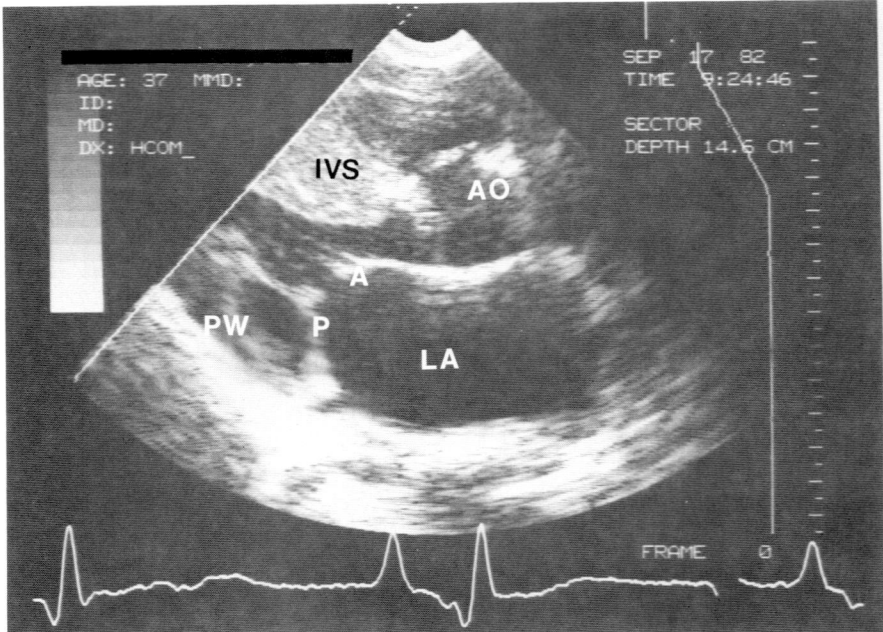

Figure 1–14. Hypertrophic cardiomyopathy (HCOM). 2-D echo, long axis view, depicts a markedly thickened interventricular septum (IVS) out of proportion to the posterior wall (PW). Additionally, there is a ground-glass shimmering appearance of the septum due to the reflectance pattern of the myocardial disarray typical of HCOM.

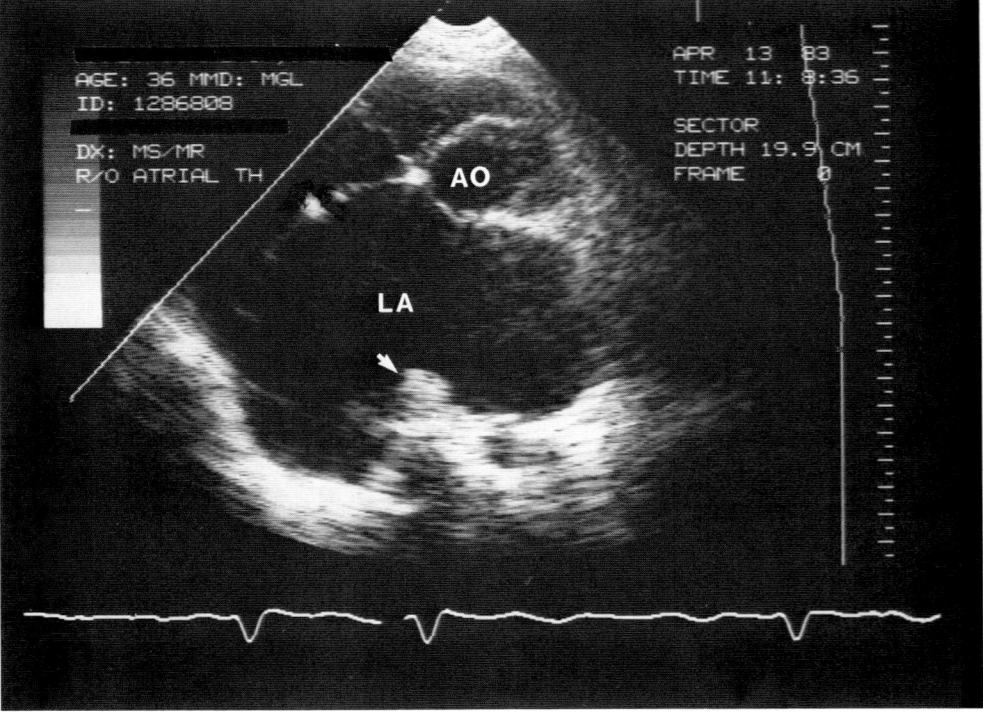

Figure 1–15. Left atrial thrombus. Short axis view of a markedly enlarged left atrium and an echo-dense oval structure, a thrombus.

Cardiac Ultrasound in Cerebrovascular Disease 13

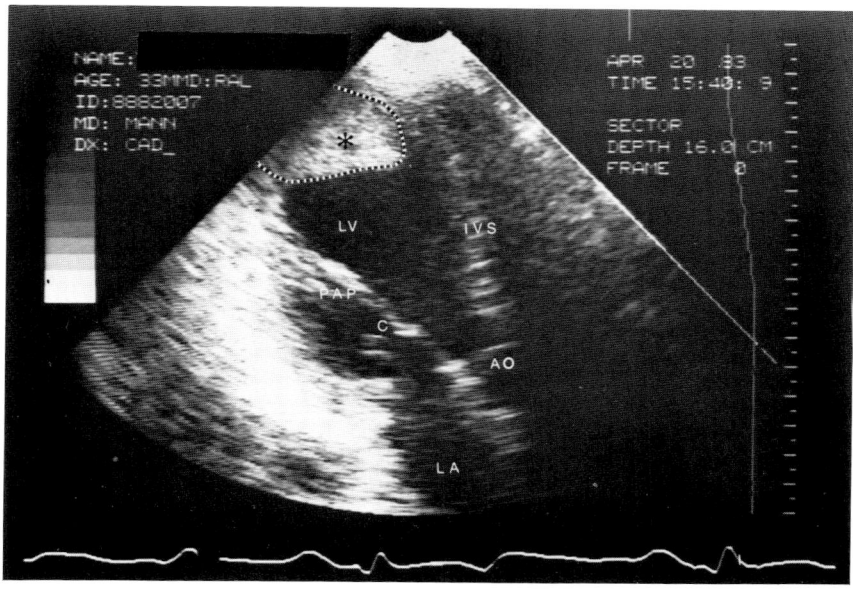

Figure 1–16. Left ventricular thrombus. Apical view demonstrating large thrombus (asterisk and outlined area) that fills the entire apex. C = chordeae; PAP = papillary muscle).

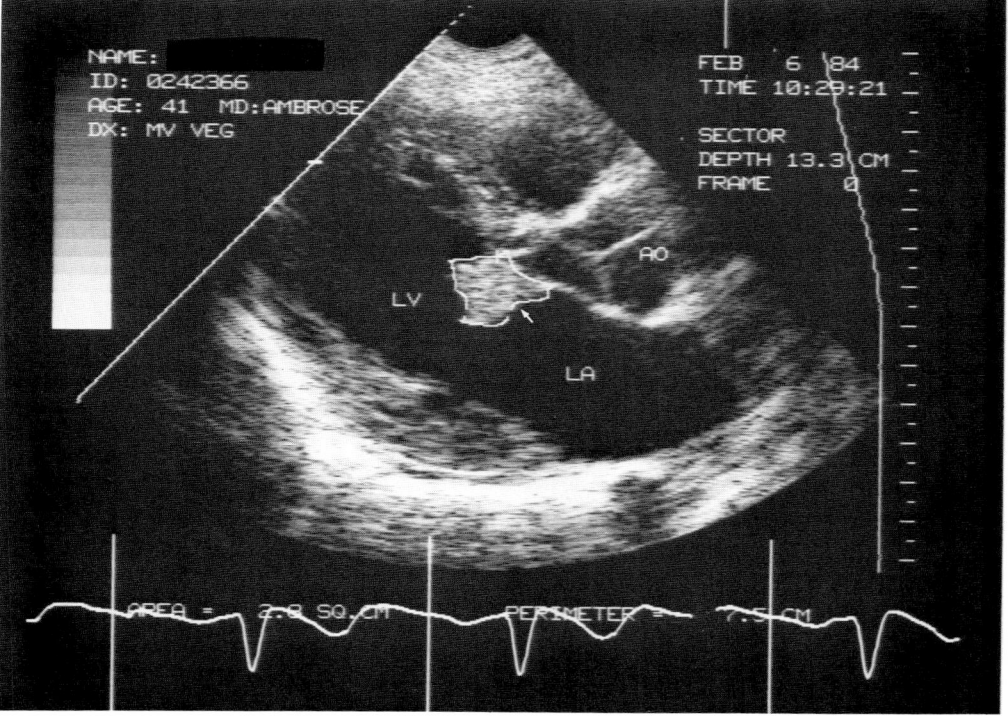

Figure 1–17. Mitral valve vegetation. 2-D long axis view of large anterior mitral valve leaflet vegetation (arrow).

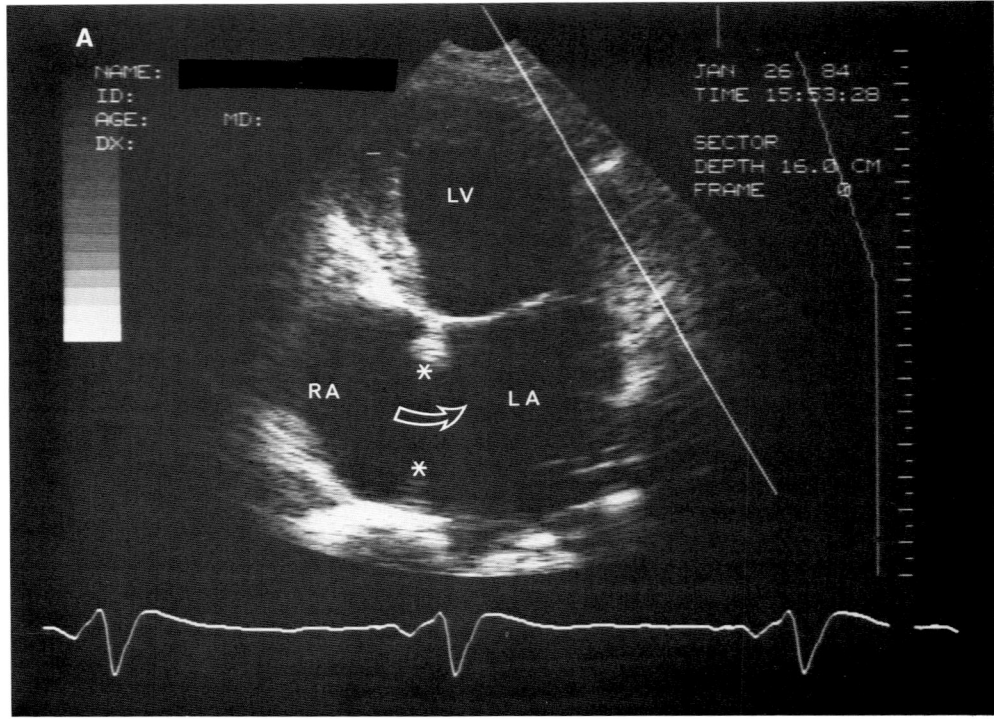

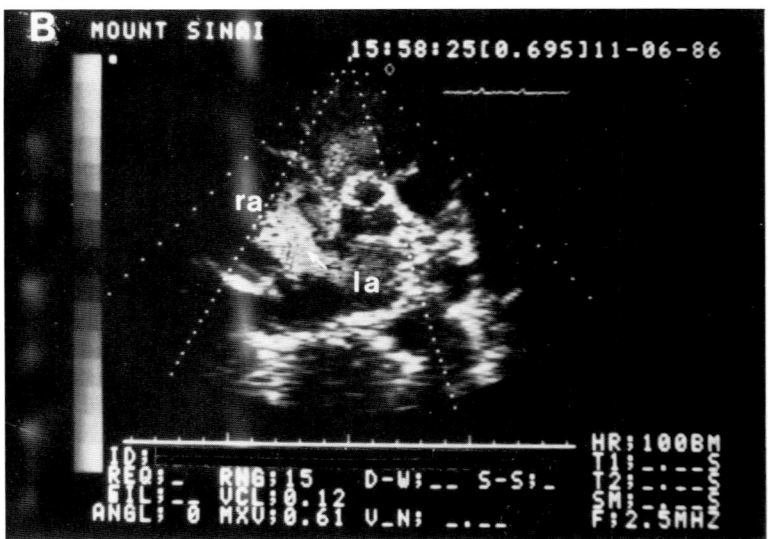

Figure 1–18. Atrial septal defect. **A:** Apical view demonstrating large area of echo dropout (asterisks), which is the location of an atrial septal defect, secundum type. Shunt flow is usually from left to right side. However, with pulmonary hypertension or even occasionally during a valsalva maneuver or coughing, the shunt can transiently flow right to left. **B:** Color Doppler of short axis view demonstrating left to right shunt (arrow, orange color) at the atrial level. (Figure 1-18B Reproduced in color on page 69.)

mation regarding cardiac function and potential valvular abnormalities. Echocardiography directly evaluates cardiac muscle function and can localize sources of thromboembolic events. Echocardiography can be repeated safely to evaluate progression or resolution of thrombi or changes in ventricular function with therapy. Color-flow echocardiography provides noninvasive quantification of valvular regurgitant lesions. Continuous-wave Doppler accurately assesses the severity of valve stenosis. Therefore, echocardiography is a valuable technique for the neurologist in assessing potential cardiac etiologies of neurologic diseases.

ACKNOWLEDGMENTS

I thank Valentin Fuster, M.D. for his critical review of the manuscript and Ms. Linda Felix for her secretarial support.

References

1. Elder I (1956) Ultrasound cardiogram in mitral valve disease. *Acta Chir Scand* 111:230.
2. Doppler CJ (1842) Uber das farbige Licht der Dopplesterne. *Ab Handlungen der Koniglishen Bohmischen Gessellschaft der Wissenchaften* 11:485.
3. Sahn DJ (1985) Real-time two dimensional echo Doppler flow mapping. *Circulation* 71:849.
4. Hatle L, Angelsen B, Tromsdal A (1979) Noninvasive assessment of atrioventricular pressure half-time by Doppler Ultrasound. *Circulation* 60:1096.
5. Currie PJ, Seward JB, Reeder GS, Vlietstra RE, Bresnahan DR, Bresnahan JF, Smith NC, Hagler DJ, Tajik AJ (1985) Continuous-wave Doppler echocardiographic assessment of severity of calcific aortic stenosis: A simultaneous Doppler-catheter correlative study in 100 adult patients. *Circulation* 71:1162.
6. Kloner RA, Parisi A (1987) Acute myocardial and prognostic application of two-dimensional echocardiography. *Circulation* 75:521.

Noninvasive Carotid Artery Testing in Cerebrovascular Disease

Jesse Weinberger, MD, and Victoria Biscarra, RN

Department of Neurology (J.W.) and Vascular Laboratory, Department of Surgery (V.B.), The Mount Sinai School of Medicine, New York, New York 10029

THE CAROTID ARTERY IN THE PATHOPHYSIOLOGY OF STROKE

The extracranial carotid artery is a potential source of cerebrovascular disease because atheroma develop at the bifurcation of the cervical carotid into the internal and external carotid arteries [1,2]. Great emphasis has been placed on atherosclerosis at the carotid artery bifurcation in the management of patients with cerebrovascular disease because the cervical carotid artery is accessible to surgical intervention [3]. Atherosclerotic disease at the carotid artery bifurcation can often be detected on routine examination of the patient prior to the occurrence of a completed cerebrovascular accident by obtaining a history of transient episodes of focal neurologic dysfunction [4] or by auscultation of a cervical arterial bruit in the asymptomatic patient [5].

The management of patients with atherosclerotic disease at the carotid artery bifurcation is controversial because while the prevalence of atheroma is quite high in the elderly population [1,2], the incidence of stroke due to an ipsilateral carotid artery lesion is from 10 to 20% [1,2], even when the patient has had an episode of transient ischemic attack [6]. In addition, many patients are diagnosed as having a transient ischemic attack when they have an episode of dizziness or syncope unrelated to carotid artery disease and may even undergo carotid endarterectomy. This may be deleterious to some patients, because angiography to define a carotid artery lesion and carotid endarterectomy are not innocuous procedures, with a complication rate of about 1% for angiography [7] and a complication rate of 1 to 15% for carotid endarterectomy [6]. The goal of noninvasive carotid artery testing is to elucidate the extent of atherosclerotic disease at the carotid artery bifurcation in patients with both symptomatic and asymptomatic lesions so that a rational judgement can be made as to the most appropriate method of treatment in each individual patient without subjecting all patients to invasive procedures.

Atherosclerotic disease at the carotid artery bifurcation can cause stroke or transient ischemic attack by embolizing thrombus to the intracranial vasculature or by reducing blood supply to the cerebral hemisphere from hemodynamic obstruction to flow. Embolization is thought to be the primary mechanism for stroke from the carotid artery bifurcation [8], because the ipsilateral cerebral hemisphere usually receives considerable collateral blood supply from the contralateral carotid artery and the posterior circulation through the circle of Willis and from the ipsilateral external carotid artery circulation.

There is considerable evidence that a combination of hemodynamic and embolic factors contribute to the occurrence of a completed cerebrovascular accident from cervical carotid artery disease, with patients having hemodynamically obstructive lesions being more prone to stroke than patients with nonobstructive lesions [5,9–11]. Noninvasive carotid artery testing must identify both nonobstructive and obstructive lesions at the carotid bifurcation as well as define hemodynamic factors in

Noninvasive Imaging of Cerebrovascular Disease, pages 17–25
© 1989 Alan R. Liss, Inc.

THE NONINVASIVE TEST BATTERY

There are several methods for identifying lesions at the carotid artery bifurcation. Indirect tests of perfusion pressure can be made by measuring ophthalmic artery pressure and assessing direction of flow from the internal to the external carotid artery by directional Doppler at the supraorbital ridge. Direct imaging of flow at the carotid artery bifurcation can be obtained using Doppler techniques, and atherosclerotic plaque can be visualized by real-time B-mode ultrasonography. Each has a role in the evaluation of the patient with cerebrovascular disease. Using a battery of tests increases the accuracy of the carotid artery evaluation and provides complementary physiologic and morphologic information that is helpful in making therapeutic decisions.

Measurement of Ophthalmic Artery Pressure

Indirect measurement of perfusion pressure in the internal carotid artery can be made by obtaining the blood pressure in the ophthalmic artery (the first intracranial branch of the internal carotid artery), by ophthalmodynamometry [12], or pneumooculoplethysmography [13]. Ophthalmodynamometry is performed by observing the pulsations of the retinal arteries in the ocular fundus while applying pressure to the globe. When the diastolic pressure is reached, the vessels begin to collapse in diastole and refill in systole. When the systolic pressure is reached, the vessels do not refill in systole. The advantage of this technique is that it can measure the diastolic pressure, which may be a more sensitive indicator of underlying carotid artery pathology. The disadvantage is that it is subjective and difficult to perform, particularly when there is retinal vasculopathy from diabetes or hypertension.

Pneumooculoplethysmography is performed by producing a vacuum on the surface of the sclera of the eye to increase intraocular pressure and recording the distortion of the eye by the pulse wave from the ophthalmic artery with a pulse volume recorder. As the intraocular pressure is reached, the pulse wave diminishes until it is obliterated. The pressure at which the pulse wave returns while reducing the vacuum is recorded as the ophthalmic artery pressure [13]. This method is less sensitive than ophthalmodynamometry because the diastolic pressure cannot be recorded, but is easier to perform and provides a reproducible objective recording.

The normal ophthalmic artery pressure is 75% of the brachial artery pressure with a standard deviation of 5% [13,14]. A pressure less than 65% of the brachial artery pressure is considered abnormal [13,14]. A reduction in pressure of 10 mmHg or more in one eye compared to the other also indicates a significant reduction in perfusion pressure [13].

Another test exists that is referred to as oculoplethysmography, in which the time for the pulse to reach the eye from the internal carotid artery and the ear from the external carotid artery are measured [15]. A delay in flow from the internal carotid artery is considered to represent hemodynamic obstruction to flow. This type of oculoplethysmography is not frequently used because so many patients have atherosclerotic disease in the carotid sinus affecting both the internal and external carotid artery that it limits the value of the test.

As a test for detecting carotid artery disease, pneumooculoplethysmography is not very sensitive because only stenosis of greater than 75% can be identified. If there is good collateral circulation, the ophthalmic artery pressure can be maintained in the normal range even with a high grade lesion. The test is quite specific for obstruction in the internal carotid artery, with false positive results when there is ophthalmic artery stenosis, which is a rare occurrence [16]. The pressure is normal with central retinal artery occlusion [16].

Measurement of ophthalmic artery pressure enhances the accuracy of the noninvasive test battery by detecting hemodynamically obstructive lesions that may be missed by direct imaging techniques. This is particularly true for lesions in the internal carotid distal to the bifurcation, lesions that are not extensive but cause high grade local narrowing of the internal carotid or complete occlusions of the internal carotid artery with normal runoff in the external carotid artery.

Pneumooculoplethysmography is also valuable as a physiologic measure of perfusion pressure in the internal carotid artery distal to a stenosis or complete occlusion and may have prognostic value as well. There is evidence that patients with carotid artery stenosis and a reduction in ophthalmic artery pressure have up to 10-fold higher risk of stroke than patients with an equivalent degree of stenosis and a normal ophthalmic artery pressure [11] and are at higher risk for stroke even when they are asymptomatic [17]. While most ischemic events secondary to atherosclerosis probably have an embolic etiology, concomitant reduction in cerebral perfusion appears to play a role in producing irreversible damage to the tissue, resulting in a completed stroke [18].

Supraorbital Directional Doppler

The direction of flow of red blood cells in an artery can be measured by Doppler ultrasonography. High frequency sound waves from 2 to 10 MHz are directed at the vessel at a fixed angle, usually 60°. The sound waves reflect back from the moving red blood cells to a receiver in the Doppler probe. The frequency of the returning sound waves is shifted by the flow of the blood, the Doppler effect. The extent of shift and direction of shift can be recorded by the receiver. Thus, the direction and velocity of flow can be measured.

Arteries in the supraorbital ridge, the supraorbital and supratrochlear arteries, form a collateral channel between the ophthalmic artery branch of the internal carotid artery and the superficial temporal and facial branches of the external carotid artery. The direction of flow is normal from the internal carotid towards the external carotid branches. Compression of the superficial temporal or facial branches of the external carotid augments the velocity of supraorbital flow from the normal internal carotid artery. When there is high grade stenosis of the internal carotid artery at the bifurcation, supraorbital flow is reversed towards the internal carotid. Compression of the superficial temporal or facial branches of the external carotid artery diminishes or eliminates supraorbital flow when flow is retrograde from the external to the internal carotid due to an obstructive lesion of the internal.

Supraorbital directional Doppler is also not an effective test for detecting carotid artery stenosis. Only high grade lesions of greater than 75% can be detected, and these can only be identified when collateral flow through the supraorbital artery is established. The sensitivity and specificity of this examination for high grade stenosis is only 75% [19]. The study is subjective and technically difficult to perform. The role of supraorbital directional Doppler is to assess the extent of collateral flow available from the external to the internal carotid artery when there is occlusive disease of the internal carotid artery. Supraorbital Doppler can also be helpful in identifying hemodynamically obstructive lesions in which the perfusion pressure at the ophthalmic artery is maintained in the normal range by collateral circulation.

Measurement of Carotid Artery Flow With Directional Doppler

The velocity of flow of red blood cells in the cervical carotid artery can be measured with continuous-wave bidirectional Doppler. The frequency shift caused by reflection of sound waves in the ultrasonic wave lengths from the red blood cells is in the audible range. Flow can be auscultated with the Doppler probe; and the frequencies of sound waves can be plotted with a frequency spectral analyzer as a waveform (Fig. 2-1) or as a histogram.

The common, internal, and external carotid arteries can be differentiated by the characteristics of Doppler flow. The internal carotid artery is a capacitance vessel, and flow continues well above zero baseline in diastole. The external carotid artery is a resistance vessel, with a shorter period of systolic flow and much lower velocity flow in diastole than the internal carotid artery (Fig. 2-2). The common carotid artery has flow characteristics intermediate to the internal and external carotid.

The velocity of flow of red blood cells through an area of stenosis is actually increased, with fewer cells traveling at a higher rate. This increases the frequency of the Doppler signal. Cells that are waiting to pass through the area of stenosis or caught in eddy currents from the obstruction are traveling at a slower than normal rate or are sometimes flowing retrograde. This causes audible turbulence and a broadening of spectral frequencies, with higher and lower frequencies than the normal velocity waveform (Fig. 2-3).

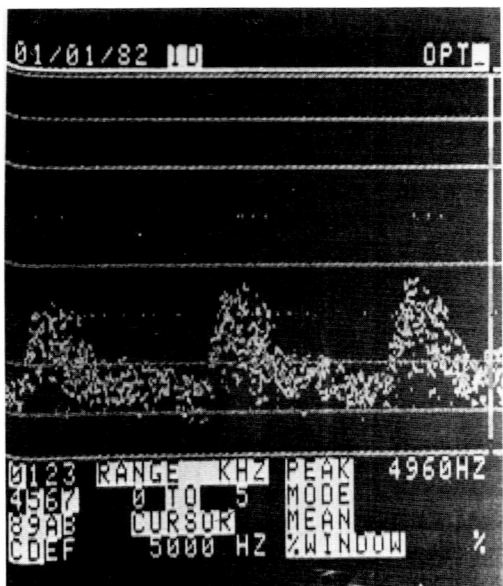 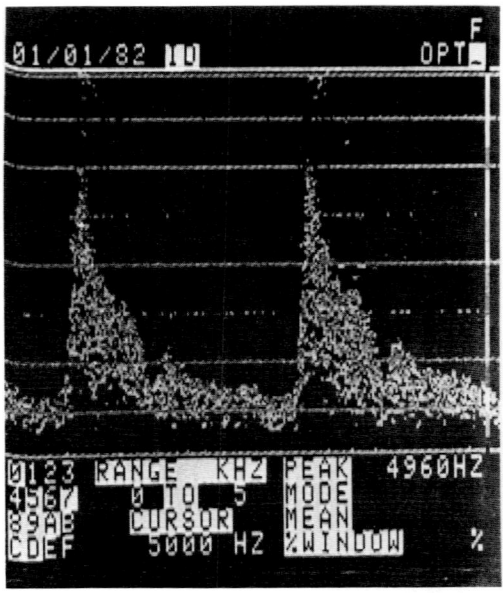

Figure 2-1. Normal velocity waveform in the internal carotid artery recorded with a 4 MHz continuous-wave Doppler probe and an Angioscan II (Unigon) spectral analyzer. The location is determined by duplex study with real-time ultrasonography. The peak velocity in systole is 2,500 Hz and the height of diastole does not fall below 1,000 Hz. Each dot represents an echo reflected from a moving red blood cell.

Figure 2-2. Normal velocity waveform in the external carotid artery recorded as in Figure 1. The systolic peak is higher and narrower than in the internal carotid artery, with rapid decline of the waveform in diastole to below 1,000 Hz.

Reduction in flow in the common carotid artery is only recorded in the case of extremely high grade stenosis or complete occlusion of the internal carotid artery (Fig. 2-4). Even in these instances, a normal flow pattern may be obtained if there is good runoff into the external carotid artery, in which case the flow wave takes on the characteristics of flow in the internal carotid artery. This makes it difficult to identify complete occlusions of the internal carotid artery when there is no turbulence identified at the bifurcation and a normal flow wave similar to internal carotid flow coming from the external carotid artery. Also, cardiac lesions, such as aortic valve stenosis that cause outflow obstruction, can cause a reduction in diastolic flow similar to the pattern seen with occlusive disease in the internal carotid. These difficulties can usually be surmounted by employing the indirect evaluations of ophthalmic artery pressure and supraorbital Doppler to help diagnose major occlusive disease in the internal carotid arteries.

More sophisticated measurements of Doppler flow can be achieved with duplex Doppler ultrasound, in which pulsed Doppler signals are recorded at a specific point along the course of the carotid artery identified by real-time B-mode ultrasonography (see Chapter 3, pp. 27–48). The advantage of using continuous-wave Doppler is that higher frequency waves can be used, increasing the sensitivity of the examination in detecting the highest velocity flow. In addition, the audible characteristics of the flow pattern are clearer. Thus, using continuous-wave Doppler is often more sensitive in identifying and quantitating the degree of stenosis at the carotid artery bifurcation, while pulsed Doppler is more valuable in specifying the location of the stenosis. Continuous-wave Doppler is also better able to detect turbulence patterns secondary to mitral valve dysfunction, such as regurgitation or prolapse that

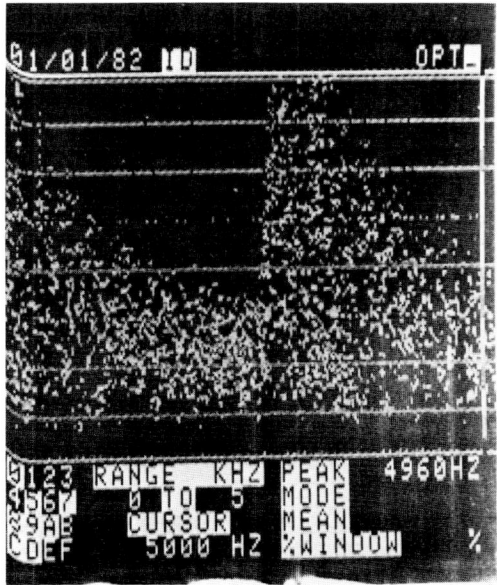 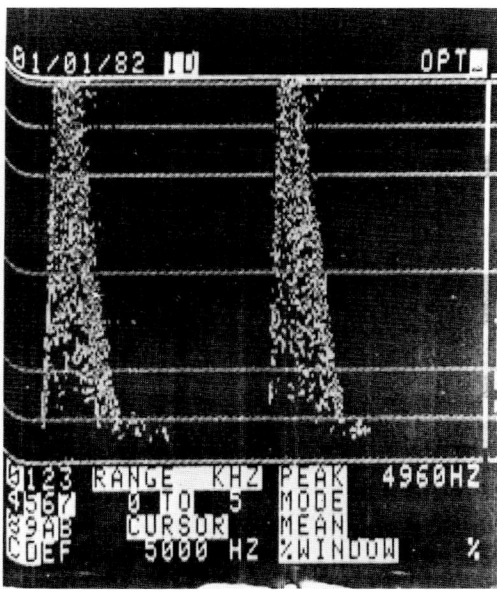

Figure 2-3. Spread of spectral frequencies in an internal carotid artery with 75% stenosis. The systolic peak is elevated to 5,000 Hz and high velocity flow continues through diastole, while low velocity flows are seen in systole, breaking up the waveform.

Figure 2-4. Reduction in flow in an occluded internal carotid artery (see Fig. 2-5). The systolic peak is high and narrow, and there is no flow velocity during diastole.

can be confused with turbulence originating at the carotid bifurcation and that in itself may be important to detect as a potential source of embolic cerebrovascular disease [20].

Real-time B-Mode Ultrasonography

Real-time B-mode ultrasonography constructs images of the carotid arteries by measuring the intensity of reflections of sound wave from structures in and around the vessel. Flowing blood produces no reflected echo, while calcium produces a high intensity echo. Plaque can be discriminated from the wall of the vessel, and the intima can be distinguished from the media. B-mode imaging of plaques in the carotid artery bifurcation provide information as to the size and morphologic character of the plaque that is not available on angiography. Lesions confined to the carotid sinus just below the bifurcation into the internal and external carotid arteries can be quite extensive and be underestimated on angiography when the plaque is not involving the origin of the internal carotid artery. B-mode ultrasonography can also determine the origin of turbulent flow detected on Doppler examination, distinguishing stenosis of the internal carotid artery from stenosis of the external carotid artery or turbulence originating from a cardiac source. This is particularly valuable when duplex scanning with concommitant Doppler measurement is performed (see Chapter 3, pp. 27–48). Complete occlusion of the internal carotid artery is difficult to visualize (Fig. 2-5), and the ancillary tests of oculoplethysmography and supraorbital Doppler are often necessary to make this diagnosis.

The main role of B-mode ultrasound in the noninvasive test battery is to visualize morphologic characteristics about atherosclerotic plaque in order to add both diagnostic and prognostic information. Plaques that have heterogeneous echolucencies intermingled with the echodensities have been shown to have intraplaque thrombus, which is associated with a higher incidence of embolic events [21,22]. Plaques that grow longitudinally along the

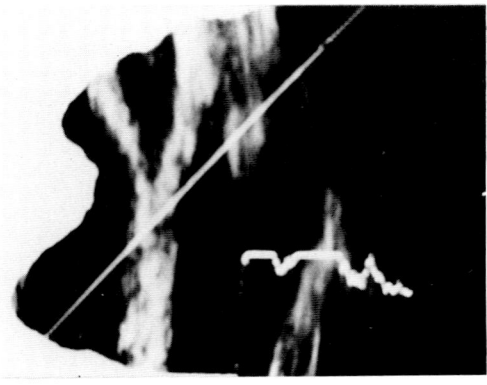 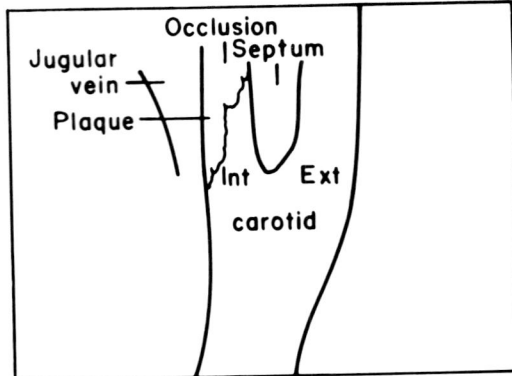

Figure 2-5. Real-time B-mode sonogram of a complete occlusion of the internal carotid artery imaged with a High Stoy SP 100B with a 7.5-MHz probe. The Doppler flow tracing from this vessel is shown in Figure 2-4.

wall of the carotid bifurcation in a mural or crescentic configuration (Fig. 2-6) are also associated with a higher incidence of neurologic symptoms than plaques forming a circular nodule (Fig. 2-7), regardless of the extent of hemodynamic obstruction to flow [10]. Mural plaques have also been demonstrated to contain a significantly higher incidence of intraplaque thrombus and intraluminal thrombus than nodular plaques [22].

In a recent study of followup B-mode examinations on patients with atherosclerotic plaques at the carotid bifurcation, new onset of neurologic symptoms ipsilateral to a carotid plaque was strongly correlated with the formation of new crescentic mural plaques, again independent of hemodynamic factors [23]. This suggests that intraplaque hemorrhage results in plaque growth and intraluminal thrombus, with resultant embolization of intraluminal thrombus to the cerebral vasculature. Plaque ulceration was not correlated with new cerebrovascular symptoms, confirming prior pathologic studies showing that symptomatology correlates with plaque hemorrhage but not plaque ulceration [24]. Thus, B-mode ultrasonography may be of value in establishing whether a carotid plaque was the source of a cerebrovascular event in patients with multiple risk factors for stroke and also may provide prognostic information as to whether the patient is liable to become symptomatic again.

Vertebral Artery Imaging

The vertebral artery can be imaged in the foramen transversarum of the cervical vertebrae from the origin at the subclavian artery (Fig. 2-8) to the fourth cervical vertebra, where it leaves the foramen transversarum to enter the cranium. In a recent study [25], the lumen diameter of the normal cervical vertebral artery on ultrasonography was 6 to 8 mm. Narrowing of the lumen below 6 mm correlates with angiographically demonstrable stenosis or occlusion of the vertebral artery with an accuracy of 85%. Duplex Doppler ultrasonography helps to determine that the structure visualized is actually the vertebral artery and documents patency of flow. Other workers have been able to identify occlusive disease of the basilar artery by demonstrating reduced Doppler flow in the vertebral arteries [26] (see Chapter 4, pp. 49–65).

Imaging the vertebral arteries is valuable in assessing elderly patients complaining of dizziness. Most patients with true rotational vertigo and no other accompanying symptoms or signs of brainstem dysfunction do not have cerebrovascular disease as the cause [27]. However, ischemic lesions in the lateral medulla can cause vertigo without other symptoms. This region is supplied by the posterior inferior cerebellar artery, the first intracranial branch of the vertebral, and the majority of patients with ischemia in this region have athero-

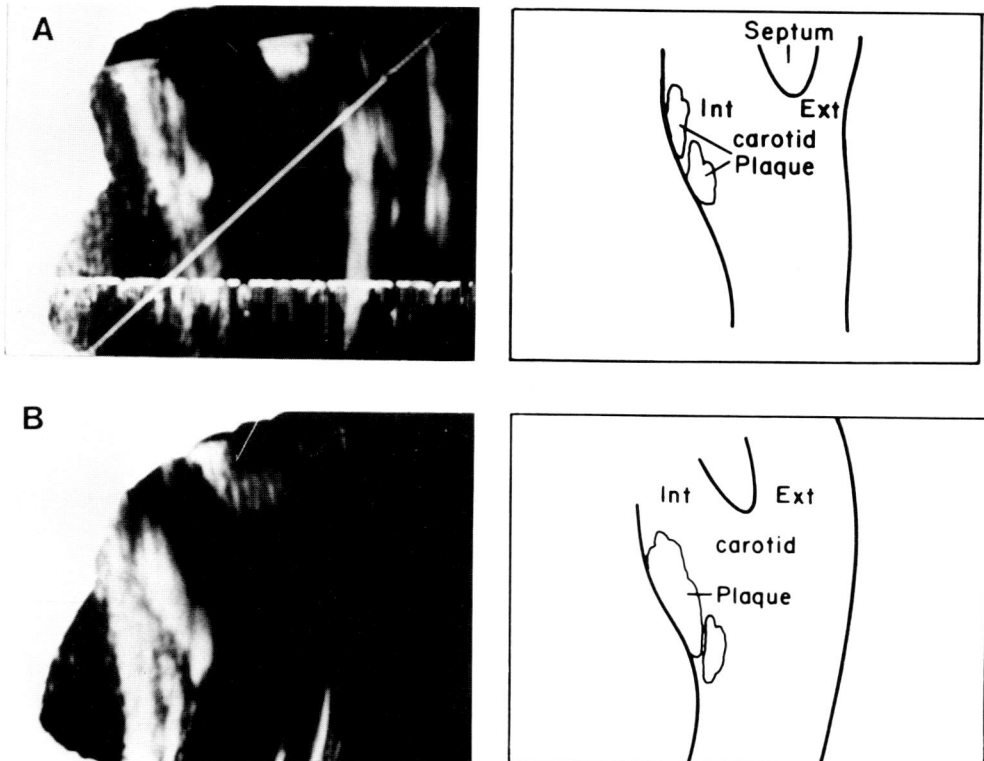

Figure 2-6. **A:** Nonobstructive mural plaque lying mainly in the carotid sinus with little involvement of the origin of the internal carotid artery. Heterogeneous echolucencies and a possible ulcer crater are seen in the plaque, suggesting thrombus formation and embolization. **B:** Large mural plaque confined to the carotid sinus which is homogeneous, but has a scalloped border, also suggesting recent thromboembolism.

sclerotic lesions in the vertebral artery [28]. Noninvasive imaging of the vertebral artery can help discriminate which patients with vertigo have symptoms on a vascular basis.

Elderly patients with syncope or lightheadedness are often thought to have circulatory insufficiency in the carotid or vertebral artery territory. Carotid or vertebral artery stenosis is found in less than 10% of patients with syncope who do not have other symptoms of cerebrovascular disease [25]. Noninvasive imaging of the carotid and vertebral arteries is valuable in screening these patients to rule out extracranial occlusive vascular disease.

SUMMARY

Noninvasive carotid artery testing has many clinical applications. It can be used to diagnose the extent of carotid artery disease in patients wtih focal cerebrovascular symptoms. It is a good screening test for patients with nonspecific symptoms suggestive of cerebrovascular disease without exposing the patients to excessive risk. By providing information of the

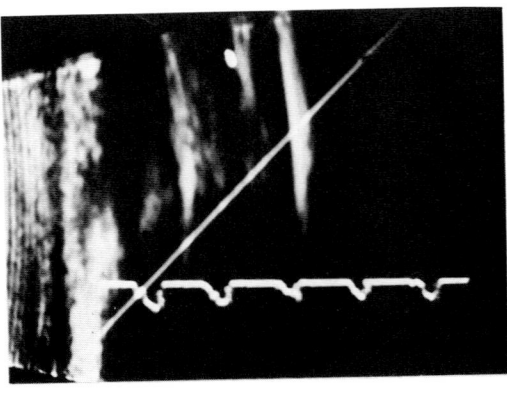 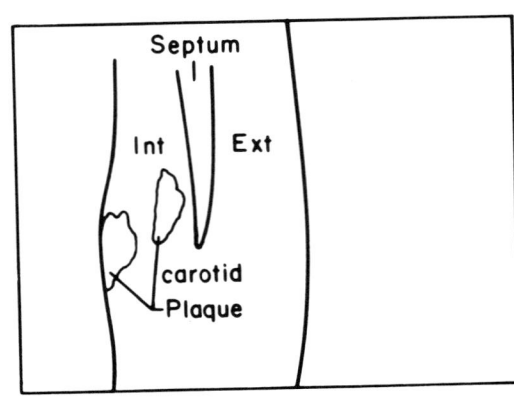

Figure 2-7. Concentric nodular plaque forming a ring at the origin of the internal carotid artery with about 70% stenosis. The plaque is not extensive, but is obstructing flow because of its location. The plaque is homogeneous, suggesting that thrombosis and possible embolization have not occurred.

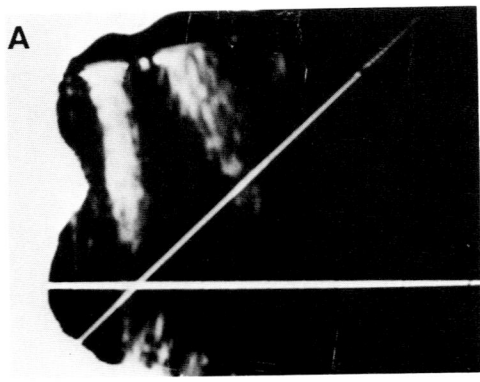 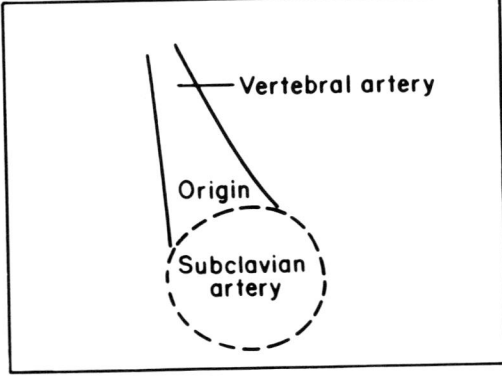

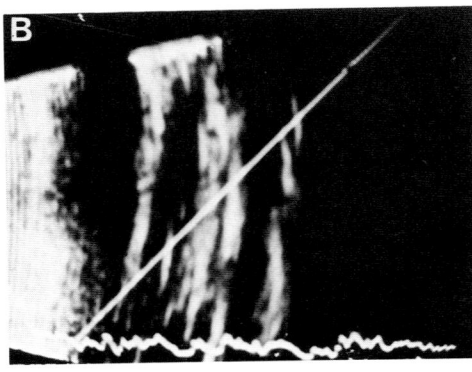 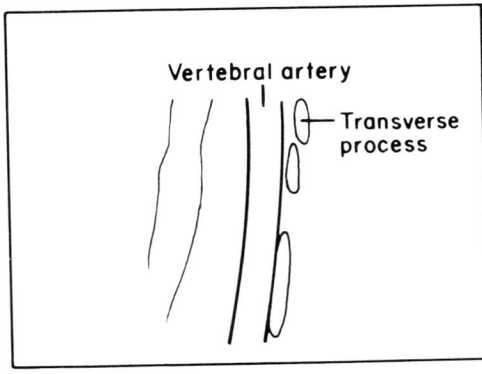

Figure 2-8. **A:** Origin of the vertebral artery is seen from the subclavian artery with normal lumen diameter distal to the origin. **B:** Cervical vertebral artery is visualized from C8 to C4 inside the foramen transversarum, outlined by the transverse processes of the vertebrae.

hemodynamics and morphologic characteristics of lesions at the carotid artery bifurcation, it can be used in the decision-making process to determine which patients with cerebrovascular disease should be managed medically and which patients would benefit from surgical intervention.

References

1. Fisher CM, Gore L, Okabe N, White PD (1965) Atherosclerosis of the carotid and vertebral arteries: Extracranial and intracranial. J Neuropathol Exp Neurol 24:455–476.
2. Schwartz CJ, Mitchell JR (1961) Atheroma of the carotid and vertebral arterial systems. Br Med J 2:1057–1063.
3. Thompson JE, Talkington CM (1976) Carotid Endarterectomy. Ann Surg 184:1–15.
4. Fisher CM (1952) Transient monocular blindness associated with hemiplegia. Arch Ophthalmol 47:167–203.
5. Chambers BR, Norris JW (1986) Outcome in patients with asymptomatic neck bruits. N Engl J Med 315:860–869.
6. Fields WS, Maslenikov V, Meyer JS, et al. (1970) Joint study of extracranial arterial occlusion. V. Progress report of prognosis following surgery or nonsurgical treatment for transient cerebral ischemic attacks and cervical carotid artery lesions. JAMA 211:1993–2003.
7. Faught E, Trader SD, Hanna GR (1979) Cerebral complications of angiography for transient ischemia and stroke: Prediction of risk. Neurology 29:4–15.
8. Moore WS, Hall AD (1970) Importance of emboli from carotid bifurcation in pathogensis of cerebral ischemic attacks. Arch Surg 101:708–711.
9. Weinberger J, Biscarra V, Weitzner I, et al. (1981) Noninvasive carotid artery testing: Role in management of patients with transient ischemic attacks. NY State J Med 81:1463–1468.
10. Weinberger J, Robbins A (1983) Neurologic symptoms associated with nonobstructive plaque at carotid bifurcation: Analysis by real-time B-mode ultrasonography. Arch Neurol 40:489–492.
11. Busuttil RW, Baker JD, Davidson RK, et al. (1981) Carotid artery stenosis: Hemodynamic significance and clinical course. JAMA 245:1438–1441.
12. Cogan DG (1961) Blackouts not obviously due to carotid occlusion. Arch Ophthalmol 66:180–187.
13. Gee W, Oller DW, Amundsen DG (1977) The asymptomatic carotid bruit and the ocular pneumoplethysmography. Arch Surg 112:1381–1388.
14. Weinberger J, Biscarra V, Weisberg MK (1981) Hemodynamics of the carotid artery circulation in the elderly "dizzy" patient. J Am Geriatr Soc 29:402–406.
15. Kartchner MM, McRae LP, Crain V, et al. (1976) Oculoplethysmography: An adjunct to arteriography in the diagnosis of extracranial carotid occlusive disease. Am J Surg 132:728–732.
16. Weinberger J, Bender AN, Yang WC (1980) Amaurosis fugax associated with ophthalmic artery stenosis: Clinical simulation of carotid artery disease. Stroke 11:209–293.
17. Meissner I, Weibers DO, Whisnant JP, O'Fallon WM (1986) The natural history of asymptomatic carotid artery occlusive lesions. Ann Neurol 20:122.
18. Sundt TM, Sharbrough FW, Piepgras DG, et al. (1981) Correlation of cerebral blood flow and electroencephalographic changes during carotid endarterectomy. Mayo Clin Proc 56:533–543.
19. Bone GE, Barnes RW (1976) Clinical implications of the Doppler cerebrovascular examination: A correlation with angiography. Stroke 7:271–274.
20. Weinberger J, Goldman M (1985) Detection of mitral valve abnormalities by carotid Doppler flow study: Implications for the management of patients with cerebrovascular disease. Stroke 16:977–980.
21. Reilly LM, Lusby RJ, Hughes L, et al. (1983) Carotid plaque histology using real-time ultrasonography: Clinical and therapeutic implications. Am J Surg 146:188–192.
22. Weinberger J, Marks SJ, Gaul JJ, et al. (1987) Atherosclerotic plaque at the carotid artery bifurcation: Correlation of ultrasonographic imaging with morphology. J Ultrasound Med 6:363–366.
23. Weinberger J, Ramos L, Ambrose JA, Fuster V (1988) Morphology and dynamic changes of atherosclerotic plaque at the carotid artery bifurcation: Sequential imaging by real time B-mode ultrasonography. J Am Coll Cardiol 11(Suppl A):52.
24. Imparato AM, Riles TS, Mintzer K, Baumann FG (1983) The importance of hemorrhage in the relationship between gross morphologic characteristics and cerebral symptoms in 376 carotid artery plaques. Ann Surg 197:195–203.
25. Weinberger J (1987) Evaluation of the elderly dizzy patient. Medical Times 115:47–52.
26. Ringelstein EB, Zeumer H, Poeck K (1985) Noninvasive diagnosis of intracranial lesions in the vertebrobasilar system: A comparison of Doppler sonographic and angiographic findings. Stroke 16:848–854.
27. Fisher CM (1967) Vertigo in cerebrovascular disease. Arch Otolaryngol 85:529–534.
28. Fisher CM (1970) Occlusion of the vertebral arteries. Arch Neurol 22:13–19.

3

Continuous-Wave Doppler Sonography of the Extracranial Brain-Supplying Arteries

Erich Bernd Ringelstein, MD

Department of Neurology, Technische Hochschule, 5100 Aachen, Federal Republic of Germany

INTRODUCTION

The clinician who applies continuous-wave (CW) Doppler sonography as a diagnostic tool on the extracranial cerebral arteries must be aware of the fact that his final, morphologic diagnosis is exclusively based on his interpretation of functional abnormalities of blood flow. During CW Doppler sonography, these flow disturbances are predominantly recognized by means of acoustic phenomena, whereas visible displays of frequency spectra and flow mapping deliver only ancillary information. For a visually trained generation of physicians, this seems to limit the clinical applicability and usefulness of Doppler ultrasound. Clinical experience has demonstrated that CW Doppler sonography of the neck vessels is highly accurate and reliable when compared to cerebral arteriography [1–3]. In an experienced laboratory, Doppler diagnoses are even superior to intravenous digital subtraction angiograms or poor-quality arch aortographs.

TERMINOLOGY AND PHYSIOLOGIC BACKGROUND

The examiner's information about blood flow conditions is based mainly on three parameters: flow direction, momentary mean flow velocity, and changes of flow velocity (or even direction) in time during each cardiac cycle. Vibration phenomena of the vessel walls and/or the surrounding tissue occur at arterial high flow velocity segments. This noise may overcome the high-pass filters of the device and may serve as an additional audible aid for the diagnosis of stenotic lesions (Fig. 3-1).

From a physiologic and didactic standpoint, the terminology proposed by Spencer is particularly helpful. He categorized the various Doppler phenomena in primary, secondary, and tertiary changes [4]. Primary changes refer to locally circumscribed, direct effects of a stenosis on blood flow, such as acceleration within the stenotic channel ("jet"), poststenotic disturbed flow (so-called "turbulences"), and, less frequently, high frequency harmonic vessel wall vibrations at the site of subtotal stenoses due to Karmann's eddy formation, i.e., so-called musical murmurs or sea gull phenomena. Secondary changes refer to far downstream effects of "hemodynamically relevant" upstream vessel lesions (dampened flow and flow velocity reduction due to energy loss within a tight stenosis) (Fig. 3-1), or, conversely, upstream changes of blood flow caused by a far downstream subtotal stenosis or occlusion (increased pulsatility due to increased peripheral resistance or even reverberating flow within blind loops [5] (Fig. 3-2). Tertiary findings refer to more indirect consequences of high-grade stenoses or occlusions on the extra- and intracranial circulation, such as recruitment and formation of collateral channels or reversal of physiologic flow direction in segments of the circle of Willis, the basal arteries, and other preformed anasto-

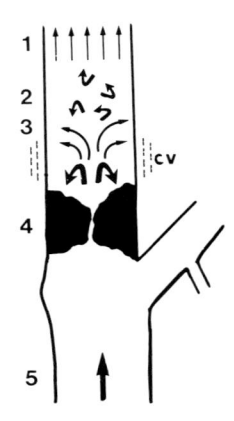

Figure 3–1. Diagram of downstream, intrastenotic, and upstream flow changes in internal carotid artery stenoses. **1:** Reduced flow velocity and pulsatility (dampened flow) far downstream after relaminarization of disturbed flow. **2:** Zone of disturbed flow (so-called turbulences). **3:** Zone of reflux phenomena and co-vibration (CV) of vessel walls and surrounding soft tissue, producing low-frequency noise. **4:** Jet within the stenotic channel with maximal flow velocity, i.e., high-frequency noise. **5:** Upstream increased pulsatility due to increased peripheral resistance (increased pulsatility = pronounced dichrotic notch, reduction or loss of diastolic blood flow velocity, rapid deceleration of blood column in early diastole).

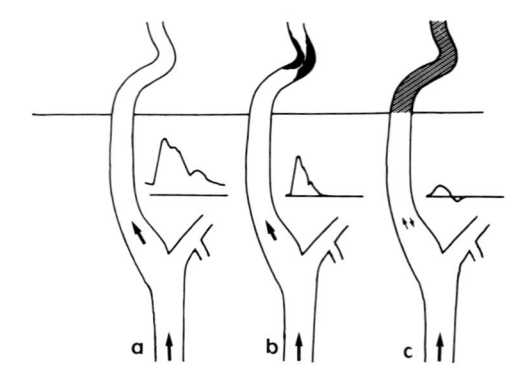

Figure 3–2. Modulation of carotid flow profiles by peripheral resistance. **a:** In normal conditions, internal carotid artery flow velocity signal reveals gradual deceleration of the blood column during early diastole, moderate dichrotic notch, and preserved diastolic flow. **b:** With high-grade siphon stenoses, extracranial flow velocity is reduced and pulsatility of carotid flow signal is increased, indicated by rapid deceleration of the blood column during late systole and loss of diastolic blood flow. **c:** If the distal internal carotid artery is occluded, the remaining blind loop reveals to-and-fro movement of the blood column during systole and early diastole. This finding is pathognomonic.

moses. A well-known example is reversal of flow within the periorbital branches of the ophthalmic artery in ICA occlusion (Fig. 3-3). Primary alterations have a higher diagnostic impact than secondary or tertiary ones and permit a topographically and quantitatively more precise diagnosis. Not infrequently, however, the vessel lesions cannot directly be approached by CW Doppler sonography for anatomic reasons. In these cases, the diagnosis must be based exclusively on secondary or tertiary flow abnormalities.

A few general remarks should be added about the insonation angle during CW Doppler studies with a pen-like probe. Theoretically, a coaxial insonation (angle between probe and flow axis of the blood column = 0°) would deliver the strongest signal. For anatomic reasons, however, this is not possible in the neck arteries. If one insonates an artery with a 90° angle, no signal can be achieved. Scattering of the ultrasound beam from the blood corpuscles also plays an important role. Thus, the insonation angle of the probe providing maximal echo strength is always a compromise. In practice, an insonation angle of 30 to 50° is adequate.

Doppler screening of a patient's neck arteries should always be complete and include indirect as well as direct approaches to all vessels [3]. This means a certain redundancy in many cases. However, this redundancy is an important intrinsic test of the diagnosis. As a rule of thumb, a diagnosis that is made when there are discrepancies between the findings in various steps of the examination must be considered highly doubtful.

APPLICATION IN THE CAROTID SYSTEM
Periorbital Doppler Flow Studies

The indirect approach to the carotid circulation should be the first step of the entire procedure. It is the easiest part of Doppler examination and gives an overall initial impression

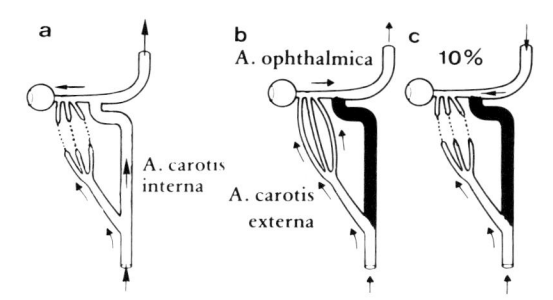

Figure 3–3. Role of ophthalmic artery as a collateral channel in high-grade internal carotid artery lesions. **a:** Under normal conditions, flow within the ophthalmic artery is directed antegrade, i.e., from the carotid siphon to the periorbital branches. **b:** If blood flow within the proximal internal carotid artery is hindered by high-grade stenoses or occlusion, the ophthalmic artery can work as a collateral pathway, channelling blood retrogradely from the facial branches of the external carotid artery via the periorbital branches of the ophthalmic artery to the carotid siphon and the cerebral arteries. **c:** If the collateralizing capacities of the circle of Willis are good, flow within the ophthalmic artery remains antegrade. This artery may be fed from a retrogradely flooded carotid siphon. In this situation, recruitment of the periorbital collateral network is not needed.

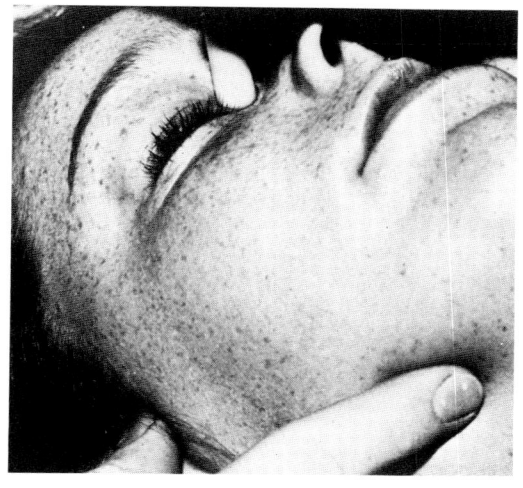

Figure 3–4. Directional Doppler sonography of the supratrochlear artery. The supratrochlear artery is insonated at the medial angle of the eye with the probe placed on the upper eye lid. The probe is held with the examiner's left hand, simultaneously stabilizing the head (not shown). Thumb and index of the examiner's right hand perform simultaneous compression tests of the facial artery (index) and superficial temporal artery (thumb). In normal cases, periorbital Doppler flow increases or remains unchanged during this compression. In pathologic cases, compression leads to striking reduction of flow velocity, alternating flow direction or reversal of flow.

of the integrity of the carotid circulation [6,7]. It is sufficient to insonate the supratrochlear artery (i.e., A. frontalis media) in the upper inner angle of the eye (Fig. 3-4). Because the supratrochlear artery may form a loop, flow direction indicated on the screen of the device is only a relative measure. In order to clarify whether blood flow has antegrade (from the carotid syphon via the ophthalmic artery to its extracranial periorbital branches) or retrograde direction, compression tests of the external carotid artery are necessary. In high-grade internal carotid artery lesions, the ophthalmic artery and its periorbital vascular tree act as a collateral pathway that is fed from branches of the external carotid artery. These vessels channel blood from the external carotid territory retrograde to the carotid syphon and, consequently, to the brain (Fig. 3-3). Compression tests of the external carotid artery branches should be performed routinely in order to define the true flow direction within the periorbital vasculature. Both the superficial temporal (STA) and facial arteries are simultaneously compressed using thumb and index finger. The contralateral hand, holding the probe, stabilizes the head during the compression maneuver in order to avoid movement artifacts (Fig. 3-4).

Side-to-side differences in flow velocity of the supratrochlear arteries are often not diagnostic of carotid artery disease. However, reduced pulsatility (for definition, see above) or even reversal of periorbital flow are suggestive or indicative of severe perfusion pressure reduction in the distal carotid system [7]. Only rarely does reversal of periorbital Doppler flow occur due to isolated ophthalmic artery occlusion [8]. An example of increased diastolic flow velocity and reversal of flow direction within the supratrochlear artery due to ICA occlusion is shown in Fig. 3-5b. In rare cases,

30 Ringelstein

so-called shuttle flow can be observed. This term refers to a regular change in flow direction during each cardiac cycle due to changing pressure gradients (Fig. 3-5c). In complete ICA occlusions, clear-cut abnormalities of periorbital Doppler flow are to be expected in 80% of the cases, less frequently in subtotal and high-grade ICA stenoses. ICA lesions causing a less than 80% lumen reduction, as a rule, do not affect periorbital Doppler flow. But even in a considerable number of cases with ICA occlusion, the collateralizing potential of the circle of Willis is so strong that the syphon distal to the occluded ICA is irrigated retrogradely and feeds the ophthalmic artery in an antegrade direction.

The Direct CW Doppler Approach to the Carotid Axis

The common (CCA), internal (ICA), and external (ECA) carotid arteries are directly insonated by tracking them with the probe along their course in the neck [2] (Fig. 3-6a). When a stenosis of the origin of the CCA or innominate artery is presumed, a retrograde insonation is also recommended. At the carotid bifurcation, it is most practical to insonate the ECA first (before switching to the ICA), because this vessel can more easily be identified. When approaching the carotid bifurcation with the probe from below, flow velocity is suddenly reduced (lower frequencies) as soon as the widened lumen of the carotid bulb is reached. This also indicates the site where in approximately 85% of the cases a more pulsatile, whiplash-like signal can be found medially and anteriorly to the CCA. This flow echo signifies increased peripheral resistance and belongs to the ECA. Repetitive compression of the STA induces a tremolo-like modulation of the ECA flow signal, thus permitting its unequivocal identification (Figs. 3-6b, 3-7A–C). Subsequently, the probe is moved slightly downward and back to the CCA. Under repetitive STA compressions, the modulation of the ECA signal will disappear abruptly (or become weaker) as soon as the CCA is reached. The probe is now moved cephalad again but more laterally and posteriorly (Fig. 3-6c). In young individuals, the origins of the ICA and ECA often lie close to each other or overlap. In the elderly, the ICA often swings 1 or 2 centimeters laterally before resuming a cephalad direction.

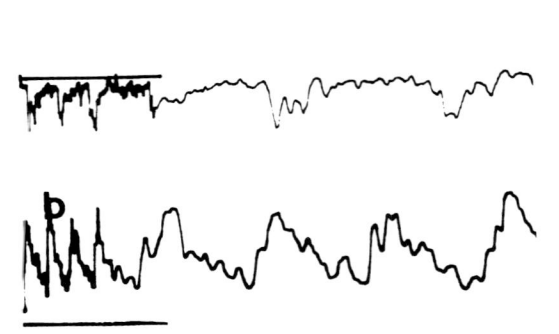

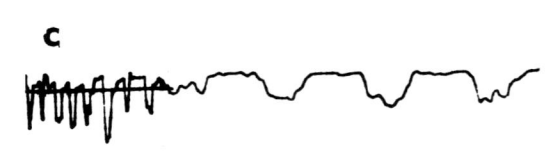

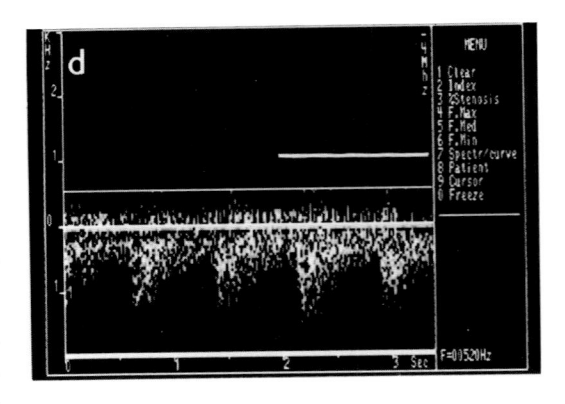

Figure 3–5. Normal and abnormal flow findings at the supratrochlear artery. **a:** Normal flow signal of the supratrochlear artery. Downward deflection of curve indicates flow towards probe. **b:** In ICA occlusion, reversal of flow direction and increased diastolic flow velocity is seen. The latter is not an obligatory finding. **c:** If the watershed area between the external and internal carotid artery territories, by chance, lies in the vicinity of the eyelid, flow with alternating directions during each cardiac cycle may occur. Horizontal bar indicates zeroline. For calibration see Figure 3–7. **d:** Normal flow signal during frequency analysis. White bar indicates compression of superficial temporal and facial arteries, which leads to slight increase of flow velocity.

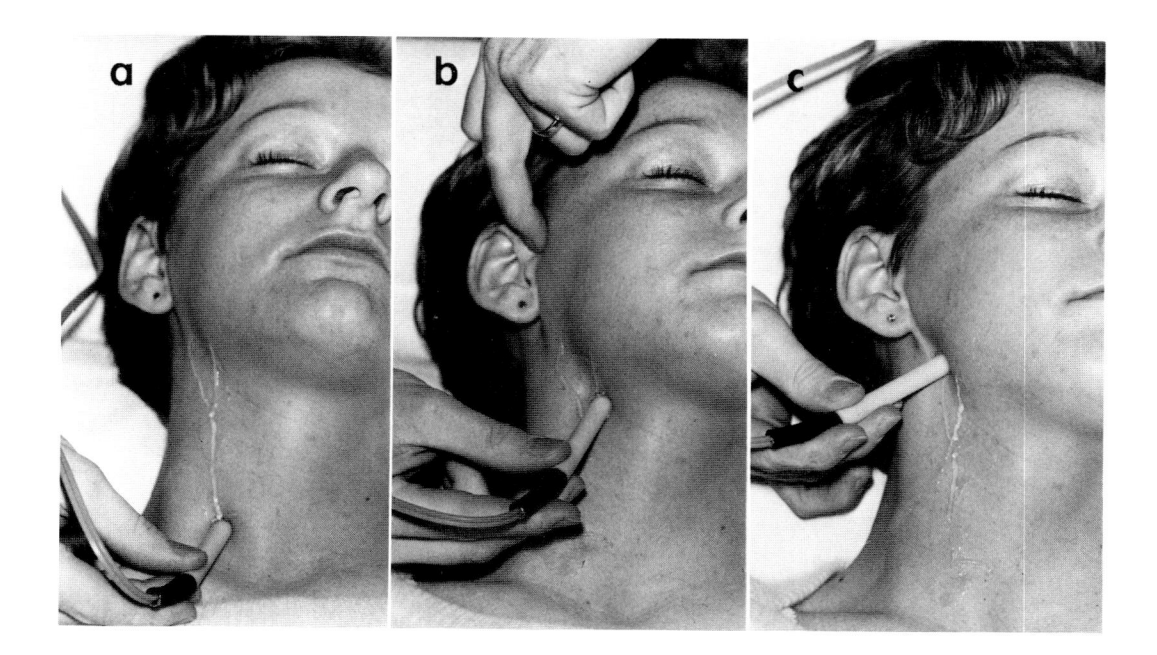

Figure 3–6. Direct Doppler sonography of the carotid arteries. **a:** The probe is placed medial to the sternocleidomastoid muscle and gradually shifted laterally until the flow signal of the common carotid artery appears. The common carotid artery is then tracked cephalad, as indicated by the gel. **b:** At the carotid bifurcation, flow velocity drops slightly due to widening of the vessel (carotid bulb). The stem of the external carotid artery is insonated just anteriorly, medially and rostrally from it. Rhythmic compression of the superficial temporal artery allows reliable identification of the vessel. **c:** After having moved the probe back to the common carotid artery, the origin of the internal carotid artery is found more laterally and posteriorly. This vessel is then tracked as far cephalad as possible.

Once the ICA is found, it is tracked cranially and as far cephalad behind the mandible as possible. This is particularly important in patients with high carotid bifurcations or in cases where a dissecting aneurysm of the carotid artery is suspected.

Flow signals are recorded on a strip chart as zero-crossing meter flow velocity curves or, with a frequency analyzer, as frequency spectra on photoprints or videotapes (Figs. 3-7A–F).

Diagnosis of Carotid Stenoses and Occlusions

In many European hospitals and private practices, CW Doppler devices use a zero-crossing meter, whereas in the United States most laboratories use a fast Fourrier frequency analyzer to visualize and document the flow signals. Thus, both types of data are provided here. Qualitative and quantitative criteria are considered when describing the characteristic Doppler phenomena of carotid stenoses (Table 3.1).

The most impressive Doppler finding in arterial stenoses is a circumscribed acceleration of blood within the stenotic channel indicated by an audible high frequency flow signal. This is shown in Figure 3-8 for both a zero-crossing meter outprint and a FFT frequency analysis of a medium-grade ECA stenosis. Another important phenomenon is a reflux during early systole. In our experience, this local reflux (de-

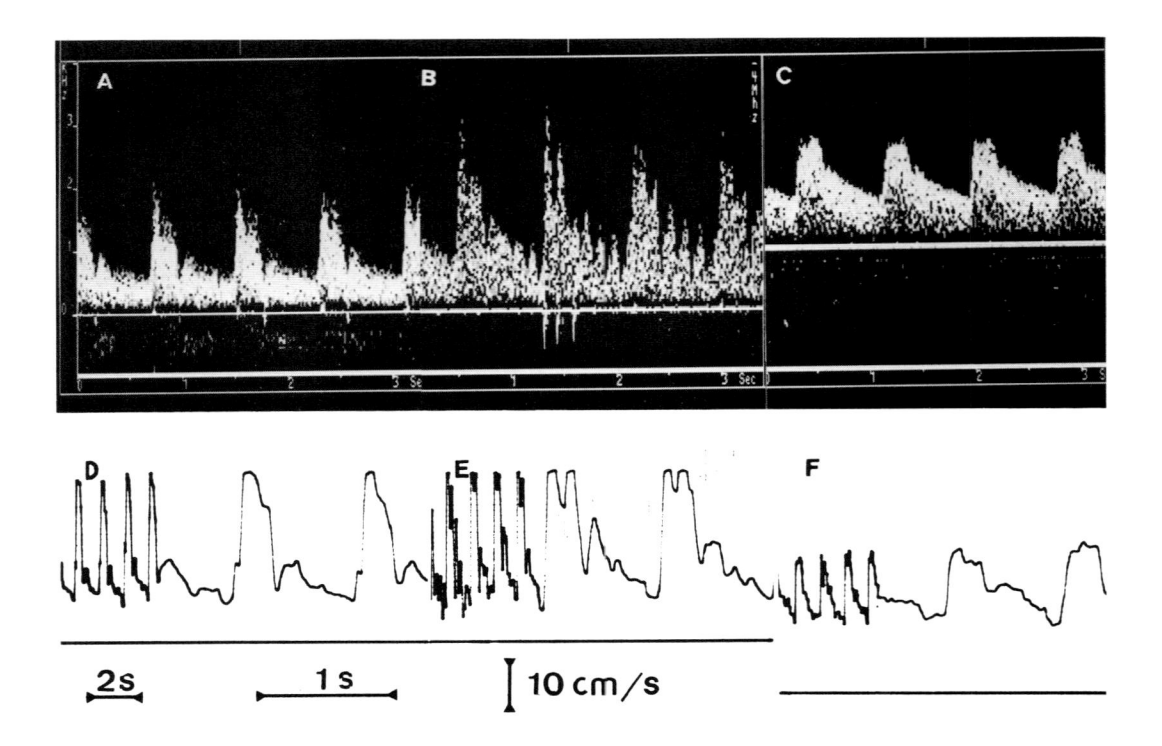

Figure 3–7. Normal flow velocity signals of the carotid arteries. **A–C:** The common external and internal carotid artery flow signals are displayed after subjecting the echo to FFT frequency analysis. Horizontal bar indicates zeroline. The increased pulsatility of the CCA and ECA signal is indicated by a deep dichrotic notch. Spikes in (B) indicate modulation of the ECA flow signal by rhythmic compression of the superficial temporal artery. Less pulsatility of the ICA is demonstrated by minimal dichrotic notch and high diastolic flow velocity. **D–F:** The corresponding display of the flow signal on a zero-crossing meter is also shown.

spite a net antegrade blood flow) indicates that the degree of the underlying stenosis has reached at least 80% lumen reduction. Higher stenoses can be further differentiated according to their frequencies (Table 3.1) using either a commercially available frequency analyzer or, more precisely, although less objectively, the ear of an experienced examiner. In subtotal stenoses and pseudoocclusions of the ICA, the stenotic flow signal loses its pulsatility and presents as a (nearly) continuous high-frequency jet signal.

In occlusion, the flow signal is missing at the site where it is expected to occur normally. In cases with a blind stump of the ICA, a faint pendulum-like (i.e., reverberating) flow signal can be recorded indicating to-and-fro movement of the blood column within the blind loop (Fig. 3-9). This finding is always suggestive of an embolic occlusion of the ICA, with the embolus lodging in the tapering segment of the retromandibular and/or petrous part of the artery (compare Fig. 3-2). Dissections of the ICA may produce similar findings. Arteriosclerotic lesions, by contrast, are nearly always located immediately at the origin of the vessel. Chronic ICA occlusions may remain undetected, if the maxillary artery operates as a major collateral pathway. This artery runs behind the ascending part of the mandible and is not eas-

Table 3.1
Evaluation of the Degree of ICA Stenosis by Doppler Sonographic Criteria

Degree of stenosis (%)	Doppler sonographic findings					
	Primary flow changes		Secondary flow changes		Tertiary flow changes	Systolic peak frequencies
	Intrastenotic	Immediately poststenotic	Prestenotic	Far down-stream		
Non stenosing plaque (0–49)	No or minimal flow changes	No or minimal flow changes	—	—	—	—
Slight stenoses (50–65)	Slight circum-scribed acceler-ation of flow	Slightly disturbed flow	—	—	—	< 5 kHz
Moderate ste-noses (66–79)	Severely acceler-ated blood flow	Severely disturbed flow without systolic reflux	—	—	—	5–7 kHz
Severe stenoses (80–89)	Severely acceler-ated blood flow	Systolic reflux phenomena; considerable covibrations	Diminution of dia-stolic blood flow velocity possible	Slight reduction of pulsatility possible	Rarely reversal or to-and-fro movement of periorbital blood flow	> 7 kHz
Subtotal stenoses (90–99)	Extremely high flow velocities; jet echo may be faint; pulsa-tility of jet re-duced or abol-ished	See previous cat-egory; massive turbulence	Increased pulsa-tility due to in-creased peripheral re-sistance; reduction of diastolic flow velocity	Turbulent flow still audible; flow velocity considerably reduced; sys-tolic accelera-tion slowed	Ophthalmic col-lateral pathway often recruited	> 8 kHz if signal strong enough
Occlusion (100)	No signal avail-able	No signal avail-able	High resistance flow profile; loss or severe reduction of diastolic veloc-ity in the CCA; reverberating flow of ICA, if proximal blind stump	No signal avail-able	Reversal of pe-riorbital blood flow in majority of cases	—

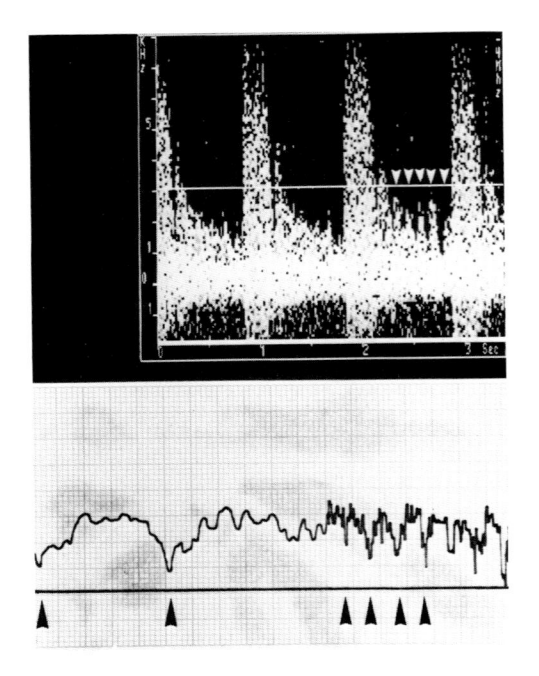

Figure 3–8. Flow signal of 80% external carotid artery stenosis. **Upper:** High systolic flow velocity (approximately 8 kHz) and low frequency systolic noise. Small white arrowheads indicate modulation of the stenotic signal by rhythmic compression of the superficial temporal artery, which proves identity of this vessel. **Lower:** The corresponding zero-crossing meter printouts demonstrate relative reflux of blood during each systole (black arrowheads), with a net antegrade flow direction (for calibration see Fig. 3–7).

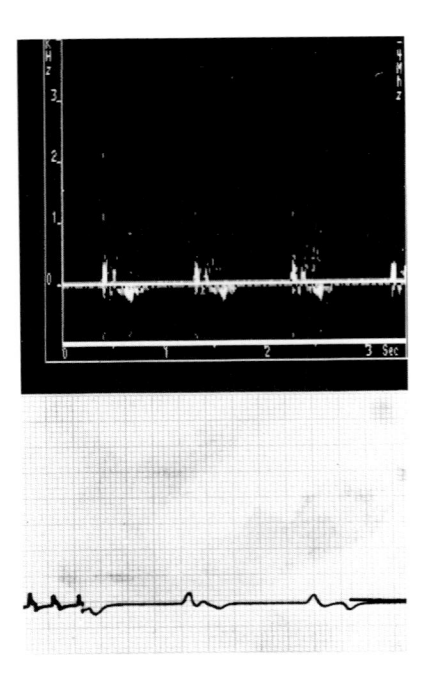

Figure 3–9. Reverberating flow in blind internal carotid artery stump. **Upper:** Rapid forward movement of the blood column into the blind stump of the distally occluded internal carotid artery is represented by the upward deflection of the signal, followed by a slower, short-lasting reflux movement of the blood column during early diastole. No blood flow is registered during most of the diastolic period. **Lower:** The same phenomenon is registered by zero-crossing meter (for calibration see Fig. 3–7). This to-and-fro type of blood movement is also called pendulum-like or reverberating flow (compare Fig. 3–2c). Horizontal bar indicates zeroline. For calibration see Figure 3–7.

ily accessible to a compression test. This artery may mimic a patent ICA. In this situation, periorbital Doppler flow studies are of particular importance. In some cases, transcranial Doppler studies of the middle cerebral artery blood flow velocity during common carotid artery compression tests are necessary in order to definitely clarify the extracranial situation.

Limitations and Reliability

The lower limit of the degree of stenosis that can be detected by CW Doppler ultrasound is approximately 50% lumen reduction. In eccentric lesions, this may correspond to an approximate 30% reduction of diameter. Small (i.e., less lumen-prominent) lesions cannot readily be identified. Occasionally, however, they may produce slightly abnormal flow phenomena like minimal increase of flow velocity and mildly disturbed flow. These findings are ambiguous and can also be found in coiling or slight kinking of the carotid arteries.

The overall accuracy of CW Doppler techniques to detect > 50% ICA stenoses is reported in the literature as approximating > 95%. (Table 3.2). We have performed a prospective study in our own laboratory on the accuracy of estimating the degree of stenosis by auditory and, if possible, visual interpreta-

Table 3.2
Accuracy of CW Doppler Sonography in the Detection of Internal Carotid Artery Stenoses (> 50% lumen reduction) and Occulsions

Reference	Accuracy compared to angiographic findings (%)
Bes et al., 1978 [24]	96
Franceschi and Jardon-Fauconnet [25]	100
Reggi et al., 1979 [26]	77 (18% false positive)
Keller et al., 1979 [6]	92
Büdingen et al., 1982 [11]	97
von Reutern and Thron, 1980 [27]	100
Ringelstein (unpublished data)	97.2% sensitivity, 92.3% specifity (N = 231 carotid arteries); 99.2% sensitivity, 91.2% specificity (N = 154 patients)
Correct differentiation of ICA stenoses and occlusions	
Reggi et al., 1979 [26]	85

tion of the flow signals. A series of 187 patients was studied both sonographically and angiographically by selective intraarterial examinations. The arteriographic degree of stenosis was measured according to the technique described by Zwiebel et al. [10]. There was good agreement of the Doppler findings with angiograms, with an increasing reliability of Doppler sonography in high-grade and subtotal stenoses (Fig. 3-10).

Clinical Usefulness

Continuous-wave Doppler sonography of the extracranial brain arteries is a very effective and reliable screening technique for the detection of carotid artery occlusive disease. In high-grade internal carotid artery stenoses and occlusions it is superior to B-mode imaging techniques for both diagnosis and quantification of the lesions [11,12]. An experienced technician/physician can perform the examination even in stuporous and restless patients.

One of the two main indications for CW Doppler sonography in clinical practice is the rapid screening of the acute stroke patient, including patients with TIA (Fig. 3-11). In connection with CT imaging of the brain, CW Doppler sonography allows for selection of those patients who require carotid endarterectomy, while another subgroup of mostly elderly individuals suffering from hypertension-related cerebral microangiopathy and simultaneously from dilatative arteriosclerosis of the large extracranial arteries can be separated for nonsur-

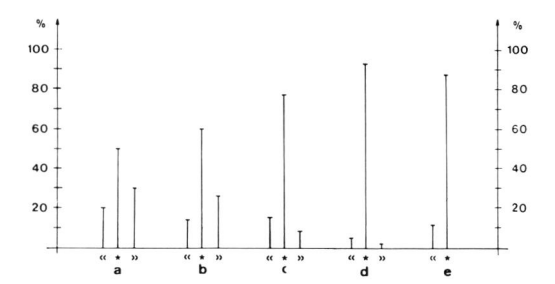

Figure 3–10. Accuracy of CW Doppler estimation of degree of ICA stenoses compared to selective cerebral angiography. With increasing degree of stenosis, accuracy of Doppler sonographic determination of severity of the stenotic process improves considerably. Abscissa indicates degrees of stenoses in percentage of lumen reduction. Ordinate indicates percentage of a correct Doppler determination of degree of stenosis in comparison to angiograms (tall middle bars). Shorter bars indicate percentage of over- (**right**) or underestimation (**left**) of degree of stenoses within neighboring categories. N = 187 angiographically two-plain verified ICA stenoses; the angiographic degree of stenosis was calculated according to Weinberger [9]. **a–e:** to approximately 60 (50–65), 70 (66–79), 90 (80–89), > 90% (90–99) stenoses and occlusions, respectively.

gical treatment. Acute stroke patients with normal extracranial Doppler findings have to be scheduled for further diagnostic procedures. Aside from CT scanning, they require a thor-

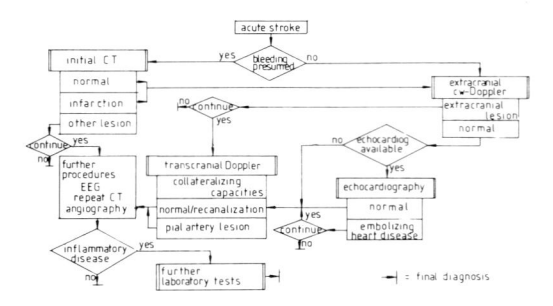

Figure 3–11. Flow chart of initial diagnostic workup of acute stroke patients. Extracranial continuous-wave Doppler screening and computerized tomography of the head are the main initial diagnostic procedures, the results of which may prompt further diagnostic steps.

ough cardiac screening with echocardiography. Next, their large intracranial cerebral arteries should be carefully examined with transcranial Doppler sonography for stenosing lesions of the middle cerebral artery and/or the vertebrobasilar axis.

Due to its noninvasiveness and its qualitative and quantitative diagnostic potential, CW Doppler sonography is the ideal tool for followup studies in patients with asymptomatic extracranial carotid artery disease. Clarification of the natural history of occlusive carotid artery disease has led to a new view on surgical procedures in these patients and, presumably, to a more adequate (i.e., nonsurgical) type of treatment. Limitations of CW Doppler sonography concerning the state of the intracranial cerebral arteries have been compensated for by the detection of transcranial Doppler techniques (Chapter 5). Its inability to detect stenoses of less than 50% lumen reduction can easily be overcome by B-mode imaging of the carotid bifurcation for visualization of nonstenosing plaques.

APPLICATION OF CW DOPPLER SONOGRAPHY TO THE VERTEBROBASILAR SYSTEM
Methodology

EXTRACRANIAL VERTEBRAL ARTERIES: EXAMINATION AND DIAGNOSIS OF LESIONS AND FLOW ABNORMALITIES

Several parts of the subclavian-vertebrobasilar arterial axis can be directly insonated (proximal subclavian artery, origin and proximal part of the vertebral artery, mastoidal slope of the vertebral artery). Other segments are only indirectly accessible (intraosseous part within the cervical segments C2 to C6, intracranial part of the vertebral artery, basilar artery). CW Doppler sonography of the hind circulation should always start with the insonation of the vertebral arteries at the mastoidal slope. The practical approach is demonstrated in Fig. 3-12a–e. The probe is placed at a flat triangular deepening between the origin of the sternocleidomastoid muscle and the mastoidal process and is aimed at the contralateral eye or ear. Some moderate pressure on the probe is necessary to compress interfering branches of the external occipital artery. Due to looping of the vertebral artery around the transverse process of the atlas, its course is unpredictable and flow can be directed both away or towards the probe (Fig. 3-13). Reversed flow (or shuttle flow) within one vertebral artery due to subclavian steal mechanism can be demonstrated by using hyperemia tests of the ipsilateral arm (see below).

The proximal vertebral artery segment is detected by moving the probe in the supraclavi-

Figure 3–12. Mode of extracranial Doppler ultrasound examination of the subclavian-vertebral circulation. **a:** Insonation of the mastoidal slope (atlas loop) of the vertebral artery. The probe is pressed into the deepening between mastoidal process and sternocleidomastoidal muscle. **b:** Insonation of the origin of the vertebral artery. Modulation of the flow signal by rhythmic compression of the distal vertebral artery at the mastoidal region helps to identify the vertebral artery at its origin in the supraclavicular fossa. **c:** By contrast, modulation of the vertebral flow signal should not occur if the superficial temporal artery is compressed. It is important to differentiate the vertebral from common carotid artery; the latter may be modulated by compression of the external occipital artery during the procedure in (b). **d,e:** The parent vessel is also examined by insonating the subclavian (d) artery distally and proximally (e) from the vertebral origin.

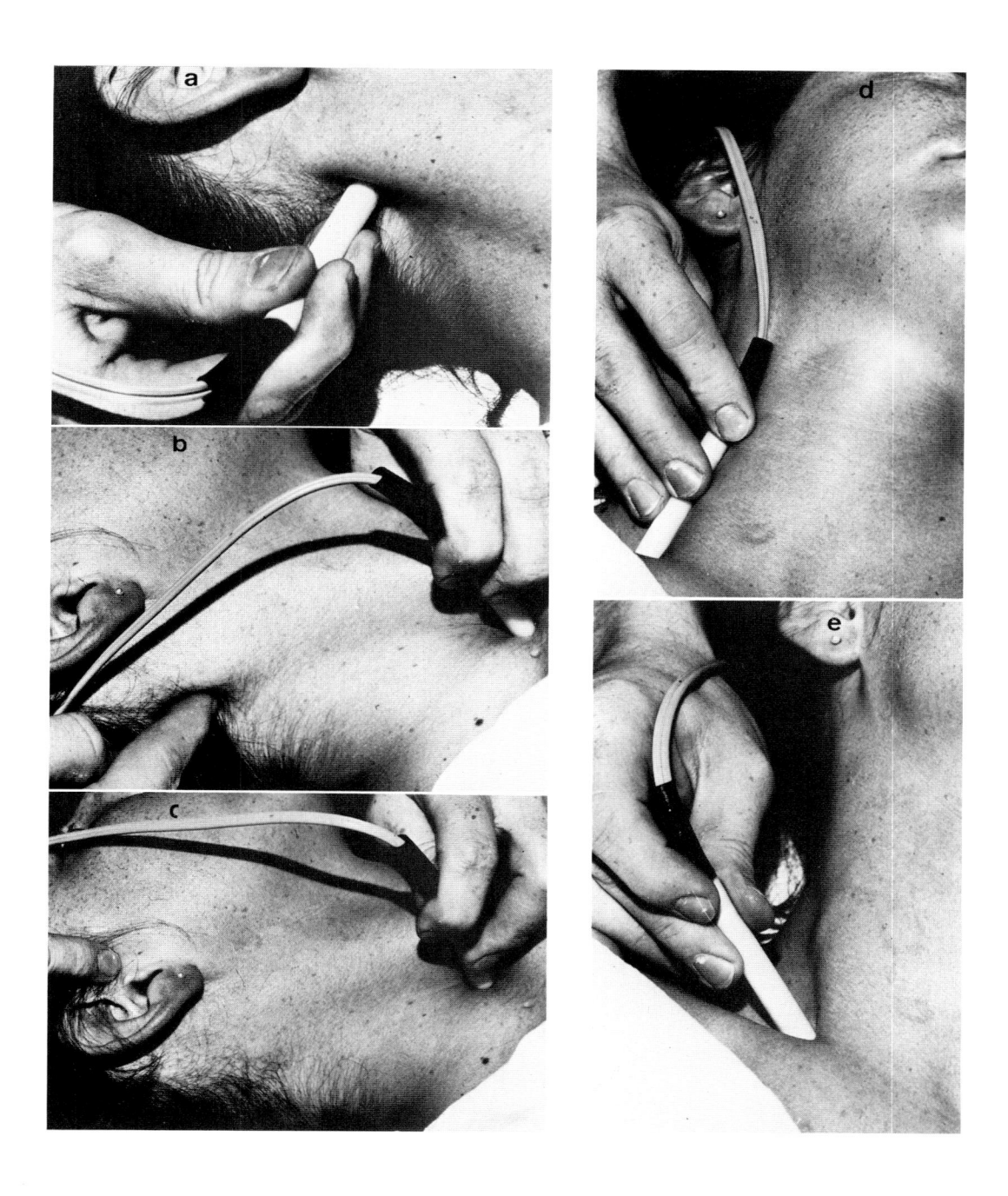

CW Doppler Sonography 37

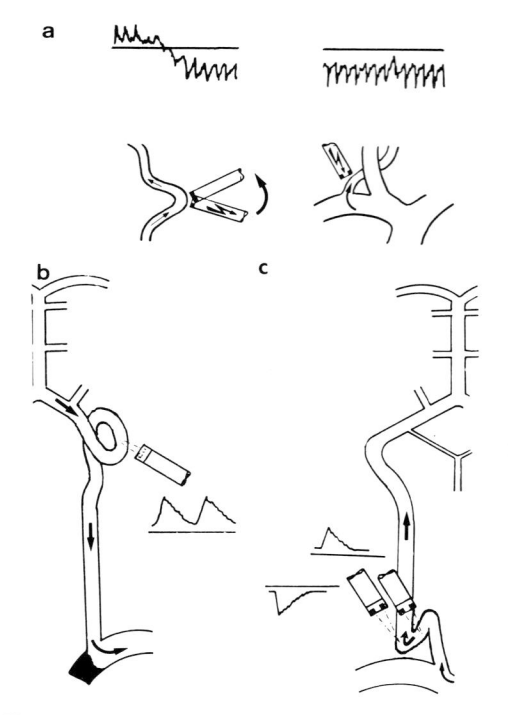

Figure 3–13. Schematic demonstration of unpredictable blood flow directions in the vertebral artery during CW Doppler examination. **a:** Normal flow signals at the mastoidal slope and origin of the vertebral artery. In ideal anatomic conditions, the cephalad-directed probe insonates the upper part of the mastoidal slope of the vertebral artery and flow is directed away from the probe. **b:** In patients with elongated arteries or arterial coiling and looping, the true flow direction within the vertebral artery cannot be determined by the deflection of the curve. In the example shown here, vertebral artery flow is directed downward due to subclavian steal mechanism although deflection of the flow signal masquerades cephalad blood flow. The final decision can only be made by compression tests on the arm. **c:** At the origin of the vertebral artery, blood flow normally is directed towards the probe, indicated by a downward-deflected curve. In a few cases, however, kinking of the vessel may simulate downward blood flow (upward-deflected curve).

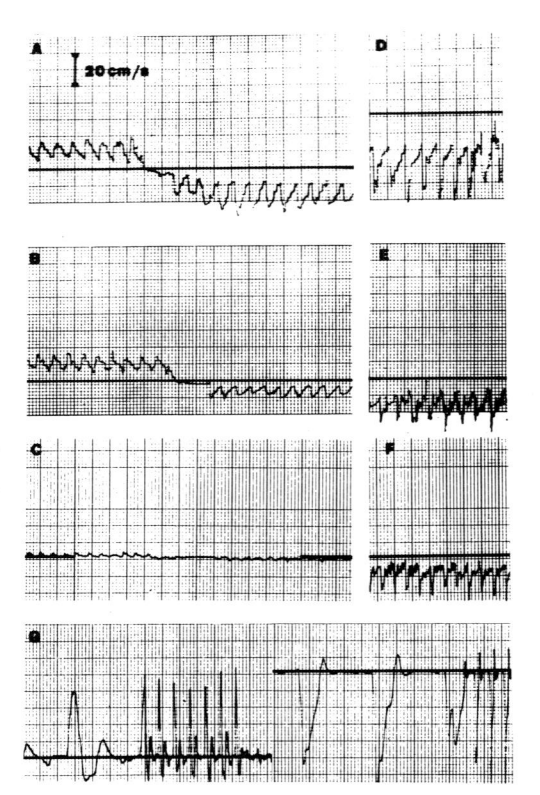

Figure 3–14. Normal continuous-wave Doppler flow signals in the vertebral and subclavian arteries. **A–C:** At the mastoidal slope of the vertebral artery, normal flow signals can be registered with strikingly different intensity of the echo. Despite a poor display on the chart (C), however, acoustic judgment of the flow signal is still sufficient. **D–F:** In most cases, flow signals from the proximal vertebral artery segment are stronger and more realistically represent the true channelling capacity of the vertebral artery. **G:** Normal flow profile of the subclavian artery during distal (left side) and proximal (right side) insonation (for calibration of the time axis see Figure 3–7).

cular fossa in a lateromedial direction angulating the beam posteriorly, medially and caudally (Figs. 3-12, 3-13c). Rhythmic compression of the soft tissue at the mastoidal slope modulates flow echos if the insonated vessel is the vertebral artery. No modulation effect, however, occurs if another neck artery (thyrocervical trunk, ascendent cervical artery, common carotid artery) is insonated. For further details of the examination technique see Ringelstein et al. [13]. Normal vertebral artery flow signals are demonstrated in Fig. 3-14a–f.

The above-described technique permits detection of medium- and high-grade stenoses at

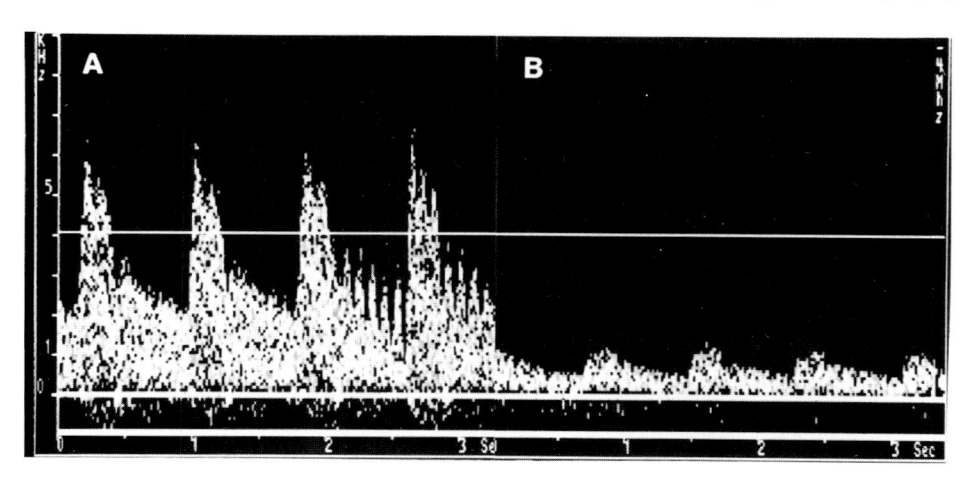

Figure 3–15. Continuous-wave Doppler flow signals of proximal vertebral artery stenoses. **A,B:** Increased flow velocity at the origin of moderately stenosed vertebral artery. Spikes are due to rhythmic compression of the vertebral artery at the mastoidal process. Normal flow velocity of the intact contralateral proximal vertebral artery is shown on the right (deflection of curves inverted for technical reasons). **C,D:** Upper left: Findings with zero-crossing meter device at the origin of vertebral artery with an approximately 80% stenosis. Three cm downstream of the vertebral artery (VA) origin, flow signal is normal. Upper right: When approaching the stenosis with the probe, a systolic reflux phenomenon occurs (arrowheads). Dotted line indicates rhythmic compression of the vertebral artery at the mastoidal slope for identification of the vessel. Lower left: High velocity flow signals occur when passing the stenotic channel with the probe from cephalad to caudad. Lower right: More proximally, the flow signal of the subclavian artery (SA) occurs. Horizontal bar indicates zeroline; for calibration see Figure 3–7.

the origin of the vertebral arteries. Stenoses with 50 to 75% lumen reduction are indicated by a circumscribed acceleration of blood flow and a more or less pronounced component of hissing noise within the flow signal. Stenoses with 80% and higher lumen reduction produce high-frequency hissing sounds (> 6 kHz), local poststenotic reflux phenomena, and low-frequency covibration of the peristenotic tissue, which causes a gruff systolic noise (Fig. 3-15). In patients with subclavian steal mechanism (see below), a stenosis at the origin of the feeding vertebral artery may be overestimated because blood flow within this artery is increased for compensation of the steal volume. In proximal vertebral artery occlusions, flow signal may either be absent, or more frequently, another neck artery functions as a collateral channel between the subclavian and more distal vertebral segment mimicking normal conditions. This situation, however, can be identified by 1) the presence of more than one supraclavicular flow signal that may be

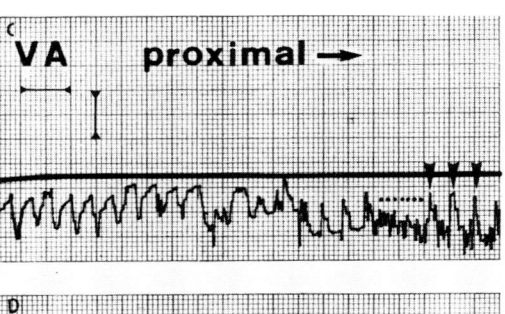

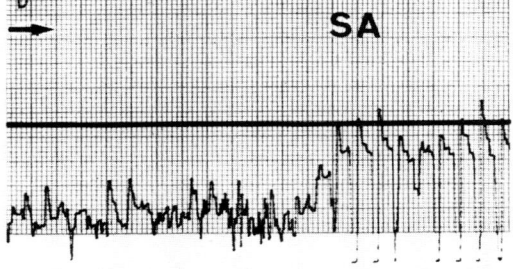

Figure 3–15 C,D.

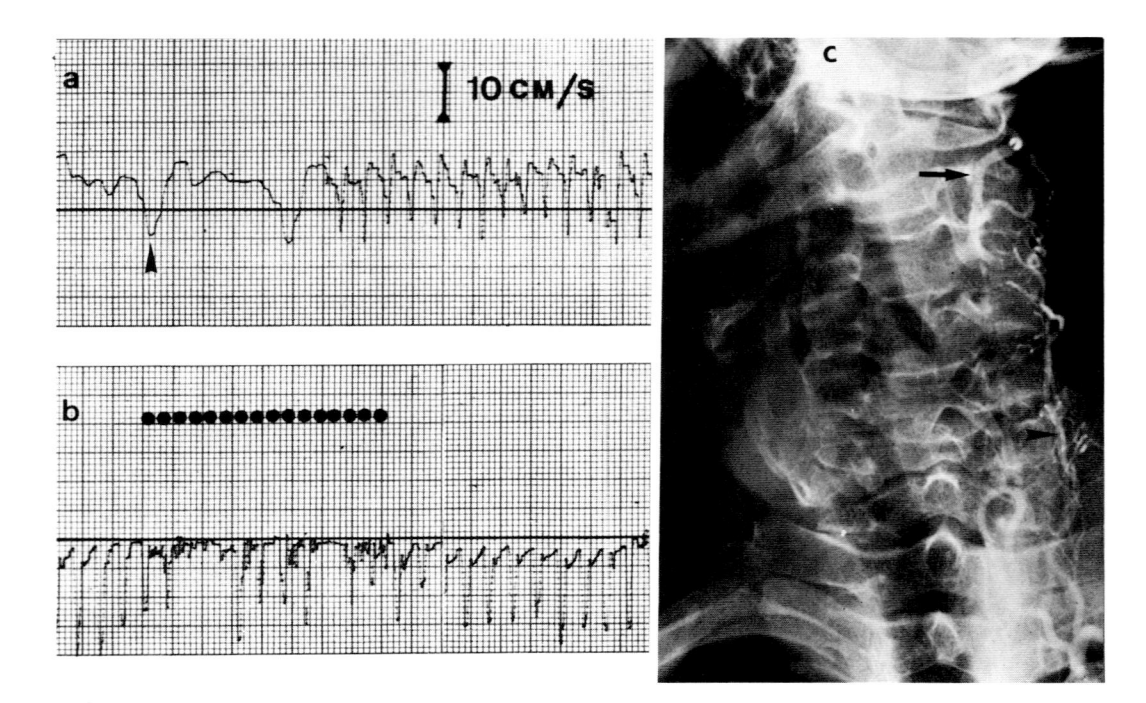

Figure 3–16. Discrepant pulsatility of vertebral artery flow signals at its origin and at the mastoidal slope due to segmental vertebral artery occlusion. **a:** At the mastoidal slope, a very soft flow signal could be registered with a "shuttle flow" signal. Reflux of the blood column occurred during early systole, indicating reduced and abnormally changing perfusion pressure (for explanation of this phenomenon see von Reutern et al. [2]. **b:** By contrast, a signal with increased pulsatility could be registered at the origin of the vertebral artery and could be modulated by compression tests at the mastoidal slope (dotted line), representing either the proximal stump of the vertebral artery itself or the thyrocervical trunk feeding extracanalicular collateralizing arteries. **c:** The angiogram showed slow filling of the distal vertebral artery (arrow) via several branches (arrowhead) of the thyrocervical trunk. The cervical vertebral artery is segmentally occluded.

modulated by perimastoidal compression tests and/or 2) compression of the lateral neck tissue surrounding the lower cervical segments. If the latter test modulates the vertebral flow echo at the mastoidal slope, collateralizing arteries run outside the transverse foramina of the spinal column and feed the vertebral system (compare Fig. 3-16c).

A mismatch in size and flow volume within collaterals bridging proximal vertebral artery occlusions may simulate stenosis of the vertebral artery itself. These overloaded channels, however, can also be modulated by compression of the lateral neck. In a few cases, hyperdynamic flow in proximal, solitary collateral channels and true vertebral artery stenosis cannot be differentiated by means of CW Doppler sonography alone.

Low- and medium-grade lesions within the intraosseous vertebral segment cannot be detected with Doppler techniques. High-grade lesions and occlusions in this location, however, lead to characteristic secondary flow changes. Due to numerous vertebral artery branches, a segmental occlusion is almost always collateralized and propagation of thrombus remains limited. Thus, a flow signal of the proximally occluded vertebral artery is regularly preserved at the mastoidal slope but provides low-flow velocity with reduced pulsatility and slowed acceleration (or even deceleration) during early systole (Fig. 3-16). These findings are often associated with compressible collateral channels in the lateral neck tissue, permitting a more reliable diagnosis (Fig. 3-16).

The easiest part of vertebrobasilar Doppler tests is the diagnosis of subclavian steal mechanism (SSM) [14]. Depending on the shape of the vertebral flow velocity profile at rest and during induced hyperemia of the stealing arm, the severity of the steal mechanism can be evaluated [15] (Fig. 3-17). With some experience, the diagnosis is absolutely reliable, and Doppler sonography is even more sensitive than any angiographic imaging technique. Due to injection of contrast medium, angiographic procedures always intervene with the labile perfusion pressures in latent or partial subclavian steal mechanism, thus mimicking vertebral artery occlusion or even antegrade vertebral artery flow. CW Doppler sonography also allows identification of the sources of blood from which the stealing vertebral artery is fed. A vertebro-vertebral overflow is less frequently found than expected (in approximately two-thirds of the cases with manifest steal), and very complex networks involving the carotid system or the contralateral neck arteries may occur. Sometimes, however, neither sonography nor angiography permit precise definition of the hidden anastomotic pathways. Intrathoracic and transnuchal anastomotic channels can hardly be assessed by means of ultrasound techniques. Increase of flow velocity in the contralateral vertebral artery or ipsilateral external carotid artery during hyperemia of the ipsilateral arm proves vertebro-vertebral or externo-vertebral steal supply, respectively. Flow curtailment within the basilar artery due to SSM can be evaluated by additional transcranial Doppler sonography (Chapter 5.) For monitoring of vertebral artery flow velocity during neuroradiologic interventions see Ringelstein and Zeumer [14].

SUBCLAVIAN ARTERIES

Finally, the subclavian arteries are also directly insonated from a supraclavicular posi-

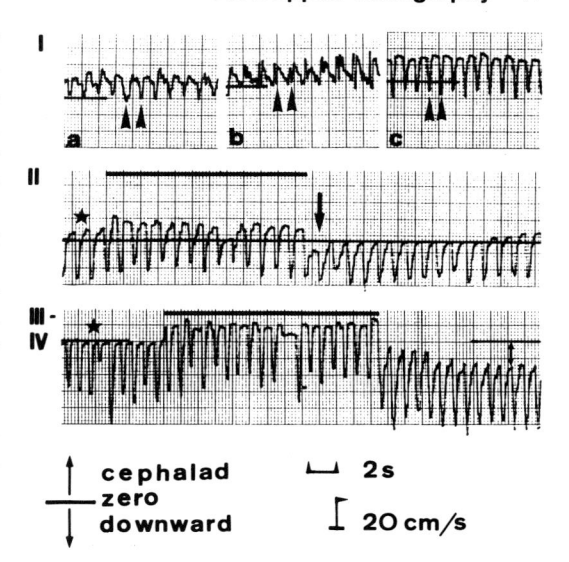

Figure 3–17. Staging I–IV of subclavian steal mechanism according to Doppler sonographic findings. **I:** Cephalad blood flow is more (b) or less (a) decelerated (arrowheads) during early systole. (c) During hyperemia of the homolateral arm following brachial artery compression, an intermittent caudal blood flow may occur (arrowheads) but net flow is still cephalad (latent or intermittent steal). **II:** Predominantly caudally directed, to-and-fro flow (*) is present at rest. Shuttle movement of the blood column is enhanced during compression of the brachial artery (black bar). Hyperemia of the arm immediately leads to a manifest subclavian steal (arrow) with gradual return to the initial labile level (partial steal). **III, IV:** Manifest steal (*) changes to-and-fro flow (or is at least diminished) during brachial compression (black bar). Hyperemia induces marked increase of flow within the stealing vertebral artery. Note high flow velocity during diastole (double-headed arrow). From Ringelstein and Zeumer, 1984 [14].

tion of the probe (Fig. 3-12d,e) (for technical details see Ringelstein and Zeumer [14]). For rapid identification of the vessel, it is recommended to insonate the distal segment first and then to angulate the tip of the probe medially by a 90° rotation in order to insonate the proximal part of the subclavian artery. Distal and proximal refers to the segments before or beyond the origin of the vertebral artery. Slight and moderate stenoses can only be detected during direct insonation of the proximal subclavian artery, whereas severe stenoses and occlusions also lead to striking abnormalities of flow within the distal segment (Fig. 3-18).

INTRACRANIAL VERTEBROBASILAR SEGMENT

The most difficult part of the vertebral Doppler examination, although the clinically most relevant, is the diagnosis of intracranially located occlusions and subtotal stenoses of the distal vertebral and basilar arteries. As the intradural part of the vertebrobasilar system cannot be directly insonated by conventional Doppler techniques, the diagnosis of these lesions must rely on secondary, extracranial flow abnormalities alone (Figs. 3-19, 3-20). The above-mentioned reverberating flow (see carotid siphon occlusions in Fig. 3-2) is pathognomonic for distal vertebral artery thrombosis (if unilaterally present, Fig. 3-19) or basilar thrombosis (if bilaterally present, Fig. 3-20). The same phenomenon occurs in brain death [5,13,16]. In unilateral intracranial VA occlusion, the non-affected vertebral artery presents a strong hyperdynamic low-resistance flow velocity profile, thus increasing the discrepancy between the affected and nonaffected side and facilitating the diagnosis. Differentiation of unilateral distal occlusion from severe hypoplasia of the vertebral artery may be difficult. The final decision is made by compression of the nonaffected vertebral artery at the atlas loop. If this prompts an increase of flow velocity on the critical side, a distal occlusion is excluded and hypoplasia is the correct diagnosis. In basilar thrombosis, flow is bilaterally disturbed and side-to-side comparisons are not conclusive. As a rule of thumb, the combination of high-resistance flow profile (reverberating flow) on one side with lack of flow signal on the other side supports the diagnosis of basilar artery thrombosis. In patients with subclavian steal mechanism, the Doppler sonographic assessment of basilar artery occlusion is impossible by an extracranial approach (for explanation see Fig. 3-21). Normal extracranial vertebral artery findings do not exclude an embolic occlusion of the distal end of the basilar artery. Absence of midbrain and occipital lobe symptoms ("top of the basilar-syndrome"

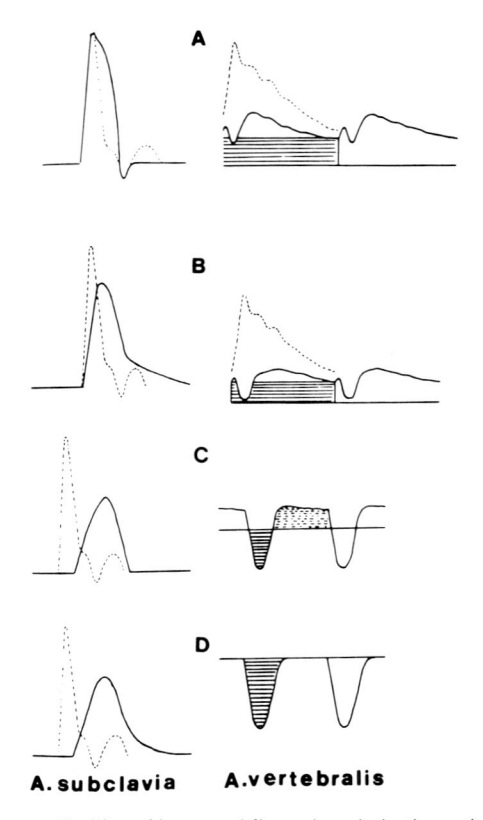

Figure 3–18. Abnormal flow signals in the subclavian and vertebral arteries due to proximal subclavian artery stenoses. **Left:** Increasingly abnormal distal subclavian artery flow velocity signals. Dotted line represents normal subclavian artery flow signal. **Right:** Increasingly abnormal vertebral artery signals (augmented) with increasing steal mechanism. Dotted line represents normal vertebral artery signal. **A:** Minimal abnormalities due to approximately 70% subclavian artery stenosis. **B:** Loss of reflux during diastole in the subclavian artery and increasing deceleration of the blood column in the vertebral artery during early systole (latent steal at rest). **C:** Early systolic reflux of blood column within the vertebral artery corresponding to approximately 90% proximal subclavian artery stenoses. **D:** Manifest steal. The shape of the subclavian artery signal is completely abnormal; blood in the vertebral artery is constantly flowing downward (manifest steal) indicating subtotal stenosis or occlusion of the proximal subclavian artery. Modified according to Marcadé [23].

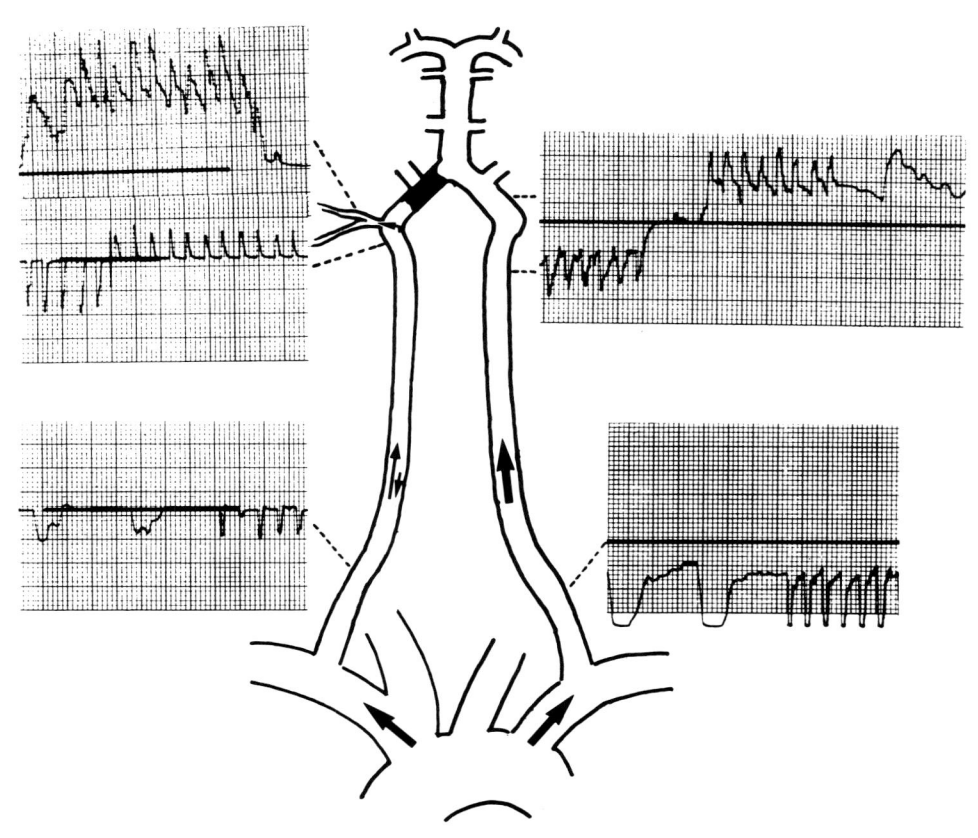

Figure 3–19. Angiographic and Doppler sonographic findings in unilateral intracranial vertebral artery occlusion (drawing made from angiogram). The right intracranial segment of the vertebral artery is thrombosed, blocking the mouth of the posterior inferior cerebellar artery. A muscle branch of the vertebral artery at the mastoidal slope gives a high velocity flow signal due to hyperdynamic flow. A high resistance flow profile with lack of diastolic flow at the mastoidal slope and reverberating flow (to-and-fro movement) within the proximal vertebral artery is registered. On the patent left side, vertebral artery flow profiles reveal compensatorily elevated flow velocity (for calibration see Fig. 3–7). From Ringelstein [16].

[17]), however, permits the resolution of this differential diagnosis.

Clinical Usefulness and Limitation

Extracranial occlusive disease of the vertebral arteries has a relative benign prognosis [16,18,19]. This is because of the peculiarities of the embryologic development of the vertebrobasilar system. Initially, a large number of arteries are present in a transverse and segmental arrangement that later merge into several major longitudinal arterial avenues, i.e., the extracranial vertebral arteries. Although not visible on angiograms, their numerous branches are still present and immediately serve as sufficient collateral pathways as soon as a drop in perfusion pressure indicates the need for collateral blood supply (compare also Fig. 3-16c). Major ancillary channels are the thyrocervical trunk (originating from the subclavian artery) and the external occipital artery (originating from the external carotid artery). Occlusions at the origin of the vertebral artery or its intraspinal part have a strong tendency to remain segmentally limited without threatening propagation of thrombus. Consequently, these lesions are asymptomatic or lead to only minor strokes or TIA. CW Doppler helps to

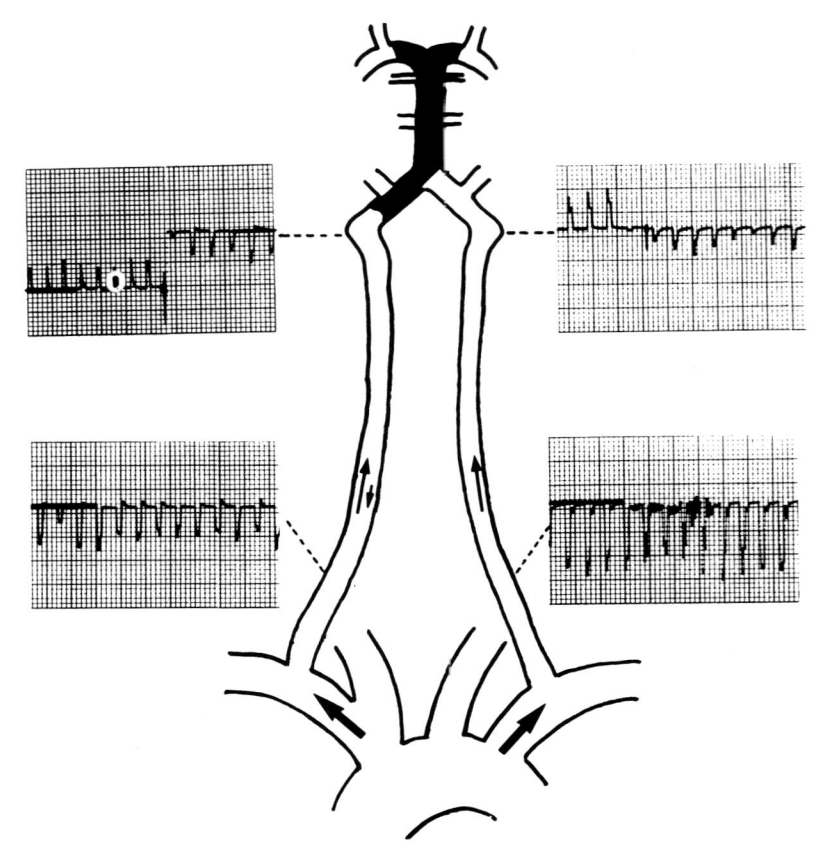

Figure 3–20. Typical Doppler sonographic findings in vertebrobasilar thrombosis (drawing made from angiogram). The original Doppler sonographic findings are demonstrated in the curves. **Left:** High resistance flow profile with reverberating flow within blind stump of vertebral artery. **Right:** Pronounced high resistance flow profile within left vertebral artery due to escape of blood via the posterior inferior cerebellar artery (for calibration see Fig. 3–7). From Ringelstein [16].

identify both the lesions, as well as the type and extent of their compensation by collateralization. Doppler techniques helped clinicians realize and understand the favorable outcome of these lesions.

In rare cases, where both vertebral arteries are severely affected, semiinvasive recanalizing techniques seem to be beneficial. CW Doppler helps to select these patients [14,20]. Percutaneous transluminal angioplasty is the method of choice for recanalization of high-grade vertebral artery stenoses if recurrent vertebrobasilar symptoms occur and the symptomatology is not related to cerebral microangiopathy.

In unilateral subtotal VA stenoses, antithrombotic treatment (acetylsalicylic acid, heparin/coumarin) is given if clinical findings suggest embolic activity of the lesions. On prospective studies, this regimen, however, has not proven to be beneficial. Heparin and/or coumarin is thought a must in patients with dissections of the vertebral arteries of either spontaneous origin or due to accidental trauma and chiropractic treatment. In dissections, segmental arterial occlusions may occur both intra- and extradurally. Doppler sonography may identify these patients, who should always be subjected to subsequent angiography for more detailed analysis and forensic proof of

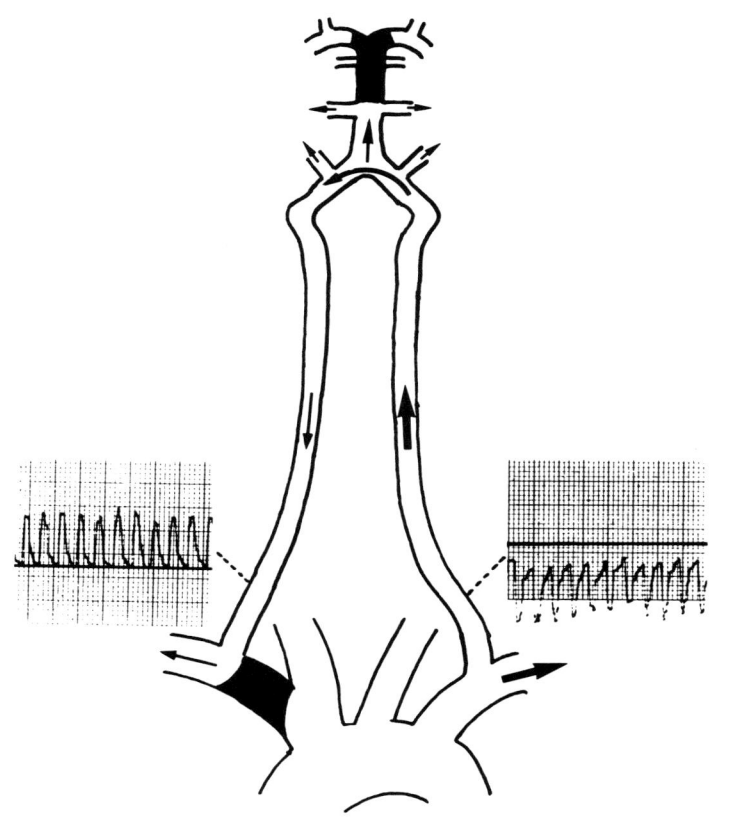

Fig. 3–21. False negative findings in basilar artery thrombosis due to extracranial subclavian steal mechanism (drawing from original angiogram). The original curves indicate normal blood flow on the left and reversed extremity-type flow signals on the right side due to subclavian artery occlusion on the right. In this constellation, basilar artery occlusion cannot affect extracranial vertebral artery flow velocities, and this remains undetected. From Ringelstein [16].

the lesions. Transcranial Doppler sonography may provide further diagnostic clues.

Subclavian steal mechanism is also a very benign condition. In our experience in a large number of cases, only half of the patients or even less are symptomatic and present either the subclavian steal syndrome (which is not clearly defined in the literature but mostly refers to a combination of mild transient vertebrobasilar symptoms) or brachial claudication. Extracranial, low-risk surgical procedures (carotidosubclavian bypass, carotidosubclavian anastomosis) are only indicated in complete subclavian occlusions provided the patients are symptomatic. A lacunar state of the brain should first be excluded as this condition may frequently better explain the patient's signs and symptoms. In high-grade subclavian artery stenoses, percutaneous transluminal angioplasty of the proximal subclavian segment is the treatment of choice [14,20] and may be applied repeatedly if necessary. In a larger series of patients with proven optimal recanalization and normalization of vertebral blood flow, only one-third became completely asymptomatic and another third reported improvement. The last third did not benefit. This clearly indicates that a close causal relationship between subclavian steal mechanism and vertebrobasilar symptoms does not exist. I have never seen a brain infarction due to subclavian steal mechanism. Arm claudication

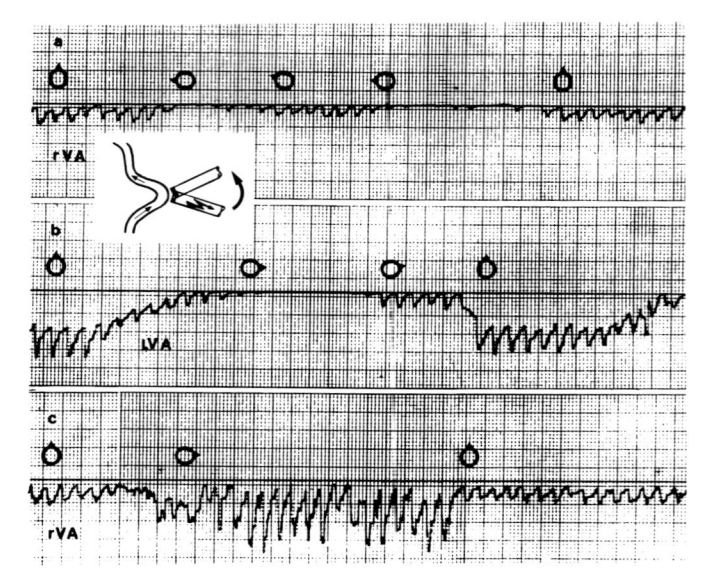

Figure 3–22. Vertebral artery flow changes during maximal head rotation. **a:** Head rotation to the left blocks blood flow within the right vertebral artery (rVA). **b:** Head rotation to the right blocks left vertebral artery (LVA) blood flow. **c:** Simultaneously, blood flow velocity within the right vertebral artery is compensatorily augmented (circles symbolize head and nose seen from above) (for calibration see Fig. 3–7). From Ringelstein Habilitation Thesis, Medical Faculty Aachen, 1984.

has a strong tendency to improve spontaneously over time due to the establishment of collateral blood flow.

Many clinicians believe that rotation of the neck can stop vertebral blood flow and thus induce vertebrobasilar symptoms such as vertigo, nystagmus, and diplopia. This view was propagated on the basis of post-mortem experiments [21] and angiographic observations in the 1960s [22]. Neck rotation can, in fact, block vertebral artery blood flow. In our experience, however, stoppage of VA blood flow occurs 1) in only a small percentage of humans, 2) most often on the side contralateral to the direction of head rotation, and 3) only during the very last degrees of maximal rotation. Furthermore, rotational clamping of VA flow is compensated for by an increase in flow velocity in the contralateral VA (Fig. 3-22). Not in a single case with otherwise intact VA Doppler findings could any vertebrobasilar symptoms be induced during maximal head rotation with and without sonographically proven stoppage of blood flow at the atlas. During the last few years, I have scrutinized a large number of patients with clinical findings and histories suggesting vertebrobasilar symptoms due to neck rotation. Only one patient was found in whom this mechanism could be demonstrated. This 52-year-old truck driver (and heavy smoker) suffered a stroke with hemihypesthesia, transient ataxia, and nystagmus. After rapid recovery, he was back on his truck; he realized attacks of severe vertigo, nausea, imbalance, and oscillating vision as soon as he turned his head to the right when driving his vehicle backwards. CW Doppler sonography revealed an intracranial occlusion of the right vertebral artery (which I attributed to the previous brainstem stroke) and a complete blockage of the left (!) VA during head rotation to the right (!). The above-mentioned symptoms occurred with a latency of 15 seconds and were reproducible.

Intracranial vertebrobasilar thrombosis is a severe condition and often leads to completed strokes or even death. In unilateral intracranial vertebral artery occlusion, dorsolateral (retro-olivary) medullary infarction is the rule, sometimes with additional infarction of the cerebellar hemispheres (due to involvement of the posterior inferior cerebellar artery arising from the occluded segment). Doppler diagnosis of this condition has further diagnostic and therapeutic consequences. If thrombus propagation can be prevented with anticoagulation, the outcome may be relatively benign although hiccups and swallowing disturbances may lead to secondary lethal complications.

Bilateral intracranial vertebral artery and basilar artery thromboses cannot be differentiated by means of extracranial CW Doppler findings. Both conditions can cause life-threatening strokes and often (in approximately 80% or more) are lethal. Rapid screening of these patients with Doppler techniques is decisive for both exclusion of vertebrobasilar thrombosis in those with coma of unknown origin, brainstem hemorrhages, and severe lacunar brainstem infarctions, as well as confirmation of the diagnosis prior to subsequent angiography and intraarterial application of fibrinolytic substances [13]. Although clinical findings are promising, this therapeutic approach has not yet been proven to be clearly beneficial or superior to heparinization.

CONCLUSIONS

Aside from history-taking and clinical examination, CW Doppler sonography of the extracranial brain-supplying arteries is the most informative and most relevant diagnostic test in every acute or chronic stroke (or stroke-prone) patient. Extracranial stroke-related occlusive macroangiopathy can be diagnosed and quantified with very high accuracy and differentiated from more benign arteriosclerosis of the dilatative type (kinking, coiling). CW Doppler sonography is of only limited value for the diagnosis of intracranial occlusive macroangiopathy, except for distal carotid occlusion and vertebrobasilar thrombosis. Correct Doppler diagnoses require considerable training and clinical experience of the examiner. For a more detailed screening of the intracranial large arteries, transcranial Doppler sonography (a new, low-frequency, pulsed Doppler technique) is the method of choice. The latter is also very helpful for the assessment of the hemodynamic effects of severe extracranial disease on the intracranial circulation. Nonstenosing plaques cannot be detected with CW Doppler sonography, but they are of less clinical relevance as compared to high-grade carotid artery disease. Additional high resolution B-mode imaging of the carotid bifurcation is necessary for plaque detection, the therapeutic and prognostic consequences of which, however, are still a matter of clinical research. In patients with lacunar infarction or subcortical arteriosclerotic encephalopathy, which are the main causes of stroke in the elderly, CT (or MR) imaging helps to prevent misinterpretation of the causal relationship between stroke symptoms and extracranial Doppler findings.

References

1. Barnes RW, Nix L, Rittgers SE (1981) Audible interpretation of carotid Doppler signals. *Arch Surg* 116: 1185–1189.
2. von Reutern G-M, Büdingen HJ, Hennerici M, Freund H-J (1976) Diagnose und Differenzierung von Stenosen und Verschlüssen der carotis mit der Doppler-Sonographie. *Arch Psychiat Nervenkr* 222:191–207.
3. Trockel U, Hennerici M, Aulich A, Sandmann W (1984) The superiority of combined continuous wave Doppler examination over periorbital Doppler for the detection of extracranial carotid disease. *J Neurol Neurosurg Psychiatry* 47:43–50.
4. Spencer MP (1986) Frequency spectrum analysis in Doppler diagnosis. In Zwiebel WJ (ed): *Introduction to Vascular Ultrasonography.* 2nd Ed. Orlando: Grune and Stratton, pp 53–80.
5. Yoneda YS, Nishimoto A, Nukada T (1974) To-and-fro movement and external escape of carotid arterial blood in brain death cases. A Doppler ultrasonic study. *Stroke* 5:707–713.
6. Keller HM, Meier WE, Zumstein B (1979) Nicht invasive Doppler-Ultraschall-Abklärung zerebro-vaskulärer Patienten: Karotis-und Vertebralis-Doppler-Untersuchung. In Kriessmann A, Bollinger A (eds): *Ultraschall-Doppler-Diagnostik in der Angiologie.* 2nd Ed. Stuttgart: Thieme, pp 90–104.
7. Müller HR (1971) Diagnosis of internal carotid artery occlusion by directional Doppler sonography of the ophthalmic artery. *Neurology* 22:816–823.
8. Weinberger J, Bender AN, Yang WC (1980) Amaurosis fugax associated with ophthalmic artery stenosis: Clinical simulation of carotid artery disease. *Stroke* 11:290–293.
9. Weinberger J, Biscarra V, Weitzner I, Sacher M (1981) Noninvasive carotid artery testing: Role in the management of patients with transient ischemic attacks. *NY State J Med* 81:1463–1468.
10. Zwiebel WJ, Zagzebski JA, Crummy AB, Hirscher M (1982) Correlation of peak Doppler frequency with lumen narrowing in carotid stenosis. *Stroke* 13:386–391.
11. Büdingen HJ, von Reutern GM, Freund HJ (1982) *Dopplersonographie der extrakraniellen Hirnarterien.* Stuttgart: Thieme, p 7.

12. Ringelstein EB, Berg-Dammer E, Zeumer H (1983) The so-called atheromatous pseudoocclusion of the internal carotid artery. A diagnostic and therapeutic challenge. Neuroradiology 25:147–155.
13. Ringelstein EB, Zeumer H, Poeck K (1985) Noninvasive diagnosis of intracranial lesions in the vertebrobasilar system. Comparison of Doppler sonographic and angiographic findings. Stroke 16:848–855.
14. Ringelstein EB, Zeumer H (1984) Delayed reversal of vertebral artery blood flow following percutaneous transluminal angioplasty for subclavian steal syndrome. Neuroradiology 26:189–198.
15. von Reutern GM, Pourcelot L (1978) Cardiac cycle dependent alternating flow in vertebral arteries with subclavian artery stenoses. Stroke 9:229–236.
16. Ringelstein EB (1984) Ultraschalldiagnostik am vertebro-basilären Kreislauf. I. Diagnose intrakranieller vertebro-basilärer Thrombosen mit Hilfe der konventionellen Dopplersonographie. Ultraschall 5:215–223.
17. Caplan LR (1980) "Top of the basilar" syndrome. Neurology 30:72–79.
18. Fisher CM (1970) Occlusion of the vertebral arteries causing transient basilar symptoms. Arch Neurol 22:13–19.
19. Hutchinson EC, Yates PO (1957) Carotico-vertebral stenosis. Lancet 1:2–8.
20. Brückmann H, Ringelstein EB, Buchner H, Zeumer H (1986) Percutaneous transluminal angioplasty of the vertebral artery. A therapeutic alternative to operative reconstruction of proximal vertebral artery stenoses. J Neurol 233:336–339.
21. Toole JF, Tucker SH (1960) Influence of head position upon cerebral circulation. Studies on blood flow in cadavers. Arch Neurol 2:616–623.
22. Sheehan S, Bauer RB, Meyer JS (1960) Vertebral artery compression in cervical spondylosis. Arteriographic demonstration during life of vertebral artery insufficiency due to rotation and extension of the neck. Neurology 10:968–986.
23. Marcadé JP (1978) L'exploration par effet Doppler des obstructions des troncs supra-aortiques (colloque tenu à Paris en Avril 1977). Actualités d'Angeiologie 30:189–207.
24. Bes A, Güll A, Braak A, Geraud G, Jannou P (1978) The contribution of Doppler sonography to the diagnosis of occlusion and stenoses of the internal carotid artery. In International Symposium on Cerebral Vascular Disorders and Stroke, Florence.
25. Franceschi C, Jardon-Fauconnet M (1978) Doppler continue des troncs supraaortiques. Actualités d'Angeiologie 3:23–29.
26. Reggi M, Bernard-Guieu D, Jausserau JM, Courbier R (1979) Exploration of extracranial arterial diseases by Doppler technique. Correlative prospective study with arteriography on a group of 435 patients. In Congress of Noninvasive Diagnostic Techniques in Vascular Disease, San Diego, California.
27. von Reutern GM, Thron A (1980) Dopplersonographie des artères carotides. Résultats et causes d'erreurs. Actualités d'Angéiologie 5:9–15.

Duplex Scanning of the Carotid Arteries

Stephen C. Nicholls, MD, R. Eugene Zierler, MD, and
D.E. Strandness, Jr., MD

Department of Surgery, School of Medicine, University of Washington, Seattle, Washington 98195 (S.C.N., R.E.Z., D.E.S.); Vascular Surgery Section, Seattle VA Medical Center, Seattle, Washington 98108 (R.E.Z.)

INTRODUCTION

Two categories of noninvasive tests have been developed for the diagnosis of extracranial cerebrovascular insufficiency [1]. Indirect tests assess carotid bifurcation disease by measuring pressure or flow changes either in the eye or the terminal branches of the ophthalmic artery. Because high-grade stenoses (greater than 50% diameter reduction) or total occlusions of the internal carotid artery are required to produce a reduction in ophthalmic artery pressure or flow, these methods have limited application. The supraorbital Doppler examination and oculopneumoplethysmography (OPG-Gee) have been the most commonly employed indirect tests.

Because of these deficiencies, tests were developed to directly obtain information from the carotid bifurcation. These direct tests include 1) quantitative phonoangiography, 2) ultrasonic arteriography, 3) real-time B-mode scanning, and 4) ultrasonic duplex scanning. There has been an evolution in these methods, and their limitations have become evident over time.

For example, phonoangiography, while theoretically attractive, was applicable only to about 20% of patients with carotid disease. Ultrasonic arteriography was the first method developed to give a two dimensional picture of the carotid bifurcation, which could also be employed to examine flow patterns [2]. It was an excellent method that gave reasonable results but has been superseded by the combined B-mode imaging and Doppler methods that have made the procedure simpler and more accurate. When carotid scanning was first developed, there was an attempt to utilize a B-mode image alone to identify disease and estimate its severity. Its drawbacks were indicated in a prospective 3-year multicenter trial that involved over 7,000 patients and demonstrated that accuracy of B-mode imaging decreased as the severity of carotid disease increased [3]. Identification of internal carotid occlusion was particularly difficult.

This study clearly pointed out the deficiencies of imaging alone and again stressed the need for both an image and a Doppler—the duplex approach. Today, all systems designed to examine the carotid artery employ both imaging and pulsed Doppler. The purpose of this chapter is to review the current status of this method as it applies to the detection of carotid artery disease.

THEORY AND INSTRUMENTATION

The duplex scanner combines in a single system real-time B-mode imaging and a pulsed Doppler flow detector. The B-mode image is generated from reflections of ultrasound at the interfaces of tissues with different acoustic impedance. The image is updated rapidly enough to provide "real-time" imaging. Doppler ultrasound may be used either as a continuous wave or a pulsed system, but the latter has several advantages. The Doppler system detects frequency shifts of ultrasound reflected from moving blood cells in the vessel lumen. Blood velocity and this frequency shift are related by the Doppler equation $Fd = F_o 2V \cos \theta / C$, where Fd is the frequency shift, F_o is the Dop-

---

Noninvasive Imaging of Cerebrovascular
Disease, pages 49–65
© 1989 Alan R. Liss, Inc.

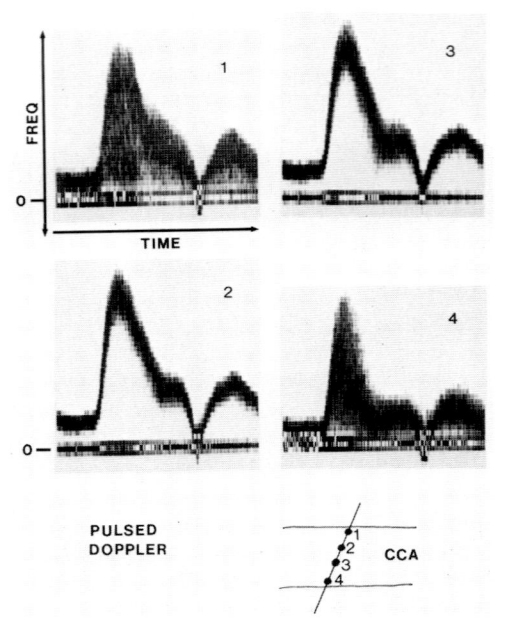

Figure 4–1. Pulsed Doppler system is used to acquire flow velocity signals across the common carotid artery. Waveforms 1 and 4 exhibit spectral broadening as a result of velocity gradients that exist near vessel walls. More central sites 2 and 3 exhibit relatively narrow band spectra. Pulsed Doppler approach is essential if spatial aspects of flow velocity field are to be appreciated. From Phillips DJ, Strandness DE (1985) Duplex scanning: Practical aspects of instrument performance. In Bernstein EF (ed): *Non Invasive Diagnostic Techniques* pp 397–408. 3rd Ed. St. Louis: The C.V. Mosby Company, with permission.

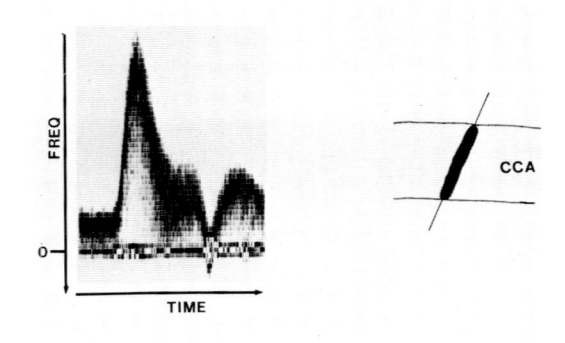

Figure 4–2. Continuous-wave Doppler system is used to acquire flow velocity signals in common carotid artery. Flow waveform is composite or superimposition of all flow velocities detected along axis of transducer. From Phillips DJ, Strandness DE (1985) Duplex scanning: Practical aspects of instrument performance. In Bernstein EF (ed): *Non Invasive Diagnostic Techniques* pp 397–408. 3rd Ed. St. Louis: The C.V. Mosby Company, with permission.

pler transmitting frequency, V is the blood cell velocity, θ is the angle between the ultrasound beam and the direction of flow, and C is the constant velocity of ultrasound in tissue.

In a pulsed Doppler system, pulses of ultrasound are transmitted into the tissues, and at a selected time following transmission the reflected signal is received by the transducer. By varying the time interval between transmission and reception one can determine the depth from which the signal is received. Thus, it is possible to selectively sample blood flow at discrete points along the path of the sound beam. If the size of the sample volume is small relative to the diameter of the artery, flow at discrete points within the lumen may be assessed (Fig. 4-1). A continuous-wave Doppler system detects all flow velocities along the ultrasound beam (Fig. 4-2). This includes not only the flow within the vessel of interest, but any adjacent vessels such as the external carotid artery and internal jugular vein that might be in the path of the sound beam. A pulsed Doppler system is essential if spatial aspects of the flow field are to be appreciated.

Modern duplex machines combine a pulsed Doppler system with real-time B-mode imaging. In addition to defining the vascular anatomy, the B-mode image also permits placement of the Doppler ultrasound beam at a specific angle with respect to the long axis of the artery. The B-mode image is displayed in real-time with the position of the Doppler beam and sample volume indicated by a superimposed line and dot (Fig. 4-3). Adjustment of the beam angle and sample volume depth enable flow to be detected at any point in the B-mode image. While audible analysis of the Doppler signal is useful for differentiating normal flow from that associated with high grade lesions, for evaluation of lesser degrees of ste-

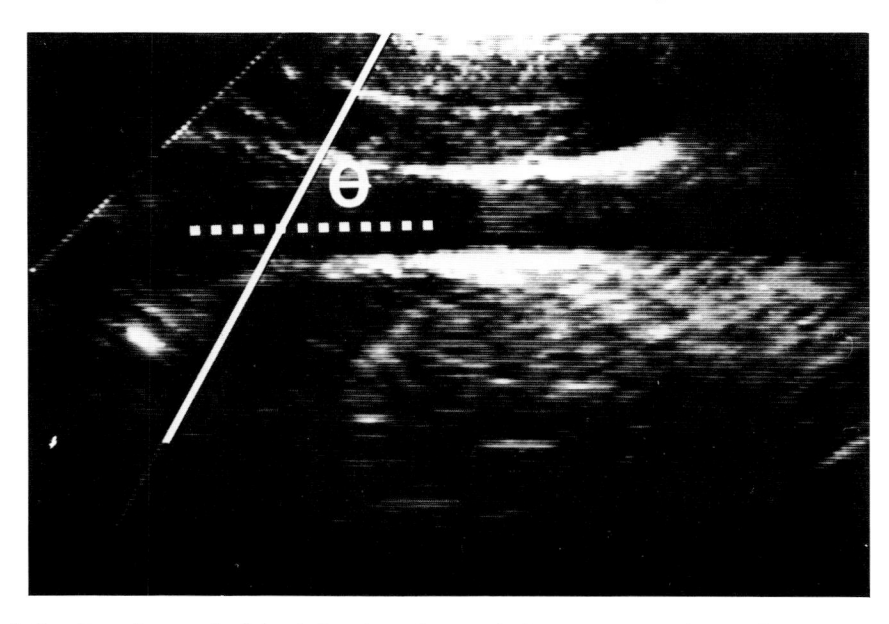

Figure 4–3. Doppler angle θ is defined as the angle between transducer ultrasound beam and blood vessel axis. It is assumed that blood flow velocity vector is parallel to vessel axis. θ is kept near 60° in studies of carotid arteries. From Phillips DJ, Strandness DE (1985) Duplex scanning: Practical aspects of instrument performance. In Bernstein EF (ed): *Non Invasive Diagnostic Techniques* pp 397–408. 3rd Ed. St. Louis: The C.V. Mosby Company, with permission.

nosis and quantification of disease, further analysis of the Doppler signal is required. The most commonly used method is spectral analysis with a digital fast Fourier transform. This displays the frequency and amplitude content of the Doppler signal with time on the abscissa, frequency on the ordinate, and amplitude as a grey scale. Frequency is directly proportional to blood cell velocity, and amplitude depends on the number of blood cells moving through the sample volume at any given time.

Experimental and clinical data have indicated that increasing degrees of intraluminal disease are associated with characteristic changes in flow patterns that can be detected by spectral analysis [4]. A normal centerstream signal produces a relatively narrow band of frequencies that represents the red blood cells moving with approximately the same speed and in the same direction. This normal laminar flow pattern is altered by intraluminal disease giving rise to disturbed flow patterns characterized by a wider range of frequencies and amplitudes referred to as spectral broadening.

With severe stenosis and marked narrowing of the lumen, high velocity jets are created that produce spectra with increased peak systolic frequencies. These quantitative changes in spectral characteristics have been compared with standard contrast angiography to define a set of criteria for classification of internal carotid artery stenosis, based on a Doppler angle of 60° and a 5-MHz transmitting frequency [5]. Prospective correlation of velocity data with angiography has enabled the following categories to be derived: A) normal, B) 1–15% diameter reduction, C) 16–49% diameter reduction, D) 50–99% diameter reduction, and E) total occlusion (Figs. 4-7). Use of end diastolic frequency has enabled further subdivision of the 50–99% category [6]. An end diastolic frequency of greater than 4.5 kHz is associated with a stenosis greater than 80% diameter reduction (Fig. 4-8). This added category is termed D+ (Table 4.1., Fig. 4-8).

The extent of agreement between angiograms and spectral data has been evaluated by the Kappa statistic. This takes into account

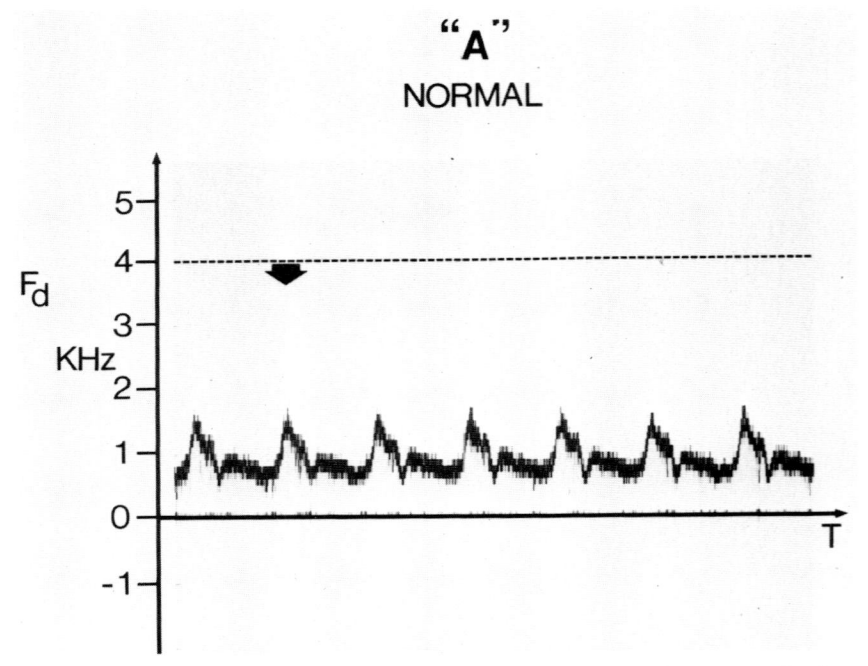

Figure 4–4. Velocity waveform from normal vessel or 0% diameter reduction.

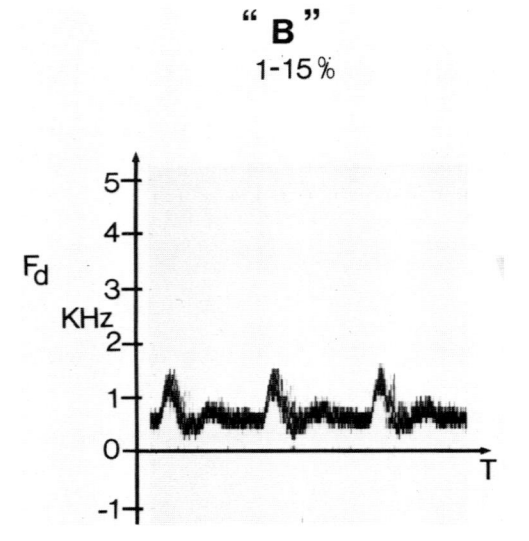

Figure 4–5. Velocity waveform from vessel with 1–15% diameter reduction ("B" lesion).

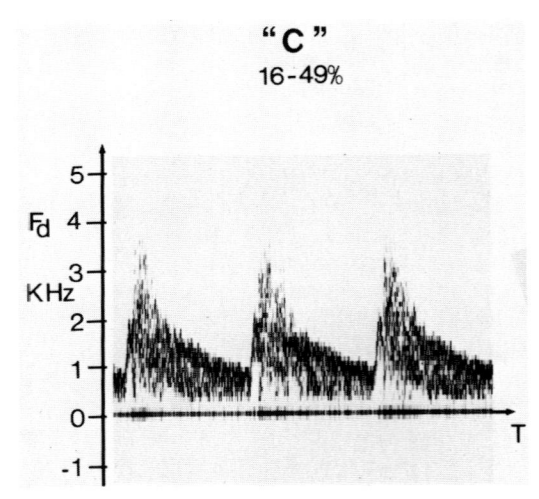

Figure 4–6. Velocity waveform from vessel with 16–49% diameter reduction ("C" lesion).

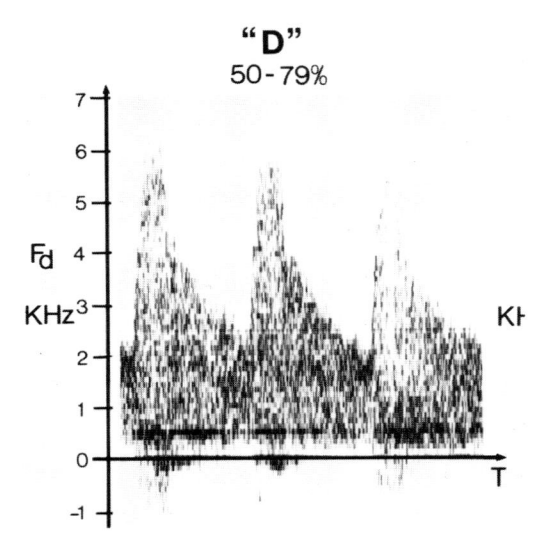

Figure 4–7. Velocity waveform from vessel with 50–79% diameter reduction ("D" lesion).

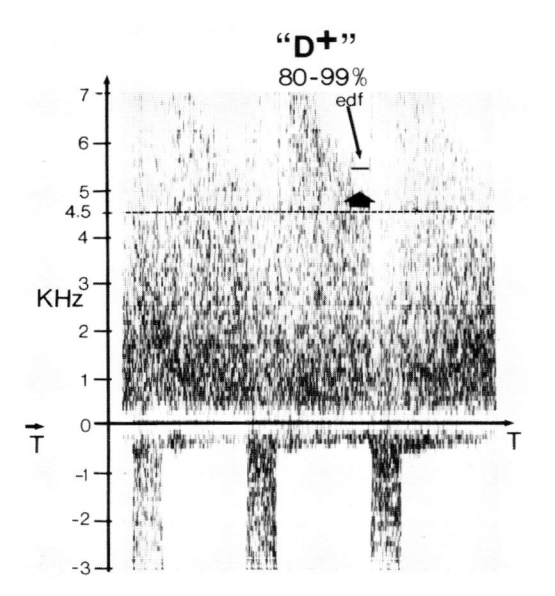

Figure 4–8. Velocity waveform from vessel with 80–99% diameter reduction ("D+" lesion).

agreement that might occur by chance alone and ranges from +1 for perfect agreement to zero for random association and −1 for complete disagreement [7]. Early results with the prototype duplex scanner yielded a Kappa value of 0.534 [8]. Progressive improvements in ultrasound hardware and experience with spectral interpretation have improved this to 0.813. It is likely that the limits of optimal agreement between duplex scanning and angiography have now been reached. For interangiographer agreement (readings of the same films by two angiographers) the Kappa value is 0.568, and intraangiographer agreement (one angiographer reading the same films at separate times) is 0.721. Variability in the duplex examination itself has also been evaluated [9]. The Kappa value between examinations by different technologists was 0.476. Variability occurred at both steps in the examination procedure: (1) obtaining the waveforms (Kappa = 0.536) and (2) using these waveforms to classify the disease (Kappa = 0.609 for interobserver variability in reading the waveforms). Intraobserver variability in rereading spectral waveforms was minimal (Kappa = 0.842). Most of this variability was accounted for in classifying minimal and moderate disease; there was little disagreement in distinguishing stenoses of hemodynamic significance.

TECHNICAL AND PRACTICAL ASPECTS OF THE DUPLEX EXAMINATION

The examination is performed with the patient supine and the head turned away from the side of interest. The technologist first surveys the vessels with the B-mode image, beginning low in the neck with identification of the common carotid artery. The carotid bifurcation is then located with the bulb being visualized as a dilatation of the artery at that level. The external carotid is usually anteromedial to the internal and can be identified by its position and typical audible velocity pattern. The internal jugular vein is easily identified because it collapses with compression. Tortuosity and anatomic variants that might influence the study may also be noted at this time. The pulsed Doppler is used to scan the plane of view to establish patency and identify any significant stenoses. Plaques containing calcium are identified by bright intraluminal echoes with posterior acoustic shadowing. Doppler signals are then obtained from standard sites: the low and high common carotid; the proximal (bulb), mid; and distal internal carotid arteries; and the external carotid (Fig. 4-9). The

54   Nicholls et al.

Table 4.1
Classification of Internal Carotid Artery Disease

Angiography[a]		Spectral waveform[b]
0% (normal)	A	Peak systolic frequency (P.S.F.) 4kHz; no spectral broadening; flow separation may be present
1–15%	B	P.S.F. 4kHz; spectral broadening in systolic downslope
16–49%	C	P.S.F. 4kHz; Spectral broadening throughout systole
50–79%	D	P.S.F. 4kHz; Spectral broadening throughout systole; end diastolic frequency 4.5 kHz
80–99%	D+	End diastolic frequency 4.5 kHz
100% (occlusion)	E	No signal in internal carotid artery; flow to zero in ipsilateral common carotid artery

[a]Percentage diameter reduction.
[b]Center stream flow sampled at a Doppler angle of 60° with a 5-MHz pulsed Doppler.

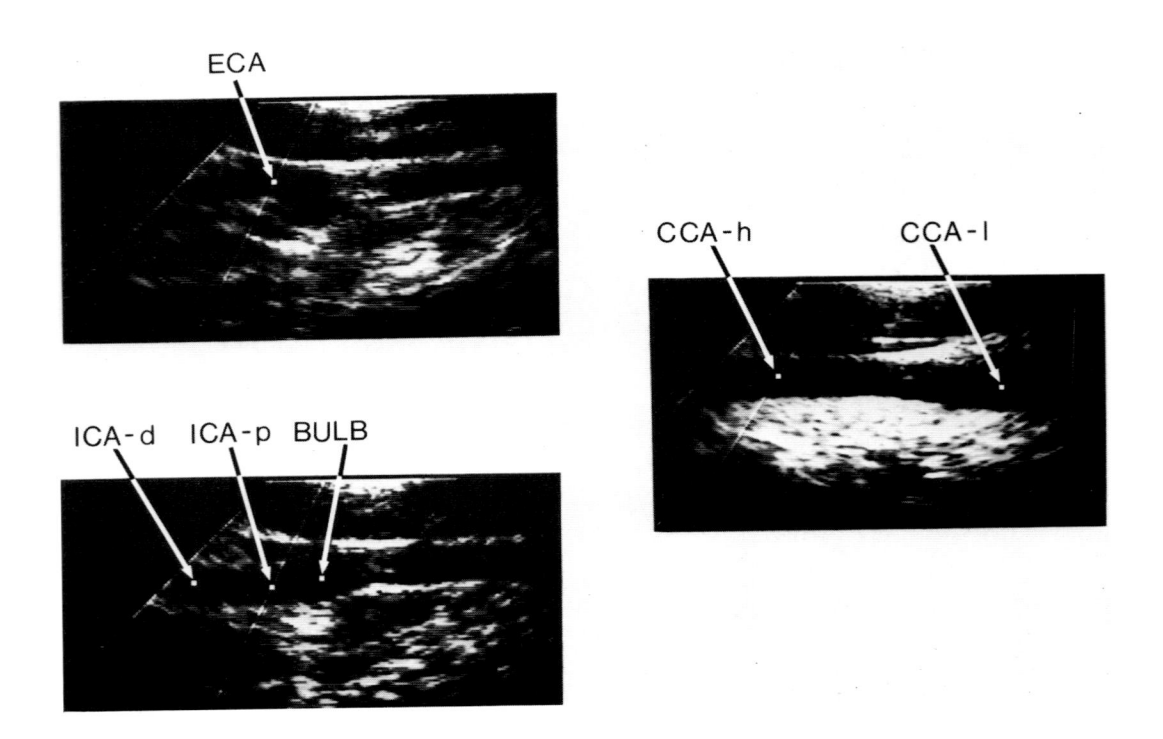

Figure 4–9. Standard anatomic sites for data acquisition in carotid system. Stenosis detected at non-standard site is also recorded. From Phillips DJ, Strandness DE (1985) Duplex scanning: Practical aspects of instrument performance. In Bernstein EF (ed): *Non Invasive Diagnostic Techniques* pp 397–408. 3rd Ed. St. Louis: The C.V. Mosby Company, with permission.

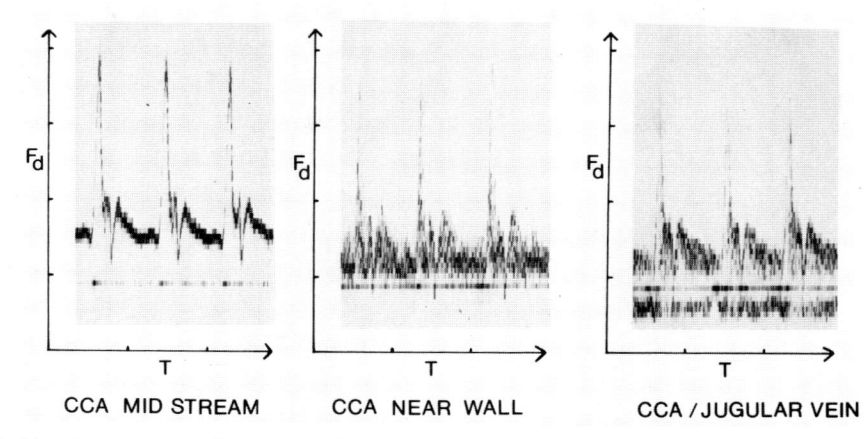

Figure 4–10. Importance of sample volume placement. In common carotid midstream, spectrum is a relatively narrow band. Near the wall, velocity gradients exist as noted by broad spectra during both systole and diastole. With sample volume placed at vessel wall, both arterial and venous flow are detected as noted by positive for the carotid and negative for the jugular vein. From Phillips DJ, Strandness DE (1985) Duplex scanning: Practical aspects of instrument performance. In Bernstein EF (ed): *Non Invasive Diagnostic Techniques* pp 397–408. 3rd Ed. St. Louis: The C.V. Mosby Company, with permission.

site of maximum velocity (greatest narrowing) is also noted. Finally, signals are evaluated in the subclavian and vertebral arteries where direction of flow is of particular interest.

The sample volume must be placed in the region of greatest flow velocity to assess the degree of narrowing. It is also essential to sample center stream velocity, because the gradients that are normally present near the wall cause apparent spectral broadening (Fig. 4-10). Respiratory movements may change the sample volume position relative to the vessel (Fig. 4-11). Sample volume size must be small in relation to the diameter of the vessel to avoid simultaneous detection of velocity gradients near the wall even when positioned in center stream. The resultant spectral broadening tends to overestimate the amount of disease present [10].

Because the detected frequency shift is directly related to both absolute velocity and the cosine of the angle of the incident ultrasound beam, the angle must be known and preferably kept constant during the examination. In the duplex scanning technique described here, the Doppler beam is kept at an angle of 60° to the long axis of the vessel. This angle is relatively easy to obtain from site to site and one examination to another. The effect of a change in the angle on the recorded frequency shift is shown in Figure 4-12. It is doubly important to be aware of this when unusual anatomic variations (as when the internal carotid is kinked) make correct angle measurement difficult (Fig. 4-13).

A significant source of error in duplex scanning is incorrect vessel identification. The branch angle and plane of bifurcation are highly variable. The low vascular resistance of the cerebral circulation results in continuous antegrade flow throughout systole and diastole in the normal internal carotid artery. In the normal external carotid, flow is reversed or goes to zero velocity in diastole, just as in any other peripheral artery. Because 70–80% of the common carotid blood flow volume passes into the internal carotid artery, the common carotid flow pattern tends to more closely resemble that of the internal carotid. However, in the presence of internal carotid artery occlusion or very tight stenosis, the common carotid flow pattern is determined by the high resis-

56   Nicholls et al.

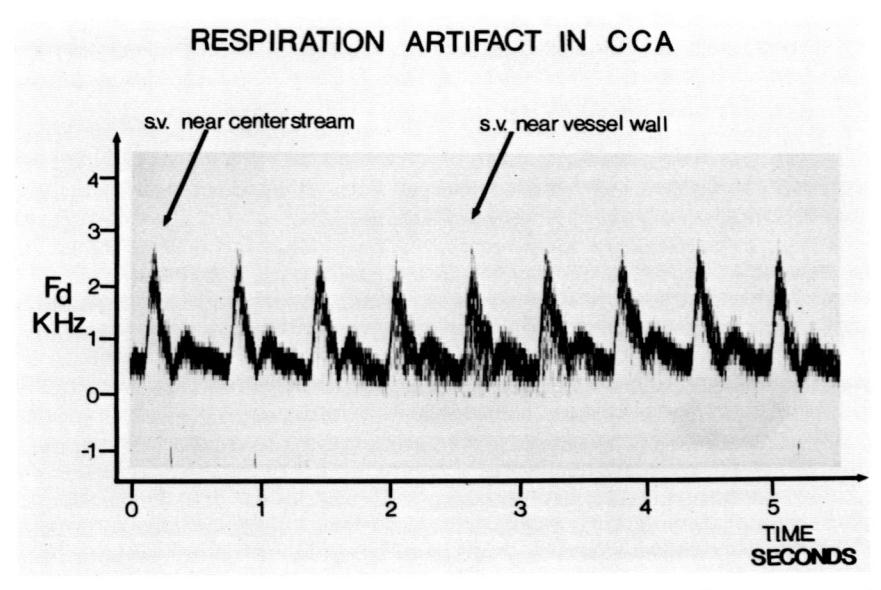

Figure 4–11. With a fixed sample volume size, respiration causes vessel movement and sampling from near the wall resulting in spectral broadening, which might be interpreted as abnormal if the obsever were not aware of the phenomenon.

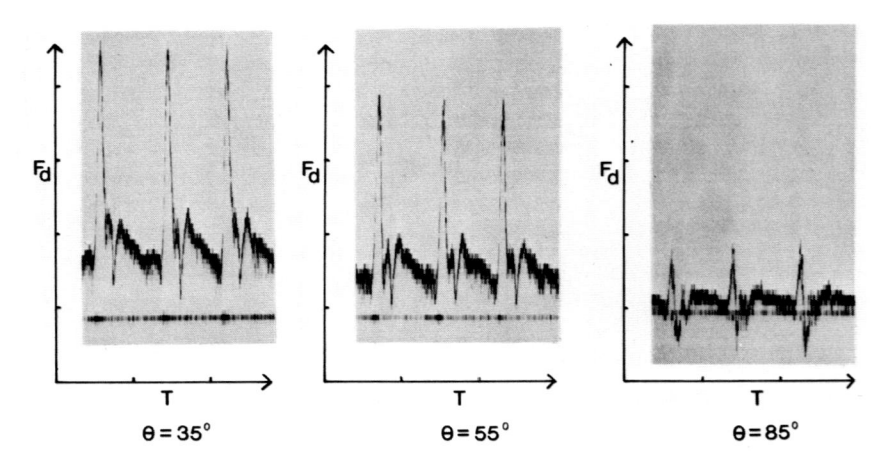

Figure 4–12. Velocity waveforms obtained from same vessel at different Doppler angles. Doppler peak frequency is directly proportional to cos θ as predicted by the Doppler equation. If signal is always acquired at 60°, then θ becomes a constant. From Phillips DJ, Strandness DE (1985) Duplex scanning: Practical aspects of instrument performance. In Bernstein EF (ed): *Non Invasive Diagnostic Techniques* pp 397–408. 3rd Ed. St. Louis: The C.V. Mosby Company, with permission.

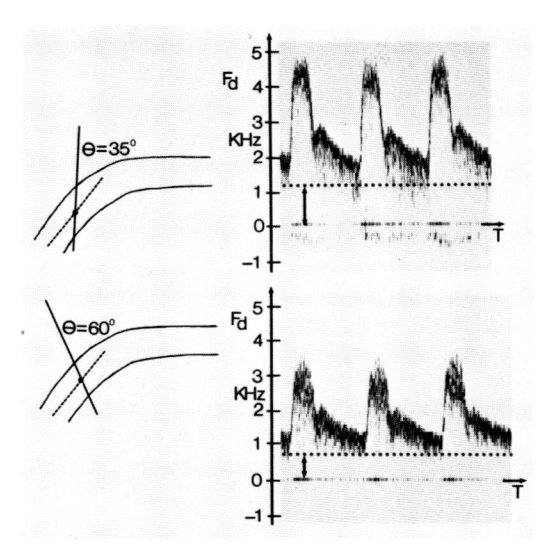

Figure 4–13. Variance in Doppler angle occasioned by difficulty in verifying axis of flow in a tortuous vessel results in significant peak frequency and spectral width differences.

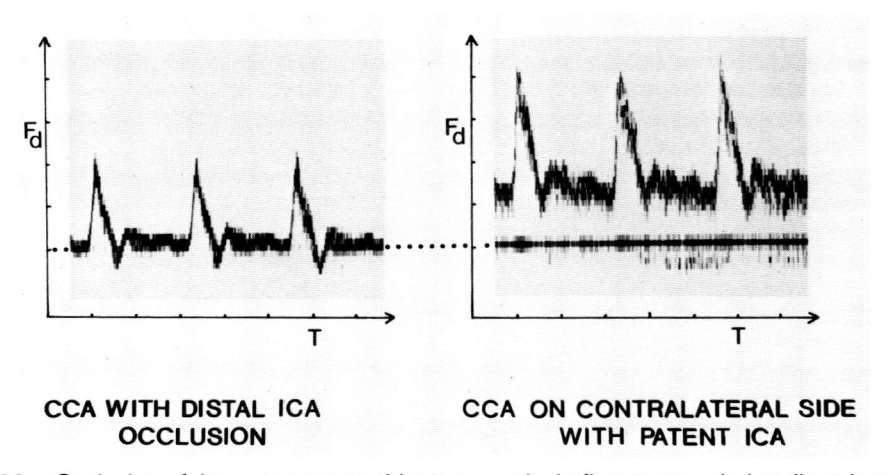

CCA WITH DISTAL ICA OCCLUSION

CCA ON CONTRALATERAL SIDE WITH PATENT ICA

Figure 4–14. Occlusion of the common carotid artery results in flow to zero during diastole on that side.

tance of the external carotid, and flow often goes to zero in diastole (Fig. 4-14). Conversely, when the external carotid artery becomes a major collateral source for the brain, the resistance to flow seen by the external carotid is very low. The velocity pattern thus recorded from the external carotid may take on characteristics seen in the internal carotid artery.

With aortic regurgitation, flow to zero may be seen in the common carotid within the presence of a patent internal carotid artery; however it will occur bilaterally. In difficult cases, identification of the external carotid may be aided by intermittent compression of the superficial temporal artery anterior to the ear. The intermittent compressions will produce

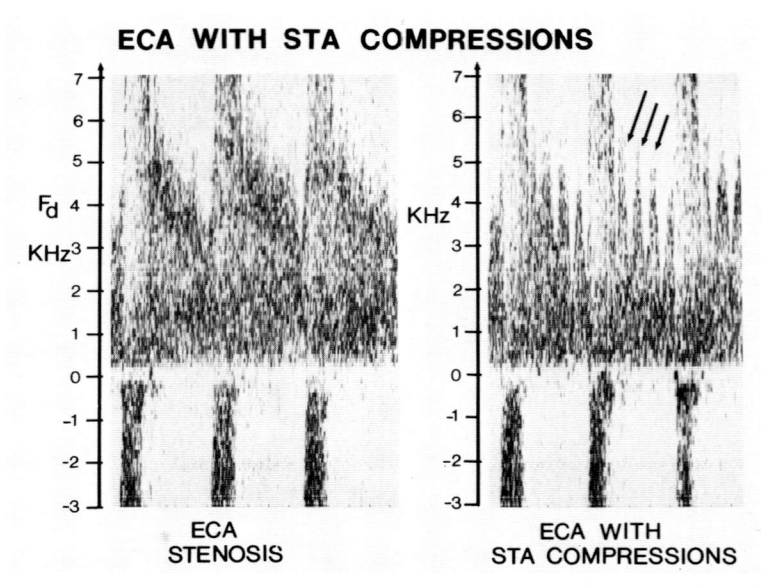

Figure 4–15. Superficial temporal artery compressions cause spikes in external carotid artery signal distinguishing it from the internal carotid artery.

spikes in the external carotid spectral waveform (Fig. 4-15).

It must also be remembered that the internal carotid artery may remain patent when the common carotid is occluded. In such cases there is retrograde flow in the external carotid as it now provides flow for the internal carotid. This clinically important situation may be difficult to evaluate with angiography, whereas it is easily recognized with the duplex scanner.

The smooth lesion of myointimal hyperplasia, which may develop in the carotid artery after endarterectomy, may result in an elevation in the peak systolic frequency and velocity but show very little in terms of spectral broadening. These stenotic arteries are different from those associated with atherosclerotic plaques (Fig. 4-16).

It must be remembered that unusual flow patterns are observed in the posterolateral region of a normal carotid bulb. These were first demonstrated in flow models and more recently in humans [11–13]. These studies have demonstrated that flow in the normal carotid bifurcation is highly complex, with isolated regions of boundary layer separation in the posterolateral part of the bulb. These were not recognized early in our experience and led to the improper classification of normals as having minimal carotid disease. However because of our studies of normal subjects, we have now come to recognize these unusual flow patterns as a good marker for the normal bulb. While there is no doubt that atherosclerosis can also lead to the generation of secondary flow patterns immediately distal to a stenosis, these should not be confused with the findings in normal subjects. In the normal, the area of boundary layer separation is localized to the outer bulb region and is not associated with a velocity increase [14]. Although it may be difficult with a single sample volume placement to distinguish these normal flow disturbances from those due to disease, sampling from multiple sites across the bulb allows recognition of these flow patterns (Fig. 4-17).

It has now been demonstrated that atheroma deposition begins in the posterolateral aspect of the carotid bulb that is adjacent to the prominent area of transient flow reversal [15]. This area has also been identified as the site of low oscillatory shear stress (Fig. 4-18) [16]. It is presumed that progressive atheroma deposition obliterates the normal configuration of the

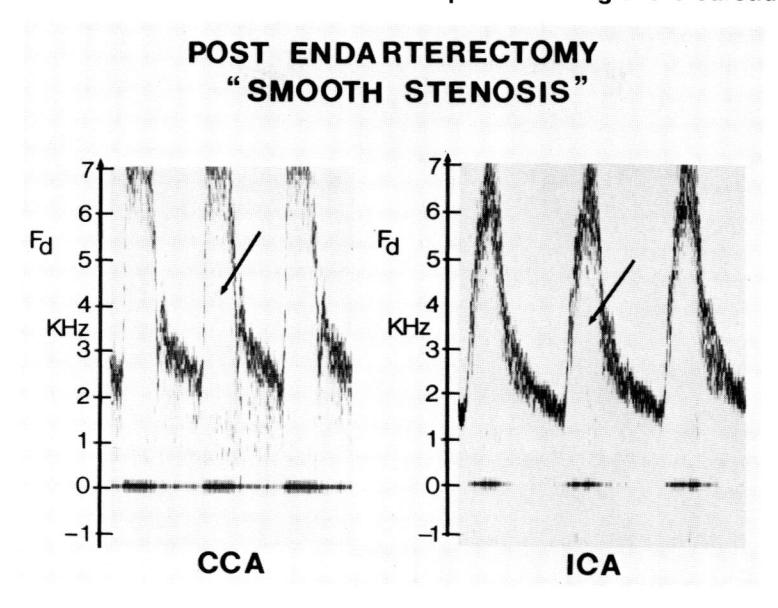

Figure 4–16. Smooth post-endarterectomy stenosis is characterized by increased peak systolic frequency without spectral broadening (arrow).

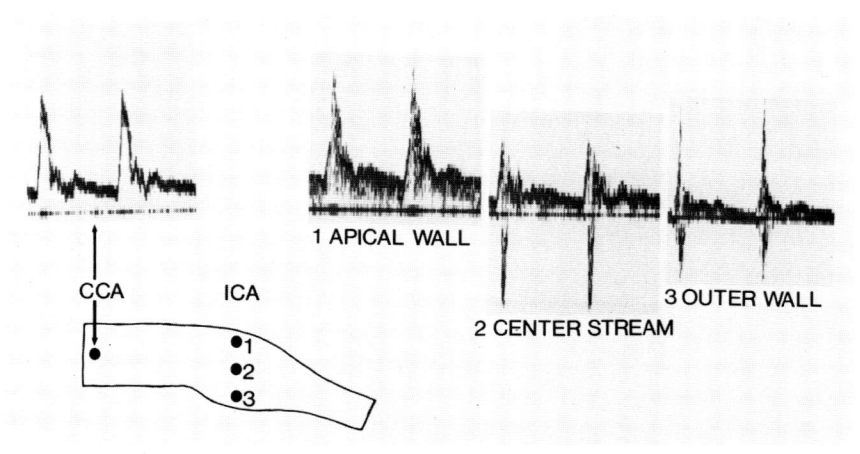

Figure 4–17. Velocity waveforms from common carotid artery and across bulb demonstrating secondary flow patterns.

bulb with consequent loss of flow separation (Fig. 4-19). The absence of flow separation is therefore associated with the earliest stages of plaque development and filling in of the bulb.

Duplex scanning has had a relatively limited role in the diagnosis of vertebrobasilar disease. Although the vertebral artery can be visualized in most cases, it has been difficult to relate these findings to any particular symptom complex. However, the vertebral artery examination can detect the presence or absence of flow, the antegrade or retrograde nature of flow, and any localized disturbances suggesting occlusive disease.

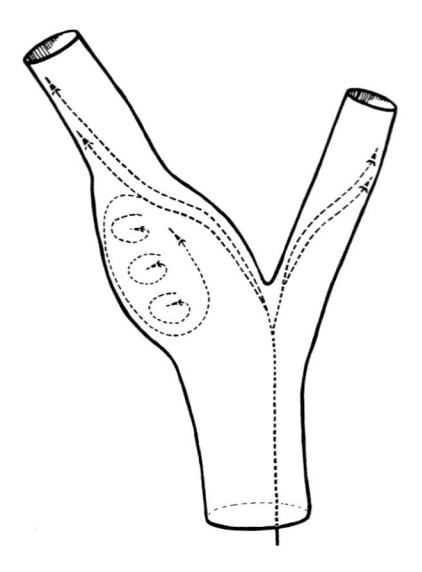

Figure 4–18. Bifurcation model demonstrating area of flow separation on lateral wall of bulb. The slow flow in this region results in low shear that oscillates during cardiac cycle.

CLINICAL APPLICATION

The role of duplex scanning in the clinical management of patients with extracranial carotid artery disease is well established [5]. It has been shown to be sufficiently sensitive to detect a wide range of carotid bifurcation disease. When used as a screening test it can identify those patients with normal or occluded internal carotid arteries who are not candidates for surgery. It is also useful for documenting disease progression because it is painless, safe, and suitable for serial examinations over time. Such a technique is essential for evaluating the natural history of carotid disease in asymptomatic patients. It is also cost-effective compared to the routine use of contrast angiography [17].

Serial testing of selected patient populations with duplex scanning has already provided important clinical information previously unobtainable with other methods. In a study of 167 patients with asymptomatic carotid bruits followed for a period of 36 months, the presence of a greater than 80% diameter-reducing internal carotid artery stenosis artery was highly correlated with the development of transient ischemic attacks, stroke, and internal carotid artery occlusion [18]. The authors concluded that it was prudent to delay surgical treatment of asymptomatic patients with carotid disease until the appearance of symptoms or progression of stenosis to greater than 80% diameter reduction by duplex scan. Similar conclusions were reached by the same group in evaluating the natural history of carotid artery disease on the side contralateral to endarterectomy [19].

Previous estimates of the rate of restenosis following carotid endarterectomy (0.5–3%) have been based on recurrence of clinical symptoms. Serial studies with duplex scanning have revealed that the incidence of restenosis is higher than previously thought (9–19%), although the different pathologic nature of the recurrent lesion confers a benign outcome [20]. While the development and validation of criteria for classification of carotid disease were based on studies of unoperated vessels, subsequent work has confirmed that the same criteria can be applied following endarterectomy [21]. Thus, duplex scanning is a suitable method for postoperative followup after operation. The pulsed Doppler approach has also been used intraoperatively before and after endarterectomy to determine adequacy of the procedure and to detect technical errors that may be clinically silent [22].

Duplex scanning has proved useful as a preoperative screening technique to identify patients with significant carotid disease who are scheduled for aortocoronary bypass or other major surgery [23]. Present clinical practice requires the performance of angiography in most patients with symptomatic cerebrovascular disease. Angiography not only visualizes the carotid bifurcation, but the common carotid origins, siphon, and intracranial circulation. However, duplex scanning may suffice as the sole preoperative test when angiography entails unacceptable risks [24,25]. It may also obviate the need for angiography in certain clinical situations that are not amenable to surgery, such as occlusion of the internal carotid artery. Duplex scanning is useful for screening patients with nonhemispheric or vague symptoms in whom surgery is rarely recommended. It is particularly useful in identifying normal bifurcations on the side of focal symptoms. In

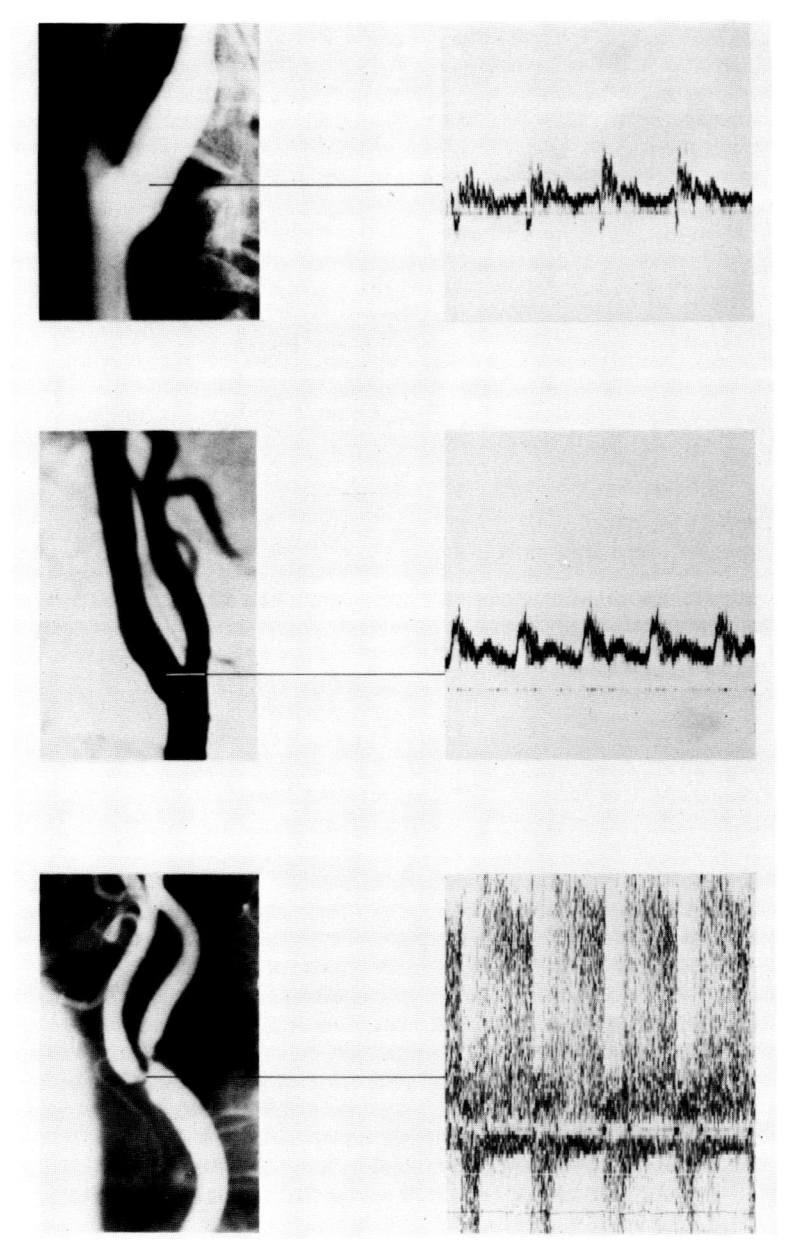

Figure 4–19. Loss of flow separation as intimal deposition occurs in the bulb. Eventually true luminal narrowing occurs.

these circumstances, diagnostic efforts may be directed towards other entities, such as cardiogenic emboli and lacunar stroke, without subjecting the patient to the risk of angiography [26].

RECENT ADVANCES

In an attempt to reduce some of the subjective elements in reading spectral waveforms, a computer-based pattern recognition program

62   Nicholls et al.

1 HEART CYCLE   4 HEART CYCLES   16 HEART CYCLES

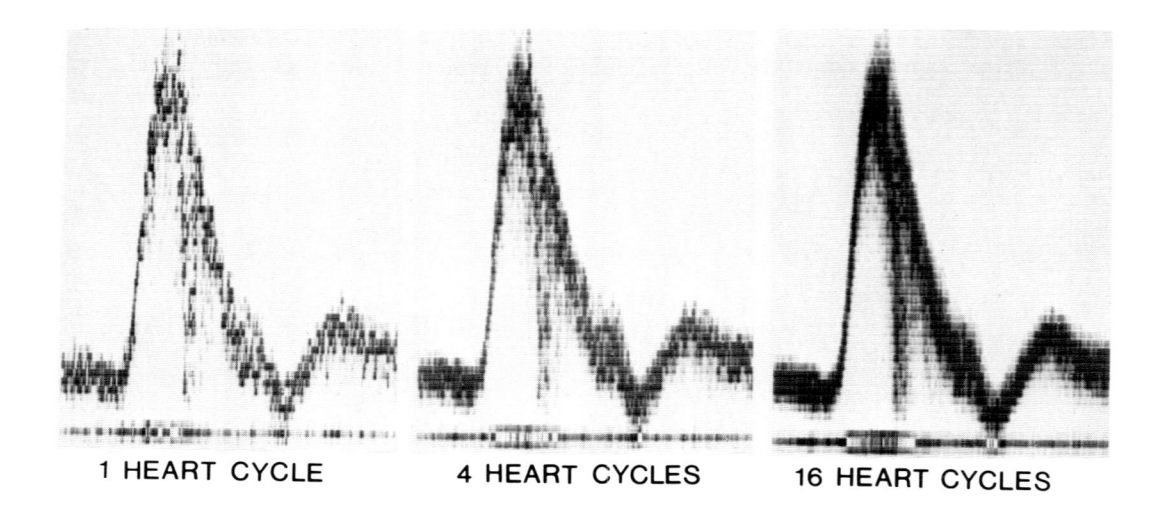

Figure 4–20. Velocity waveform of 1 heart cycle and ensemble averages of 4 and 16 cycles. Central tendency of waveform becomes increasingly evident as number of cycles is increased. From Phillips DJ, Strandness DE (1985) Duplex scanning: Practical aspects of instrument performance. In Bernstein EF (ed): *Non Invasive Diagnostic Techniques* pp 397–408. 3rd Ed. St Louis: The C.V. Mosby Company, with permission.

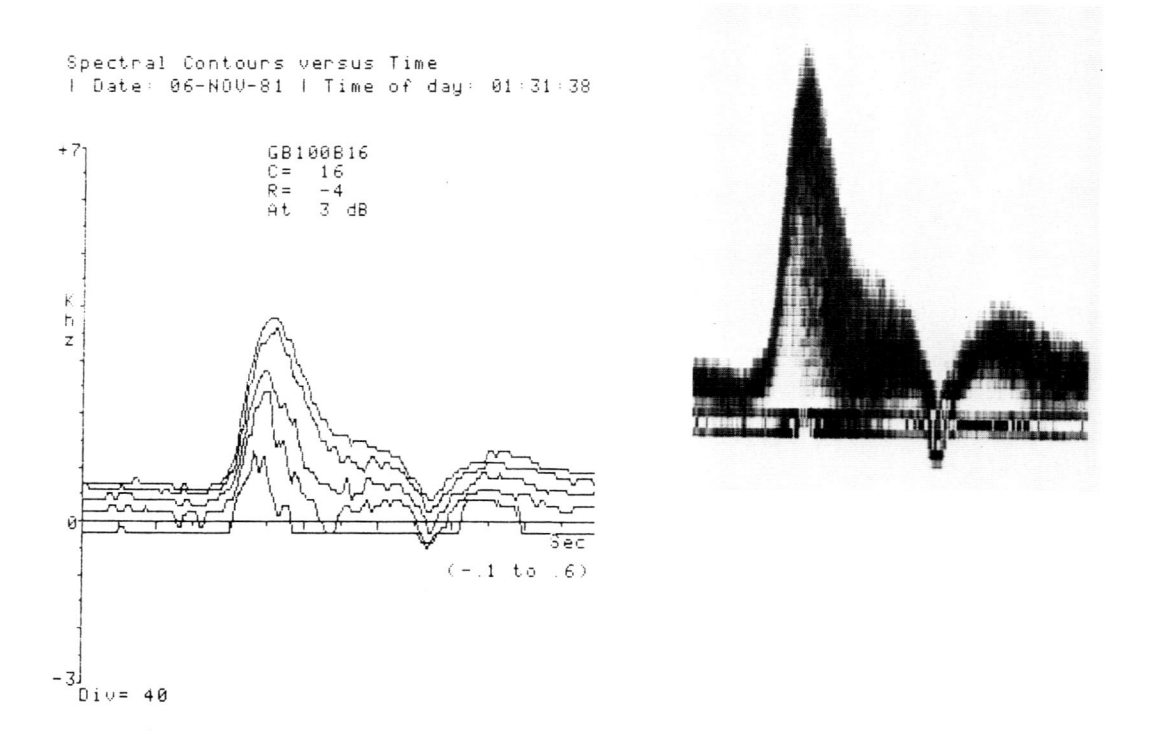

Figure 4–21. Computer-generated contour plot showing mode, 3-dB, and 9-dB bands for the ensemble waveform at right.

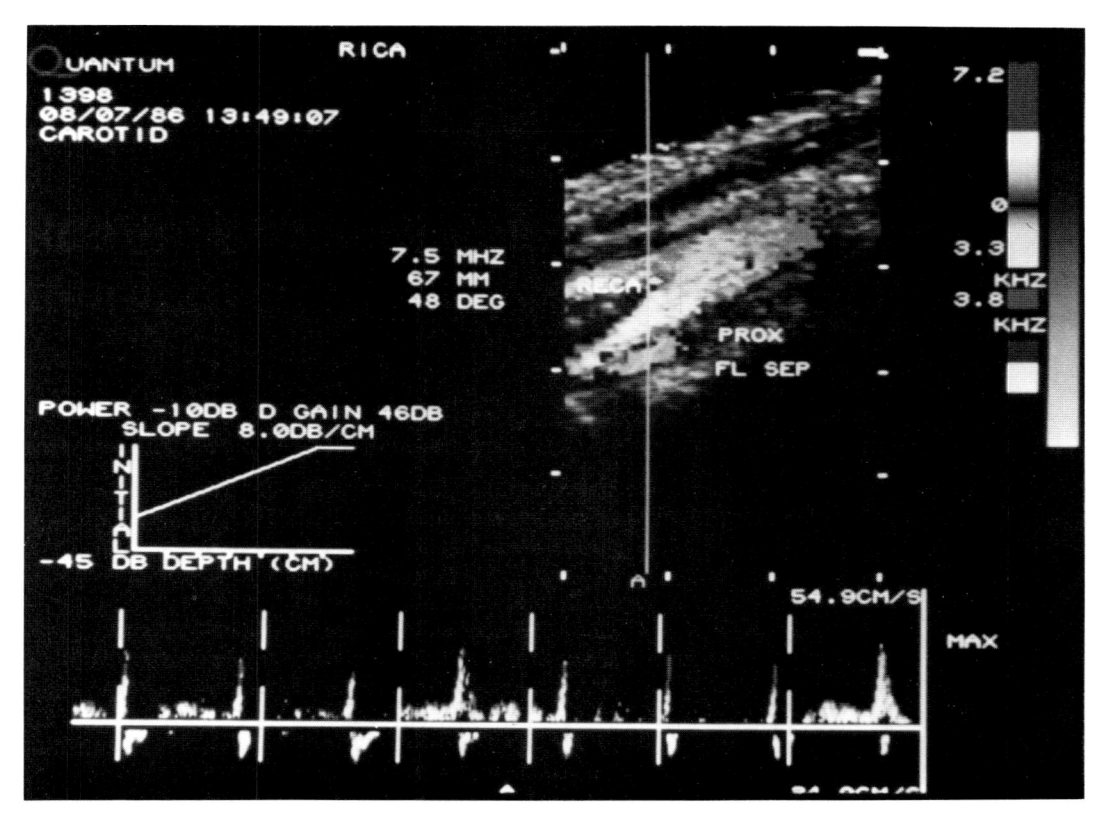

Figure 4-22. Flow separation in a normal carotid bifurcation. Flow toward the transducer is red. Higher frequencies in the same direction along the apical divider are labeled white. Flow in the separation zone (posterolateral bulb) is blue because it is away from the transducer (flow reversal). The external carotid is labeled. N.B.: The internal jugular vein has been compressed, and no flow is seen in this vessel. (Reproduced in color on page 71.)

was developed at the University of Washington [27]. Waveforms from the low common carotid and proximal internal carotid artery locations were collected using the electrocardiogram R-wave as a time reference, and the spectra from 20 heart cycles were combined and averaged. The process of ensemble averaging reinforces the constant features of the waveform while minimizing the random, nonperiodic features (Fig. 4-20). For each ensemble waveform, the mode (highest amplitude/frequency), the "half power" or 3-db point, and the 9-db point above and below the mode were plotted. This averaged waveform was then used to extract features for analysis (Fig. 4-21). Final disease classification was made by a step-wise selection algorithm. One hundred seventy vessels were prospectively evaluated by both angiography and the pattern recognition process [28]. Four categories of diameter reduction were made: normal, 1–20%, 21–50%, and 51–99%. One hundred forty-one or 82% of the vessels were classified into the same category by both angiography and the pattern recognition method. The computer and angiography differed by more than one category in only one of the 170 vessels. The level of agreement corrected for chance (Kappa) was 0.769. This level of agreement compares favorably with the agreement between the reading of the angiograms themselves [29]. It is now possible to use this method on-line at the time of the duplex scan.

A new duplex scanning system has been developed that superimposes a color-flow image

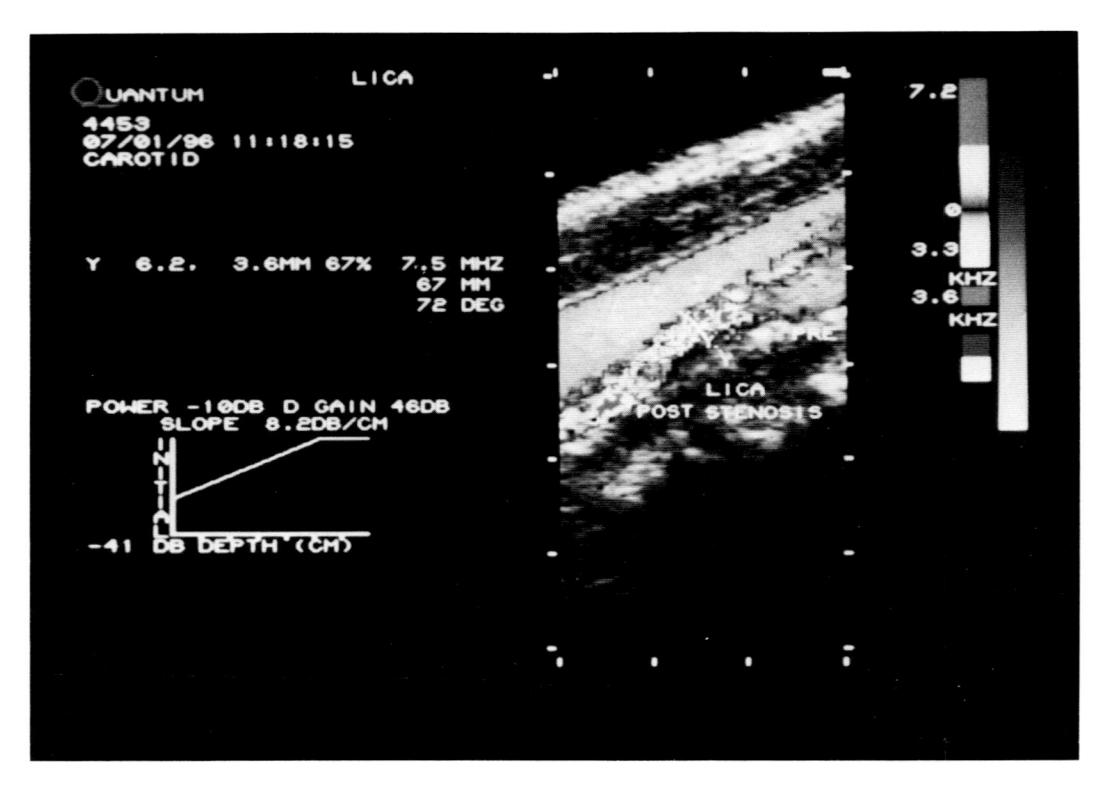

Figure 4-23. Left internal carotid artery stenosis. Red indicates flow toward the transducer. Blue indicates flow away from the transducer. Color scale (on the right) has been set by the operator so that all frequencies in the stenosis >3.8 kHZ are green. N.B.: Flow in the internal jugular vein is blue because it is away from the transducer. (Reproduced in color on page 71.)

on a real-time B-mode tissue image (Figs. 4-22, 4-23). In contrast to a conventional duplex scanner that uses a single pulsed Doppler sample volume to detect flow, this instrument detects flow throughout the entire scan field. Shades of red and blue are used to indicate direction of flow with respect to the transducer, and lighter shades represent higher Doppler shift frequencies or flow velocities. While clinical experience with the color flow system is limited, it clearly permits rapid visualization of the normal complex flow patterns in the carotid bulb. The zone of boundary layer separation along the outer wall of the bulb is seen as a blue area that changes size and shape during the cardiac cycle, while continuous forward flow along the flow divider appears as red. Flow disturbances associated with minor lesions and high velocity jets associated with severe stenoses can also be recognized. The color-flow image is particularly helpful in identifying unusual anatomic variations such as kinks, tortuous vessels, and occlusions. Work is currently in progress to elucidate specific critera for interpretation of the color-flow images.

ACKNOWLEDGMENTS

The authors wish to thank D.J. Phillips, Ph.D., and Jean Primozich, B.S., for their major role in providing the illustrations.

References

1. Nicholls SC, Strandness DE (1984) Noninvasive diagnosis of cerebrovascular insufficiency. *Int Surg* 69:199.
2. Hokanson DE, Mozersky DJ, Sumner DS, Strandness DE (1971) Ultrasonic arteriography: A new approach to arterial visualization. *Biomed Eng* 6:420.

3. Comerota AJ, Cranley JJ, Katz ML, et al. (1984) Real-time B-mode carotid imaging: A three year multicenter experience. *J Vasc Surg* 1:84.

4. Blackshear WM, Phillips DJ, Chikos PM, Harley JD, Thiele BL, Strandness DE (1980) Carotid artery velocity patterns in normal and stenotic vessels. *Stroke* 11:67.

5. Langlois YE, Roederer GO, Chan A, et al. (1983) Evaluating carotid artery disease. *Ultrasound Med Biol* 9:51–63.

6. Roederer GO, Langlois YE, Jager KA, et al. (1984) A simple spectral parameter for accurate classification of severe carotid disease. *Bruit* 8:174–178.

7. Cohen J (1960) A coefficient of agreement for nominal scales. *Educational and Psychological Measurement* 20:37.

8. Fell G, Phillips DJ, Chikos PM, Harley JD, Thiele BL, Strandness DE (1981) Ultrasonic duplex scanning for disease of the carotid artery. *Circulation* 64:1191.

9. Kohler T, Langlois Y, Roederer G, et al. (1985) Sources of variability in carotid duplex examination: A prospective study. *Ultrasound Med Biol* 11:571.

10. Knox RA, Phillips DJ, Breslau PJ, Lawrence R, Primozich J, Strandness DE (1982) Empirical findings relating sample volume size to diagnostic accuracy in pulsed Doppler cerebrovascular studies. *J Clin Untrasound* 10:227.

11. Phillips DJ, Greene FM, Langlois Y, Roederer GO, Strandness DE (1983) Flow velocity patterns in the carotid bifurcations of young presumed normal subjects. *Ultrasound Med Biol* 9:39.

12. Bharadraj BK, Mabon RF, Giddens DP (1982) Steady flow in a model of the human carotid bifurcation. *J Biomech* 15:349.

13. Ku DN, Giddens DP (1983) Pulsatile flow in a model carotid bifurcation. *Arteriosclerosis* 3:31.

14. Ku DN, Giddens DP, Phillips DJ, Strandness DE (1985) Hemodynamics of the normal human carotid bifurcation: In vitro and in vivo studies. *Ultrasound Med Biol* 11:13.

15. Zarins CK, Giddens DP, Bharadvaj BK, Sottiurai VS, Mabon RF, Glagov S (1983) Carotid bifurcation atherosclerosis. Quantitative correlation of plaque localisation with flow velocity profiles and wall shear stress. *Circ Res* 53:502.

16. Ku DN, Zarins CK, Giddens DP, Glagov S (1983) Shear stress oscillation and plaque localisation at the carotid bifurcation. *Circulation* 68(Suppl 3):301.

17. Zierler RE (1984) Cost effectiveness of non-invasive testing for carotid artery disease. *Vascular Diagnosis and Therapy* 5:12.

18. Roederer GO, Langlois YE, Jager KA (1984) The natural history of carotid arterial disease in asymptomatic patients with cervical bruits. *Stroke* 15:605.

19. Roederer GO, Langlois YE, Lusiani L, et al. (1984) Natural history of carotid artery disease on the side contralateral to endarterectomy. *J Vasc Surg* 1:62.

20. Nicholls SC, Phillips DJ, Bergelin RO, et al. (1985) Carotid endarterectomy. Relationship of outcome to early restenosis. *J Vasc Surg* 2:375.

21. Roederer GO, Langlois Y, Chan ATW, et al. (1983) Post endarterectomy carotid ultrasonic duplex scanning concordance with contrast angiography. *Ultrasound Med Biol* 9:73.

22. Zierler RE, Bandyk DE, Thiele BL (1984) Intraoperative assessment of carotid endarterectomy. *J Vasc Surg* 1:73.

23. Ivey TD, Strandness DE, Williams DB, Langlois Y, Misbach GA, Delagans AP (1984) Management of patients with carotid bruit undergoing cardiopulmonary bypass. *J Thorac Cardiovasc Surg* 87:183.

24. Blackshear WM, Connor RG (1982) Carotid endarterectomy without angiography. *J Cardiovasc Surg* 23:477.

25. Crew JR, Johnson JM, Dean MJ (1982) Carotid surgery without angiography: When and why. In *San Diego Symposium on Invasive Diagnostic Techniques in Vascular Disease*, October, 1982.

26. Nicholls SC, Phillips DJ, Primozich JF, et al. (1987) The diagnostic significance of flow separation in the carotid bulb. *Stroke* 18:10.

27. Greene FM, Beach KW, Strandness DE, Fell G, Phillips DJ (1982) Computer based pattern recognition of carotid arterial disease using pulsed Doppler ultrasound. *Ultrasound Med Biol* 8:161.

28. Langlois, YE, Greene FM, Roederer GO, et al. (1984) Computer based pattern recognition of carotid artery Doppler signals for disease classification. *Ultrasound Med Biol* 10:581.

29. Chikos PM, Fisher LD, Hirsch JH, Harley JD, Thiele BL, Strandness DE (1983) Observer variability in evaluating extracranial carotid artery stenosis. *Stroke* 14:885.

Color Figure Section

1

Cardiac Ultrasound in Cerebrovascular Disease

Martin E. Goldman, MD

Pages 1–15

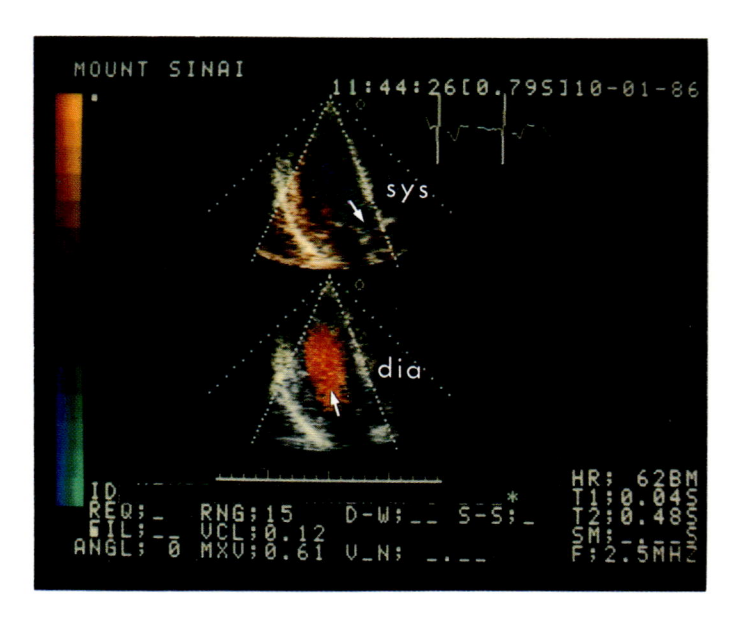

Figure 1-7. Color Doppler. During diastole (**lower**), blood moving into the ventricle (and toward transducer) is depicted in orange, while during systole (**upper**), blood moving out the aorta is depicted in blue.

Color Figure Section 69

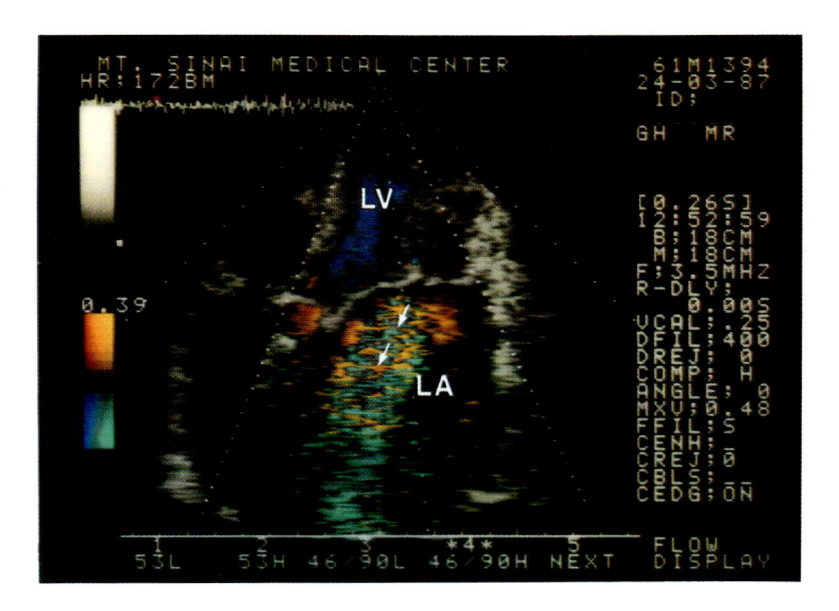

Figure 1-9. Color Doppler. Mitral regurgitation. During systole, blood moving out the left ventricle into the aortia is in deep blue, while mitral regurgitation (arrows) into a large left atrium is a turbulent mosaic pattern of turquoise and yellow. LA, left atrium; LV, left ventricle.

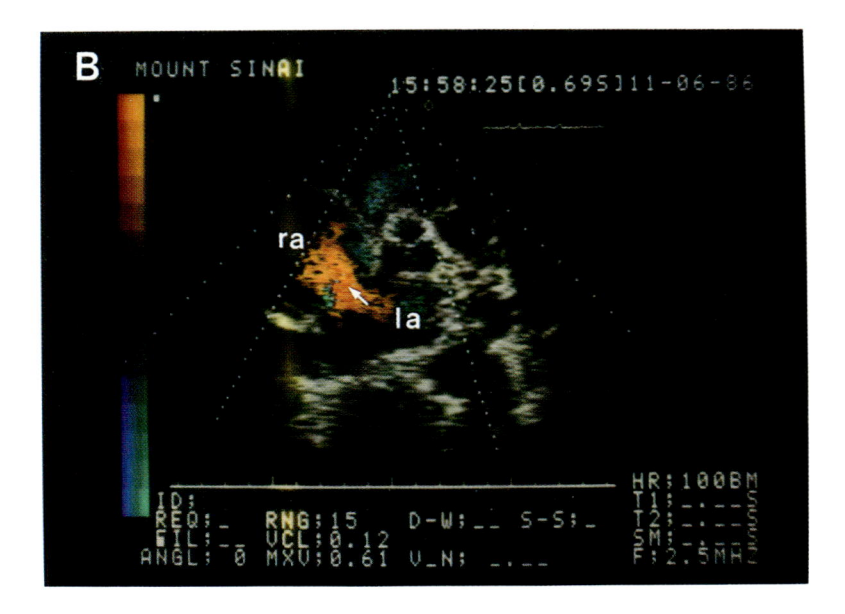

Figure 1-18. B) Color Doppler of short axis view demonstrating left to right shunt (arrow, orange color) at the atrial level.

4

Duplex Scanning of the Carotid Arteries

Stephen C. Nicholls, MD, R. Eugene Zierler, MD, and D.E. Strandness, Jr., MD

Pages 49–65

Figure 4-22. Flow separation in a normal carotid bifurcation. Flow toward the transducer is red. Higher frequencies in the same direction along the apical divider are labeled white. Flow in the separation zone (posterolateral bulb) is blue because it is away from the transducer (flow reversal). The external carotid is labeled. N.B.: The internal jugular vein has been compressed, and no flow is seen in this vessel.

Figure 4-23. Left internal carotid artery stenosis. Red indicates flow toward the transducer. Blue indicates flow away from the transducer. Color scale (on the right) has been set by the operator so that all frequencies in the stenosis > 3.8 kHZ are green. N.B.: Flow in the internal jugular vein is blue because it is away from the transducer.

Color Figure Section 71

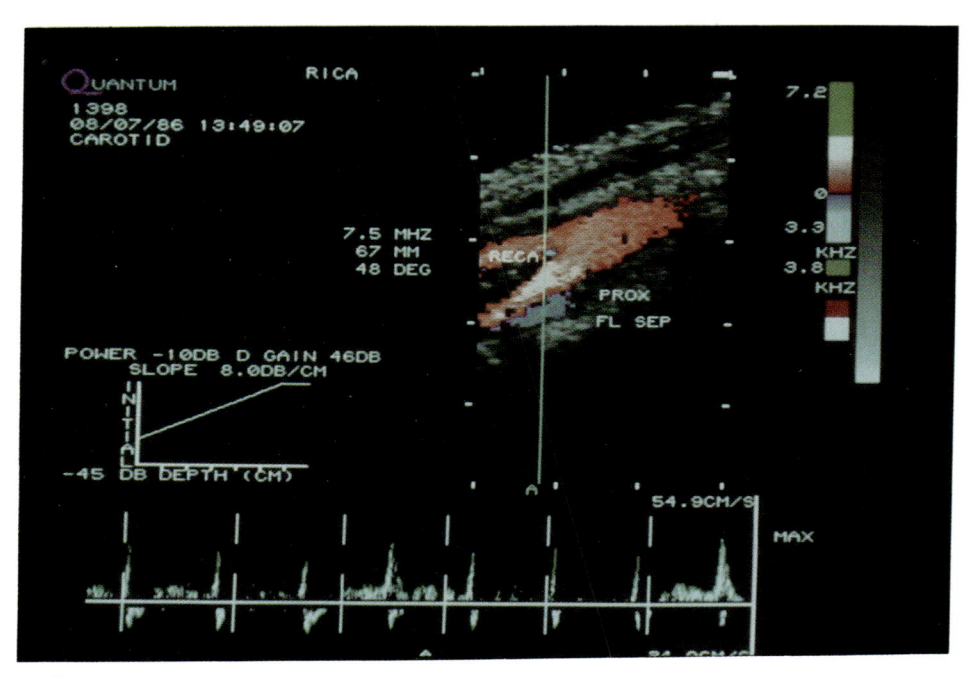

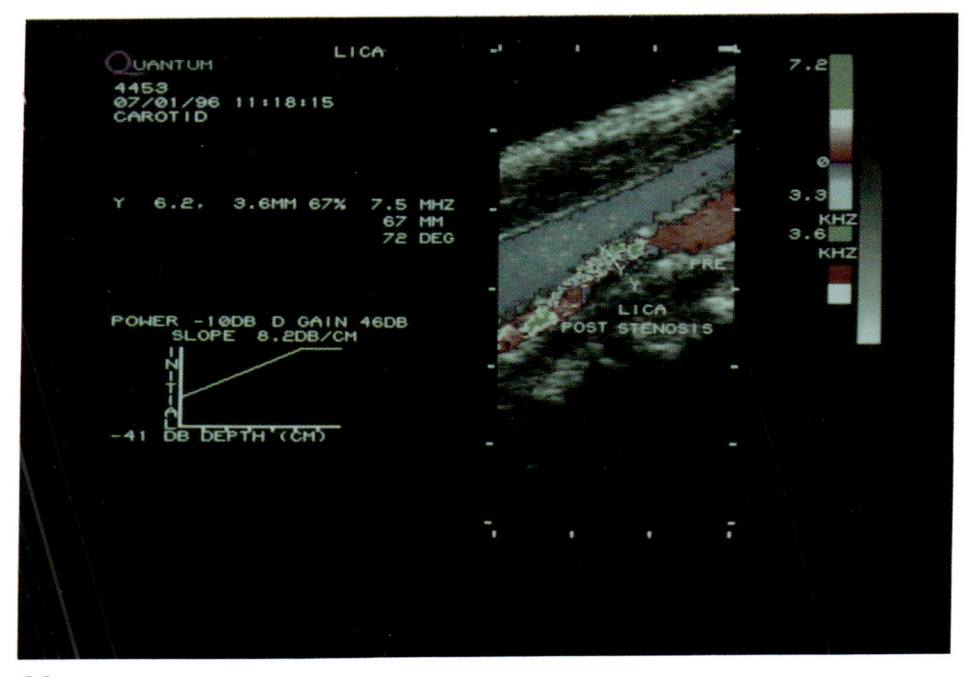

22

23

5

A Practical Guide to Transcranial Doppler Sonography

Erich Bernd Ringelstein, MD

Pages 75–121

Figure 5–12. Transcranial Doppler flow mapping of the circle of Willis in a patient with right-sided MCA stenosis. **a:** At an insonation depth of 61 mm, increased flow velocity of 121 cm/sec and severely disturbed flow are registered immediately posterior to the stenotic channel (upper part). **Upper:** Large arrow, MCA stenosis; arrow heads, carotid siphon (AP view). **Lower:** small arrows, right P1 segment; double arrow, left P1 segment (axial view). **b:** At an insonation depth of 66 mm, musical murmurs occur, indicating the maximum stenosis. Note the red-colored, band-like, symmetrical, high-energy Doppler shift phenomena during each systole indicating harmonic covibrations of vessel tissue (i.e., musical murmurs). Flow direction and flow velocity are color-coded (yellow and red = towards the probe; blue and lilac = away from the probe. The size of the spots represents signal amplitude.

Color Figure Section 73

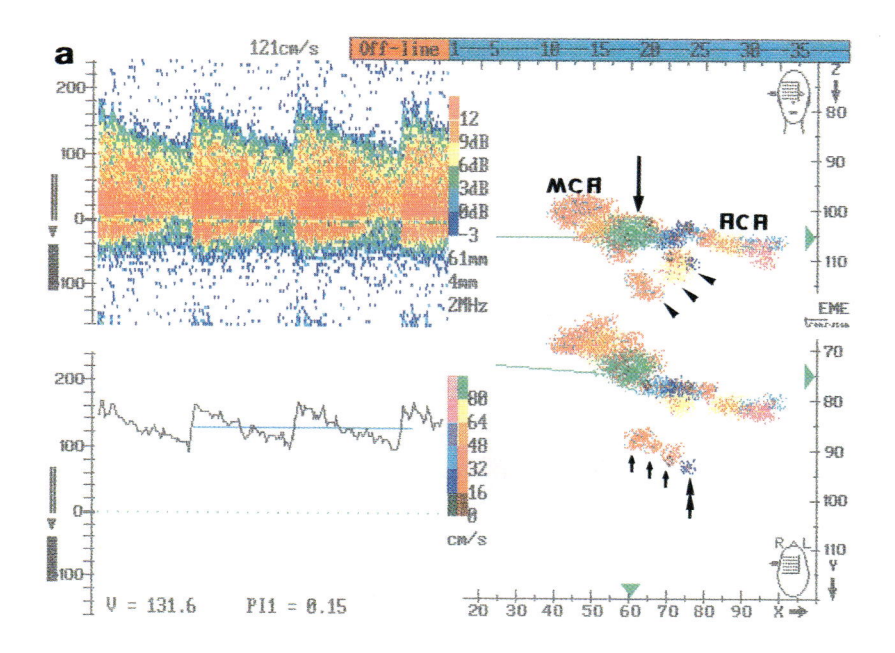

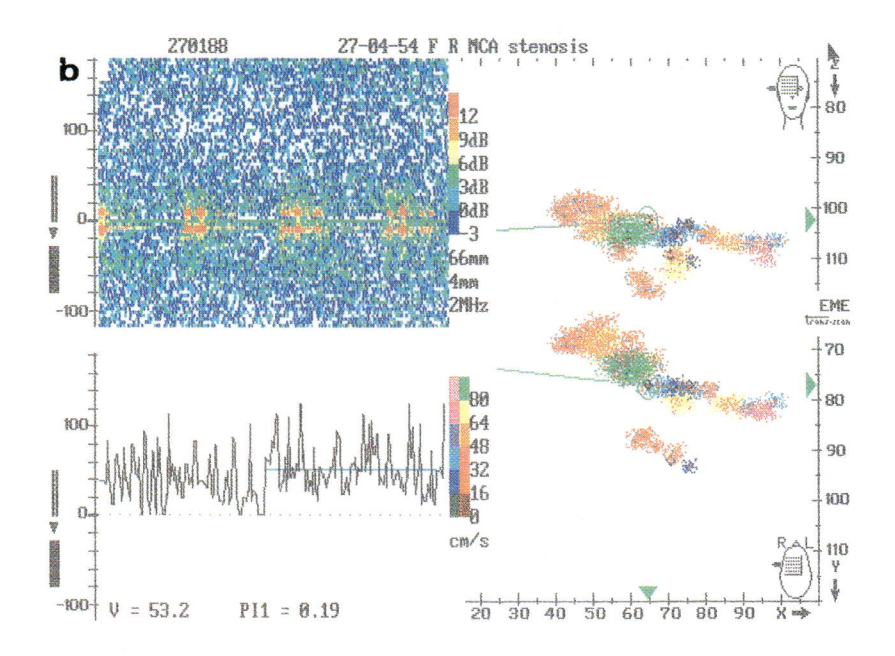

7

SPECT Perfusion Imaging in Cerebrovascular Disease

B. Leonard Holman, MD, Jean-Luc Moretti, MD, PhD, and Thomas C. Hill, MD

Pages 147–162

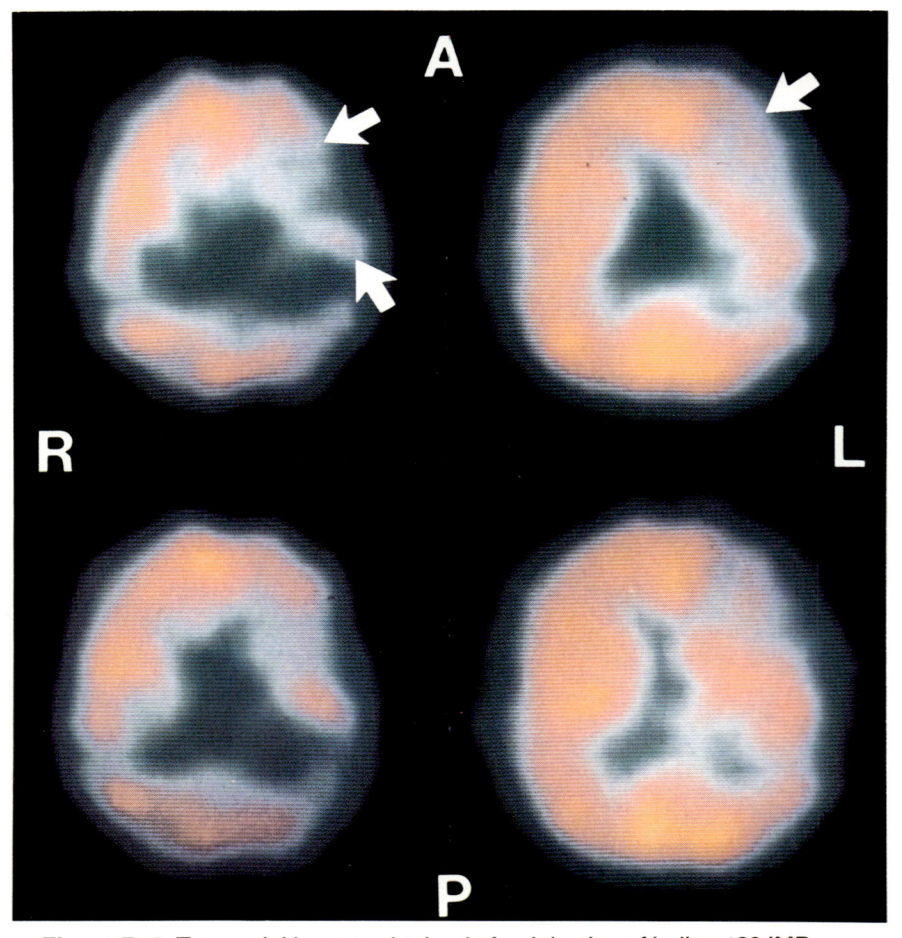

Figure 7–4. Transaxial images obtained after injection of iodine-123 IMP in patient with left internal carotid and middle cerebral artery stenoses. Left, extensive perfusion defect is noted in preoperative study (arrows). Right, after surgery, perfusion has improved to most of the hemisphere but with persistent perfusion defect at the site of surgery (arrow). Images were obtained with a rotating gamma camera. A indicates anterior; P, posterior.

A Practical Guide to Transcranial Doppler Sonography

Erich Bernd Ringelstein, MD

Department of Neurology, Technische Hochschule, 5100 Aachen, Federal Republic of Germany

INTRODUCTION

The term transcranial Doppler sonography (TCD) refers to a completely new ultrasonic technique recently introduced by Aaslid et al. [1–3] for the detection of cerebral arterial vasospasm following subarachnoid hemorrhage. During the last few years, however, this 2 MHz pulsed Doppler technique has turned out to be a useful tool in the entire field of neuroangiology for both scientific as well as practical clinical purposes [4]. Table 5.1 lists promising or already established applications of transcranial Doppler sonography in clinical and experimental settings. Further exciting applications may be expected, if TCD measurements are combined with electrophysiologic findings such as EEG [5] or SEP [6], which may lead to a better understanding of the interaction between cerebral circulation and brain function.

A principle problem in TCD application seems to be the yet not clearly defined relationship between cerebral blood flow volume and the flow velocities within the basal cerebral arteries as assessed with TCD, which makes some workers in this field hesitate to apply TCD as a regional cerebral blood flow (rCBF) measurement technique. There are in fact several fundamental limitations of TCD in this particular respect: Because the diameter of the middle cerebral artery (MCA) (3.82 ± 0.43 mm [7] as well as the volume of the MCA-dependent brain tissue, vary considerably from individual to individual, flow velocity within the main trunk of the MCA also has a wide range of normality (Table 5.2). This is even more true when individually different insonation conditions (i.e., insonation angle and attenuation of beam and echoes within the skull) or changes of cerebral blood flow during age are also considered (Table 5.2). By comparing intraindividual measurements under normo- and hypercapnic conditions, however, these limitations can be overcome [8], and relative changes in blood flow velocity (delta BFV) reflect the relative changes in regional cerebral blood flow (delta rCBF) [9].

Besides its noninvasiveness and low cost, the decisive advantage of TCD as a CBF-evaluation instrument, however, is the optimal time resolution of the measurements [10]. Aside from their limitations in precision [11], conventional rCBF techniques, as well as stable Xenon computerized tomography, are not able to measure the time course of rapid cerebral blood flow changes if the latter occur in shorter intervals than 10–30 minutes, whereas TCD provides true real-time data. Relative changes in cerebral blood flow can now be measured objectively and immediately, for as long and as often as desired. This makes TCD a very attractive tool to solve certain scientific problems and to get deeper insights

---

The author wants to express his deep gratitude to Mrs. Christiane Goebel, Uschi Tietz, Monika Schumacher, and Mary Rossman, vascular technicians; to my medical students, Andreas Holling, Eva Niggemeyer, Frank Richert, Birgit Spaar, Christoph Nielen, Sara Ecker, Simeon Matentzoglu, Carsten Sievers, Manfred Weckesser, and Susanne Weckesser for technical assistance and artwork; as well as to Drs. Wolfgang Grosse, Margret Busker, and Georg Leonhardt for important clinical and scientific contributions. The author also wishes to cordially thank Mrs. Kati Seidel for preparing the manuscript.

Ringelstein

Table 5.1
Applications of Transcranial Doppler Sonography

Diagnosis of intracranial occlusive disease
  Individual diagnostic workup
  Epidemiologic studies
Ancillary test for confirmation or exclusion of extracranial occlusive disease, (particularly for confirmation of well-collateralized chronic ICA occlusions when combined with common carotid artery compression tests)
Diagnosis and followup of dissecting aneurysms of the internal carotid artery
Evaluation of hemodynamic effects of extracranial occlusive disease on intracranial blood flow velocities in significant ICA stenoses, ICA occlusion(s), subclavian steal mechanism, combined extracranial lesions, etc.
Detection/identification of feeders of AV malformations
  Preoperative assessment
  Postoperative assessment
  Assessment before and after heavy particle radiation treatment
  Assessment of pathophysiology of AV malformations
Assessment of the collateralizing capacities of the circle of Willis
  Preoperatively in carotid endarterectomy to predict effect of clamping
  Preinterventionally in any kind of occlusive therapeutic procedure (embolization, balloon occlusion, etc.)
Intermittent monitoring and followup studies
  Vasospasm in subarachnoid hemorrhage
  Vasospasm and/or hyperperfusion in migraine
  Time-related flow alterations in acute stroke
  Time-related flow alterations in blunt head trauma
  Spontaneous or therapeutically induced recanalization of occluded basal arteries
  Flow changes in occlusive disease during anticoagulation therapy
  Cerebral flow velocity studies at high altitude and in acute mountain sickness
  Any treatment monitoring that affects cerebral blood flow
Continuous monitoring during neuroradiologic intervention acute pharmacologic trials of vasoactive drugs, carotid endarterectomy, cardiac surgery and other cardiac interventions, increasing intracranial pressure, evolving brain death
Functional tests
  Stimulation of the cerebral vasomotor response with CO_2, acetazolamide, lowering of systemic arterial blood pressure, etc.
  Increase of blood flow velocity during activation of circumscribed cortical areas. (light and mental stimulation of the visual cortex, stimulation of the motor strip, etc.)
Noninvasive ancillary tests and monitoring procedures in animal experiments
Future application during experiments in space

into the pathophysiology of cerebral circulation in acute stroke. Further, abrupt or short-lasting effects of any external mechanical manipulation at or functional stimulation of the intracranial circulation can be assessed [12–17].

This chapter should serve as a practical guideline for the beginner in TCD. Therefore, a comprehensive portion deals with the examination technique and the various TCD approaches. It should, however, also give the more advanced user information about the practical value of TCD application for the solution of certain clinical and neuroangiologic problems. Purely scientific applications are also mentioned as far as they have led to obviously useful findings. I would like the reader to share my increasing enthusiasm and excitement regarding the application of TCD within the last 5 years. The list of TCD applications is still growing, and it remains for the reader's fantasy to add new ideas as to where and how TCD can provide clues to the physiology and pathophysiology of blood flow in the brain.

EXAMINATION TECHNIQUE
General Prerequisites

There are two main anatomical difficulties the examiner has to deal with. 1) The number and extent of so-called "ultrasound windows" or foramina within the skull that can be penetrated with the ultrasound beam in order to hit the basal and/or major leptomeningeal cerebral arteries are limited and sometimes not easily identified. 2) The arteries at the base of the skull are extremely variable in terms of aplasia, hypoplasia, or normal caliber of certain segments, as well as with respect to their site and course. In patients with arteriosclerosis, displacement of brain arteries due to tortuosity is a frequent finding. Pioneers in the field of transcranial Doppler sonography have elaborated certain rules to find the windows and identify vessel segments by means of compression tests at the neck arteries [1,4,5,14,15,17–22]. For didactic purposes, identification of the vessels and examination of the brain arteries are described separately. In practice, however, this is done in one procedure.

Before performing a transcranial Doppler examination, two prerequisites should be fulfilled. 1) The status of the extracranial arteries has to be completely known (e.g., ICA occlusion, subclavian steal mechanism, etc.). 2) To avoid major fluctuation of pCO_2, the patient must lie supine in a stable position. The examiner sits behind the patient's head to permit stable positioning of the probe. The patient's head should be directed straight forward for better visual orientation of the outside of the skull. I recommend starting with a conventional TCD device before using a color-coded flow mapping system. The latter will be of advantage only for experienced examiners who know how to interpret the scanning data. Tables 5.2 and 5.3 list criteria that help the examiner orient himself within the skull. Normal flow velocities are also provided, although in clinical practice diagnoses are hardly ever made on the basis of these data (Table 5.2).

The Four Windows

Four different TCD approaches at the outside of the skull to insonate the intracranial arteries are the 1) transtemporal, 2) transorbital, 3) suboccipital (transforaminal, transnuchal), and 4) submandibular. (Figs. 5-1–7).

During the transtemporal approach, the probe is placed on the temporal plane cephalad to the zygomatic arch and immediately anterior and slightly superior to the tragus of the ear conch (Figs. 5-1a, 5-8a). This site is most promising to find an adequate ultrasound window (compare Fig. 5-8b and c). A more posterior window, immediately over and slightly dorsal to the first one, may be more appropriate only in a minority of cases, but is the optimal site for insonation of the P2 segment of the posterior cerebral arteries (PCA) (see position 2 in Fig. 5-8a). In some patients, more frontally located temporal ultrasound windows may be present (position 3 in Fig. 5-8).

With the preauricular, transtemporal approach, the beam can be angled anteriorly or posteriorly relative to a frontal plane, running through the corresponding probe positions on either side of the head. The anterior orientation of the beam allows for the insonation of the M1 and M2 segments of the middle cerebral artery (MCA), the C1-segment of the carotid siphon (very distal, supraclinoidal segment) and the A1 segment of the anterior cerebral artery (ACA) including the anterior communicating artery (ACOA), whereas the posteriorly angulated beam hits the P1 and P2 segments of the posterior cerebral artery, the top of the basilar artery (BA), and the posterior communicating arteries (PCOA). The transtemporal application of TCD is the most informative (see Figs. 5-2–4).

Due to the unpredictable course and tortuosity of the carotid siphon, the transorbital approach (Fig. 5-1b) can be very difficult. Under normal anatomic conditions, the ophthalmic artery can be insonated at depths of 45 to 50 mm, the anterior genu of the carotid siphon (corresponding to the C3 segment) is normally met at insonation depths of 60/65 mm (compare Fig. 5-5), with the C2 segment showing flow away from the probe (downward deflection of the curve) and the C4 segment showing flow towards the probe (upward deflection of the curve) at a slightly greater insonation depth of 70 to 75 mm. These statements are true for nearly sagittal angulation of the beam via the supraorbital fissure or via the infraorbital fissure with a slightly oblique approach (Fig.

Table 5.2
Identification Criteria and Normal Flow Velocities of Various Intracranial Arterial Segments (n = 106 normal subjects of different age and sex)

Arterial segment	Insonation depths Range (mm)	Reference depth (mm)	Normal flow velocity (mean ± S.D.) (cm/sec)	Changes with age (yr) (mean ± S.D.) <30	30–69	≥70	Main features for identification of vessel segment[a]
MCA	30–60	50	55 ± 12	70 ± 16	54 ± 10	41 ± 7	M1: Insonation depths 50 mm; traceability forward and backward; flow towards probe; slightly anterior angulation of beam M2: Insonation depths 40mm
M1	45–60	50	55 ± 12				
M2	30–40	35					Too variable; not systematically evaluated
ACA	60–75	70	50 ± 11	61 ± 15	47 ± 8	38 ± 6	Insonation depth; flow away from probe; traceability; slightly anterior angulation of beam; for clearcut differentiation from carotid siphon use compression tests[a]
C1 (C2) (carotid siphon transtemporal approach)	60–70	65	39 ± 9	—	—	—	Insonation depth; relatively low flow velocity compared to M1 segment; slightly anterior and caudal angulation of beam; flow direction towards probe[b]

P1 (posterior cerebral artery)	60(55)–75	70	39 ± 10	—	Insonation depth; flow towards probe (ipsilat. P1); traceability to top-of-basilar and contralateral P1'; slightly posterior and caudal angulation of beam; relatively low flow velocity compared to M1 segment; compression test necessary for unequivocal differentiation from MCA branches[a]
P1 and P1' (top-of-basilar)	70–80	75	See P1 values	—	Insonation depth; bidirectional flow; traceability backward and forward; angulation of beam (see P1); compression tests[a]
P2 (PCA) (probe placed in position 2 in Fig. 5-8a)	60–65	65	40 ± 10	—	Flow away from probe; placement of probe; posterior angulation of probe (compare Fig. 5-4a); modulation by opening and closing eyes
Extradural distal vertebral artery	40–55	50	34 ± 8	—	Suboccipital placement of probe; insonation depth; strongly lateral angulation of beam; flow towards probe

(Continued)

---

[a]For additional information from compression tests see Table 5.3.
[b]Due to anatomic variability of vessels, this is not always the case.
[c]Due to a tremendous interindividual variability of both thickness of the neck and site of VA junction or arteriosclerotic elongation of the vertebrobasilar axis, the range of insonation depths of the vertebral artery and basilar trunk strongly overlap.

Table 5.2
Identification Criteria and Normal Flow Velocities of Various Intracranial Arterial Segments (n = 106 normal subjects of different age and sex) (*Continued*)

Arterial segment	Insonation depths Range (mm)	Reference depth (mm)	Normal flow velocity (mean ± S.D.) (cm/sec)	Changes with age (yr) (mean ± S.D.) <30	30–69	≥70	Main features for identification of vessel segment[a]
Intradural distal vertebral artery	60–95 (100)[c]	70	38 ± 10	—	—	—	Insonation depth; Beam aimed at bridge of nose or slightly laterally; traceability forward and backward; compression tests at common carotid or vertebral arteries sometimes necessary[a]
Basilar trunk	70(65)–115(120)[c]	95 (100, if possible)	41 ± 10	46 ± 11	35 ± 7	32 ± 7	Insonation depth; Flow away from probe; often slight increase of flow velocity compared to vertebral artery; traceability of vertebrobasilar axis; compression tests: see vertebral artery[a]
C2 (carotid siphon, transorbital approach)	65–80	70	41 ± 11	—	—	—	Sagittal or slightly oblique angulation of beam; flow away from probe,[b] insonation depth
C3 (carotid siphon, transorbital approach)	65(60)	65 Bidirectional, not measured	—	—	—	—	Bidirectional signal; sagittal angulation of beam; insonation depth

C4 and distal part of C5 (carotid siphon, transorbital approach)	65–80 (85)	70	47 ± 14	—	—	—	Sagittal or slightly oblique and caudal angulation of beam; flow towards probe;[b] insonation depth
Ophthalmic artery	35–55	45	21 ± 5	—	—	—	Insonation depth; flow towards probe[b]
Contralateral A1 (ACA) (transorbital approach, ancillary approach if lack of temporal window)	75–80	?	Measurements in a few cases only	—	—	—	Strongly oblique angulation of beam via optic canal (see Fig. 5-9); flow towards probe; compression test necessary for separation from carotid siphon and MCA[a]
C6 and retromandibular segment of ICA (extradural ICA) (submandibular approach)	35–80 (85)	60	30 ± 9	—	—	—	Flow away from probe; medial angulation of beam; insonation depth

[a] For additional information from compression tests see Table 5.3.
[b] Due to anatomic variability of vessels, this is not always the case.
[c] Due to a tremendous interindividual variability of both thickness of the neck and site of VA junction or arteriosclerotic elongation of the vertebrobasilar axis, the range of insonation depths of the vertebral artery and basilar trunk strongly overlap.

Table 5.3
Criteria for Identification of Various Intracranial Arterial Segments During Common Carotid Artery Compression Tests

Part I: Ipsilateral CCA Compression Test

Reaction		Phenomenon can be explained by	Neuroangiologic Meaning: configuration of circle of Willis[a]
Any effects of ipsilateral compression test?	If no:	Unsuccessful compression maneuver. Try it again! Or you insonate the:	
		1. P2 or	Nonembryonal type of PCA[b]
		2. P1 or	Absence of posterior collateral pathway[c]
		3. ICA or MCA or A1 or PCoA	Ipsilateral ICA occlusion; clarify extracranial Doppler findings![a]
If yes: Go ahead! Decreased flow velocity?	If yes:	1. MCA or	Existence of collateral pathways[d]
		2. PCoA or P2 or	Embryonal type of PCA;[b] existence of collateral pathways[e]
		3. C1 (ICA) or	Existence of posterior collateral pathway
		4. A1	Existence of posterior collateral pathway only
If no: Go ahead! Flow stoppage?	If yes:	1. MCA or C1 (ICA) or A1 or	Lack of collateral pathways
		2. P2 or PCoA	Embryonal type of PCA; lack of collateral pathways
If no: Go ahead! Increased flow velocity?	If yes:	1. P1 or PCoA	Existence of posterior collateral pathway

	If no: Go ahead! Flow inversion	If yes:	1. A1 or C1 (ICA) or
			Existence of internal anterior collateral pathway[f]
			2. PCoA
			Existence of posterior collateral pathway
	If no: Go ahead! Alternating flow?[g]	If yes:	1. C1 (ICA) or A1 or
			Existence of both anterior and posterior collateral pathways
			2. PCoA
			Embryonal type of PCA; existence of both anterior and posterior collateral pathways.
	If no:		Inadequate examination technique. Try it again!
Part II: Contralateral CCA Compression Test			
Any effects of contralateral compression test?	If no:		Unsuccessful compression maneuver. Try it again! Or you insonate the:
			1. MCA or P2 or P1 or
			Further differentiation possible with flow chart I and Table 5-2.
			2. C1 (ICA) or A1
			Absence of internal anterior cross-filling[f]
	If yes: Go ahead! Decreased flow velocity?	If yes:	Artery supplied from contralateral ICA. Clarify whether a contralateral artery is insonated; compare flowchart I the ipsilateral ICA/MCA is occluded; check extracranial Doppler findings

(continued)

Table 5.3
Criteria for Identification of Various Intracranial Arterial Segments During Common Carotid Artery Compression Tests (Continued).

If no: Go ahead!		
Flow stoppage?	If yes:	Artery supplied from contralateral ICA. Clarify whether a contralateral artery is insonated; compare flowchart I the ipsilateral ICA/MCA is occluded; check extracranial Doppler findings
If no: Go ahead!		
Flow inversion?	If yes:	Artery supplied from contralateral ICA. Clarify whether a contralateral artery is insonated; compare flowchart I the ipsilateral ICA/MCA is occluded; check extracranial Doppler findings
If no: Go ahead!		
Alternating flow?	If yes:	Artery supplied from contralateral ICA. Clarify whether a contralateral artery is insonated; compare flowchart I the ipsilateral ICA/MCA is occluded; check extracranial Doppler findings
If no: Go ahead!		
Increased flow velocity?	If yes:	1. C1 (ICA) or A1 or Existence of internal anterior cross-filling[f]
		2. P1 or PCoA Existence of both posterior collateral pathway[c] and internal anterior cross-filling[f]
If no:		Inadequate examination technique. Try it again!

[a]Provided that ICA or CCA are not occluded, flow conditions in patients with residual trigeminal artery are not considered, retrograde basilar flow in proximal basilar occlusion or manifest steal mechanism is not considered.
[b]Nonembryonal type means PCA blood supply exclusively via basilar artery, in contrast to embryonal type, indicating partial or complete PCA blood supply via ICA.
[c]Refers to a collateral pathway from basilar artery via P1 segment of posterior cerebral artery and posterior communicating artery to internal carotid artery.
[d]The precise type of pathway cannot be defined yet.
[e]With the "pure" embryonal type of PCA blood supply, decrease of P2 blood flow indicates existence of both PCoA and anterior collateral pathways in this particular situation.
[f]The term internal anterior cross-filling refers to cross-flow via the anterior communicating artery to the contralateral MCA territory, in contrast to an external anterior cross-filling via the external carotid artery to the contralateral ophthalmic artery in cases with both contralateral ICA and ECA occlusion.
[g]Regular biphasic change of flow direction during each cardiac cycle due to a labile watershed situation.

5-9). By contrast, during a strongly oblique approach with the probe placed at the superior outer quadrant of the eyelids and angulating the beam medially, ultrasound penetrates the optic canal and is aimed at the contralateral anterior cerebral artery, supraclinoidal carotid siphon, and even the proximal middle cerebral artery (Fig. 5-9). Typical insonation depths are listed in Table 5.2.

The suboccipital approach (Fig. 5-1c) is essential for screening the vertebrobasilar axis in its whole length. The probe is placed exactly between the squama ossis occipitalis and the palpable spinal process of the first cervical vertebra with the beam aimed at the bridge of the nose and an insonation depth of 65 mm to start with. The distal vertebral arteries (VA) are tracked in both directions, i.e., cephalad, by joining the BA to up to 125 mm and caudad to as shallow an insonation depth as possible in order to avoid blind spots during vertebrobasilar screening. With small insonation depths (e.g., 35–50 mm) and by angulating the beam strongly to one side, the extradural part of the VAs on the posterior arch of the atlas can be screened (flow towards the probe) while the top-of-basilar is normally reached at depths of 95 to 125 mm with flow directed away from the probe (Fig. 5-6).

The submandibular approach (Fig. 5-1d) adds valuable information and completes the examination in the sense that the retromandibular and more distal extradural parts of the ICA (C5 and C6 segments) can also be checked. This step of the TCD examination is particularly helpful as a complementary test to extracranial studies and helps to find chronic ICA occlusions in cases with abundant collateralization via external carotid artery (ECA) branches. In young and middle-aged acute stroke patients, the submandibular TCD approach is a must in order to detect (spontaneous) ICA dissection(s) as the underlying cause of stroke. With the beam directed slightly medially and posteriorly to the longitudinal axis of the body, the ICA can regularly be tracked up to 80 (85) mm where it bends medioanteriorly to form the siphon (Fig. 5-7).

Other windows within the skull are present and will be penetrated with further improvement of probe technology. For example, this is true for the insonation of the calcarine artery from a paramedian occipital placement of the transducer just above the protuberantia occipitalis externa. However, this has not yet achieved practical importance.

The First Steps

Empirically, it has been most convenient to start with the MCA on either side at 50 (55) mm insonation depth (ISD) and then to track the basal arterial network step by step in various directions. Proof of "traceability" of the MCA is decisive for its unequivocal identification. This is also true for other parts of the basal vasculature (see Table 5.2). Traceability refers to the fact that the MCA (and some other arteries) can be tracked in 2-mm (Medasonics device) or 5-mm (EME and CME devices) steps from more shallow ISD (i.e., 35 mm) to deeper sites (i.e., 55 mm) without changes in character of flow profile and flow direction. When tracing the MCA medially (65/70 mm), an abrupt change in flow direction indicates insonation of the A1 segment of the anterior cerebral artery (ACA) (compare Fig. 5-3), while flow towards the probe at this depth is usually registered from the carotid siphon (compare Fig. 5-2).

When angulating the beam more posteriorly during a transtemporal approach (Fig. 5-4), the P1 segment of the posterior cerebral artery (PCA) can most easily be picked up at an ISD of 70 (65) mm and can then be tracked over the top-of-basilar (which is nearly always hit at 75 mm ISD) to the contralateral PCA (P1': 80/85 mm). Again, the criteria of traceability, display of bilateral blood flow at the top of the basilar artery and change of flow direction within the contralateral PCA, are very important features for identification of the PCAs without compression tests (Fig. 5-5).

Identification of Vessel Segments by Compression Testing

As mentioned above and specified in Table 5-2, a particular vessel segment can be identified by a synopsis of the following, partially redundant, information: 1) window or foramen used, 2) angulation of the beam relative to certain landmarks at the skull (posterior, anterior, etc.), 3) insonation depth, 4) direction of blood flow relative to probe, and 5) traceability of the vessel segment. In pathologic conditions and in elderly subjects with coiling and tortuosity of

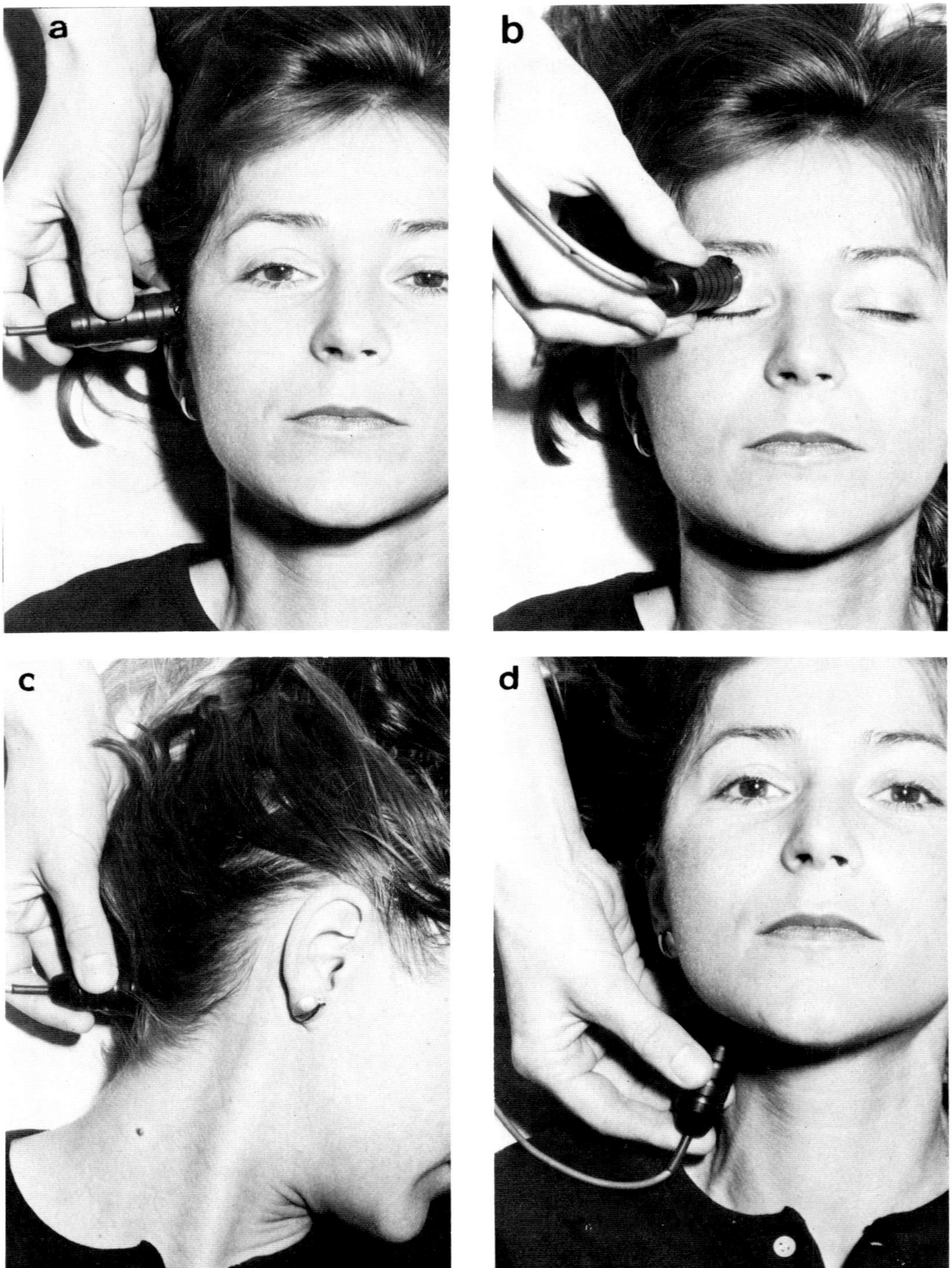
a
b
c
d

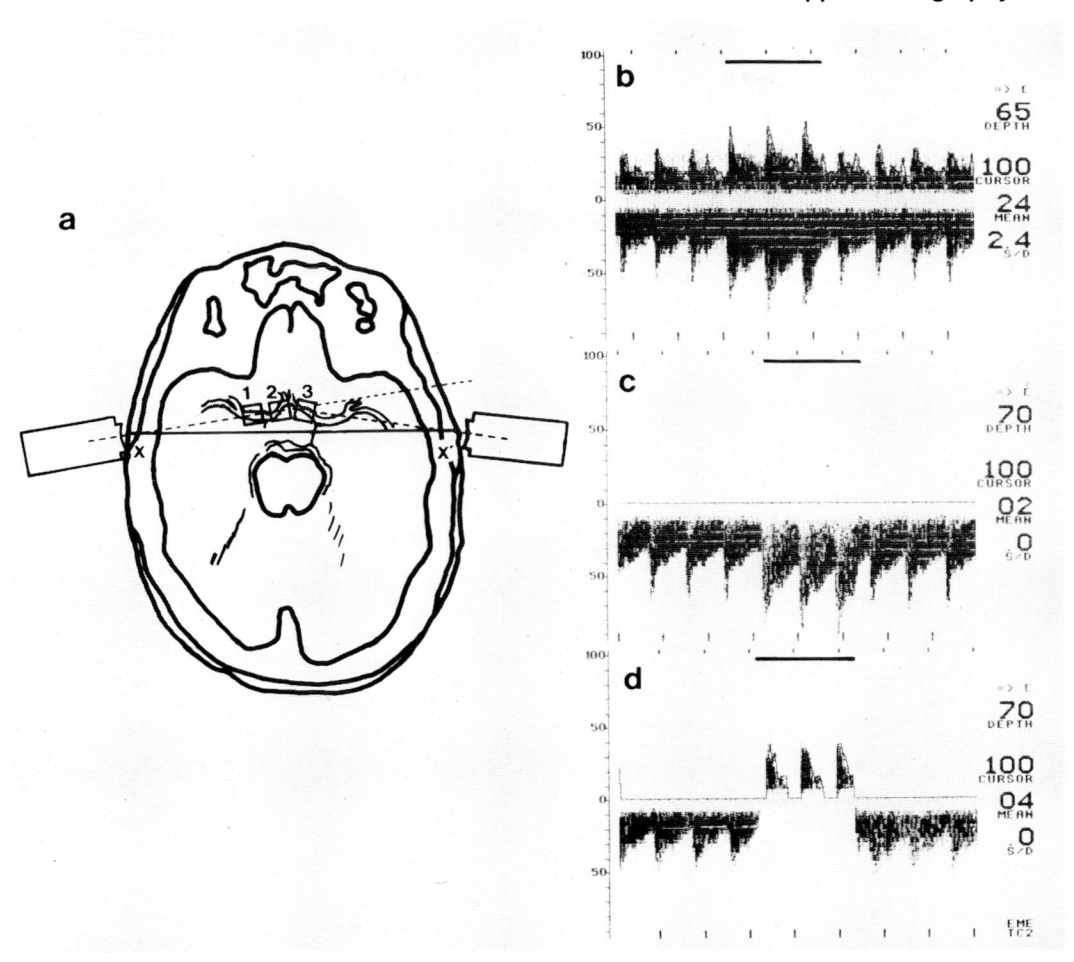

Figure 5–2. Schematic representation of the anterior part of the circle of Willis (drawing made from a contrast medium-enhanced CT). **a:** Positions 1, 2, and 3 of the sample volume correspond to the internal bifurcation of the ICA and the A1 segment of the ACA on either side. Notice the slightly anterior angulation of the ultrasound beam. **b:** At the inner bifurcation of the ICA, a bidirectional signal is obtained originating from the distal siphon (upper curve, flow directed towards the probe) and from the ACA (lower curve, flow directed away from the probe). During compression of the contralateral common carotid artery (black bar), flow velocity increases in both arteries. **c,d:** During insonation of the anterior cerebral artery, a contralateral common carotid artery compression test leads to an increase of flow velocity due to cross-filling, whereas an ipsilateral common carotid artery compression test (black bar) induces reversal of blood flow within the A1 segment due to inverted cross-filling.

Figure 5–1. The four approaches of TCD to the intracranial brain arteries. **a:** Transtemporal approach for insonation of the middle cerebral artery (M1 and M2 segment), anterior cerebral artery (A1 segment), distal carotid siphon, posterior cerebral artery (P1 and P2 segments), top of the basilar artery, and, if thick enough or working as a collateral channel, the posterior communicating artery. **b:** Transorbital approach for insonation of the various segments of the carotid siphon (C1–C4), the ophthalmic artery, and, via the optic canal, the contralateral anterior cerebral artery (compare Fig. 5-9). **c:** The suboccipital approach is necessary to insonate the distal vertebral arteries and the basilar trunk. **d:** The submandibular approach permits insonation of the retromandibular internal carotid artery and the petrous part of this vessel (C5/C6).

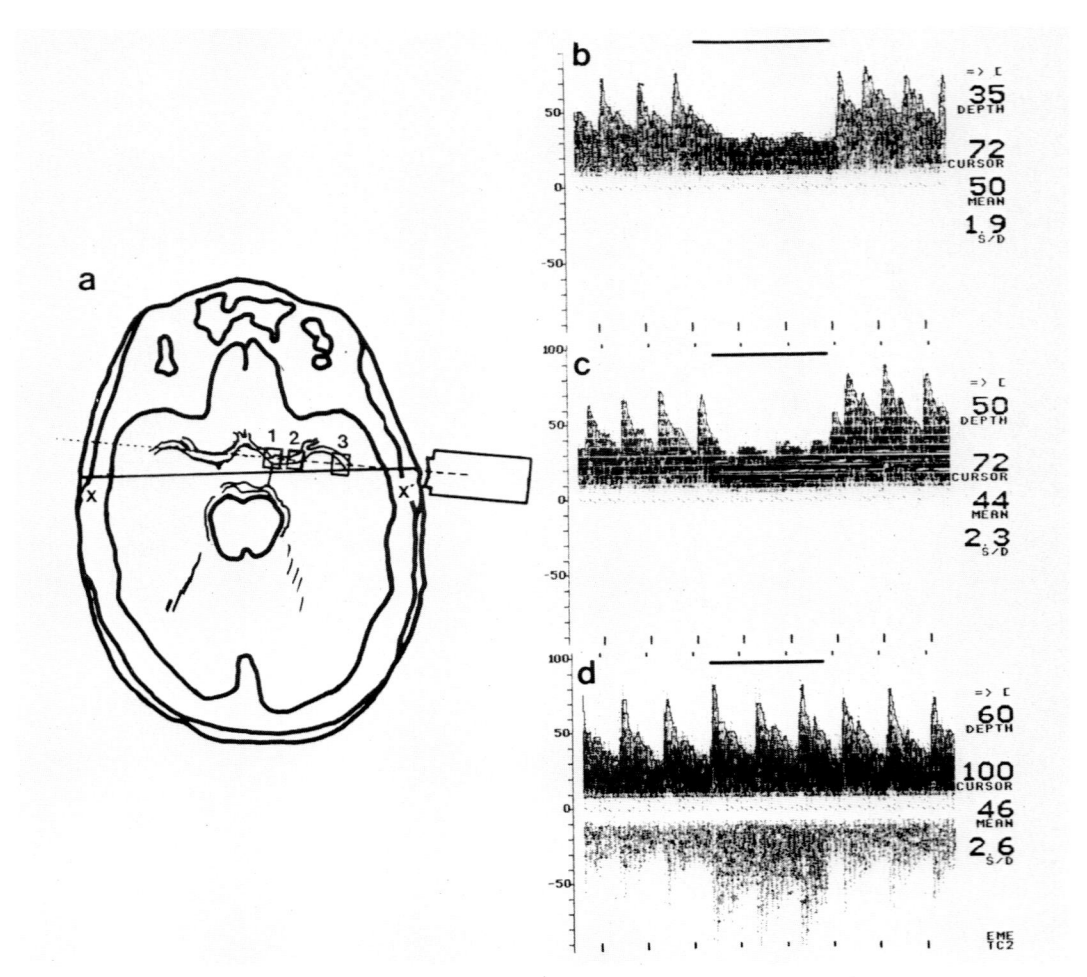

Figure 5–3. Insonation of the middle cerebral artery via a transtemporal approach. **a:** Positions 1, 2 and 3 of the sample volume correspond to the A1-M1 junction, the M1 segment, and the M2 segment of the middle cerebral artery. **b,c:** During insonation of the M2 or M1 segment of the MCA, an ipsilateral common carotid artery compression test (black bar) leads to a drop in flow velocity with recruitment of some collateral blood flow (c) and overshoot after release of the compression (c). **d:** Simultaneous insonation of the A1 (lower curve) and M1 segment (upper curve). Compression of the contralateral common carotid artery leads to an increase of flow velocity only within the A1 segment (compare Figure 5-2b).

the arteries due to arteriosclerotic elongation, compression tests may become necessary to unequivocally identify a certain arterial segment. Details of this identification process in the form of a flow chart are listed in Table 5-3. Compression tests during TCD examinations can be performed on both the common carotid arteries (CCA) low in the neck (using two fingers) or on the vertebral arteries at the mastoidal slope (using one finger tip). (For site of vertebral artery compression see the placement of the ultrasound probe in Figure 3-12a of chapter 3.) However, in the majority of cases, vertebral artery compression testing at the mastoid is ineffective due to insulation of the vessel deep within the neck muscle and bone tissue, making the degree of vessel narrowing during vertebral artery compression unpredictable.

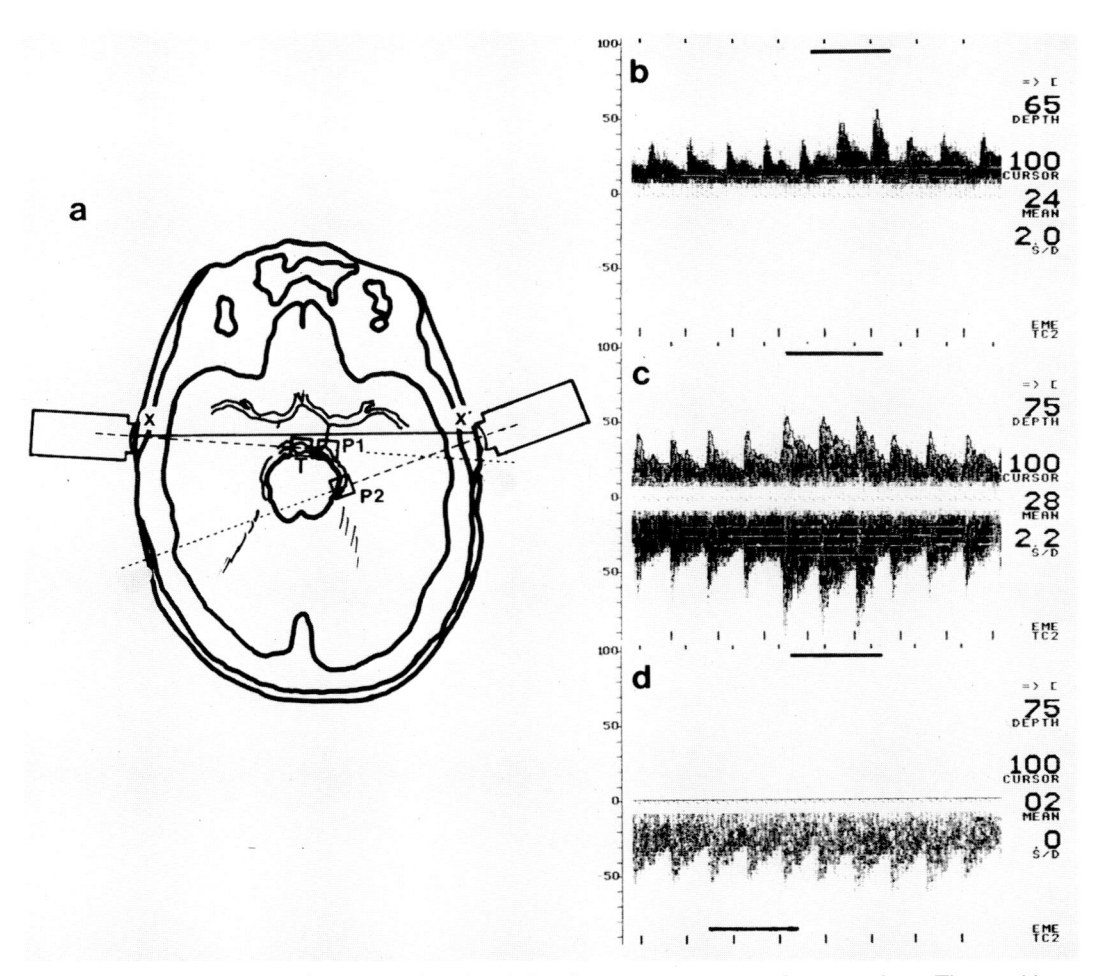

Figure 5–4. Insonation of the posterior circulation from a transtemporal approach. **a:** The positions T, P1, and P2 of the sample volume correspond to the top of the basilar artery, P1 segment, and P2 segment of the posterior cerebral artery (PCA). Note that the ultrasound beam is angulated slightly (P1, T) or strongly (P2) posteriorly. **b**: During insonation of the P1 segment at 65mm, flow is directed towards the probe. Compression of the ipsilateral common carotid artery (black bar) leads to considerable increase in flow velocity, indicating posterior cross filling to the carotid territory via the posterior communicating artery. **c**: At 57mm insonation depth, the top of the basilar artery with both branching P1 segments exhibits flow in both directions(*i.e., bidirectional flow). The lower curve corresponds to the contralateral P1 segment. Compression of the ipsilateral common carotid artery (black bar) leads to a significant increase in flow velocity in both posterior cerebral arteries, indicating bilateral posterior cross filling. **d**: Insonation of the P2 segment of the ipsilateral PCA. Flow is directed away from the probe (downward deflected curve). Compression of the ipsilateral common carotid artery (black bar) does not affect blood flow velocity.

Examples of the effect of VA compression are given in Figure 5-10.

There are six different responses of flow within intracranial arteries in response to any kind of extracranial compression maneuver: 1) no reaction at all, 2) increase of flow velocity, 3) decrease of flow velocity, 4) reversal of flow, 5) alternating flow direction (i.e., to-and-fro movement of the blood column during each cardiac cycle), and 6) complete stoppage of

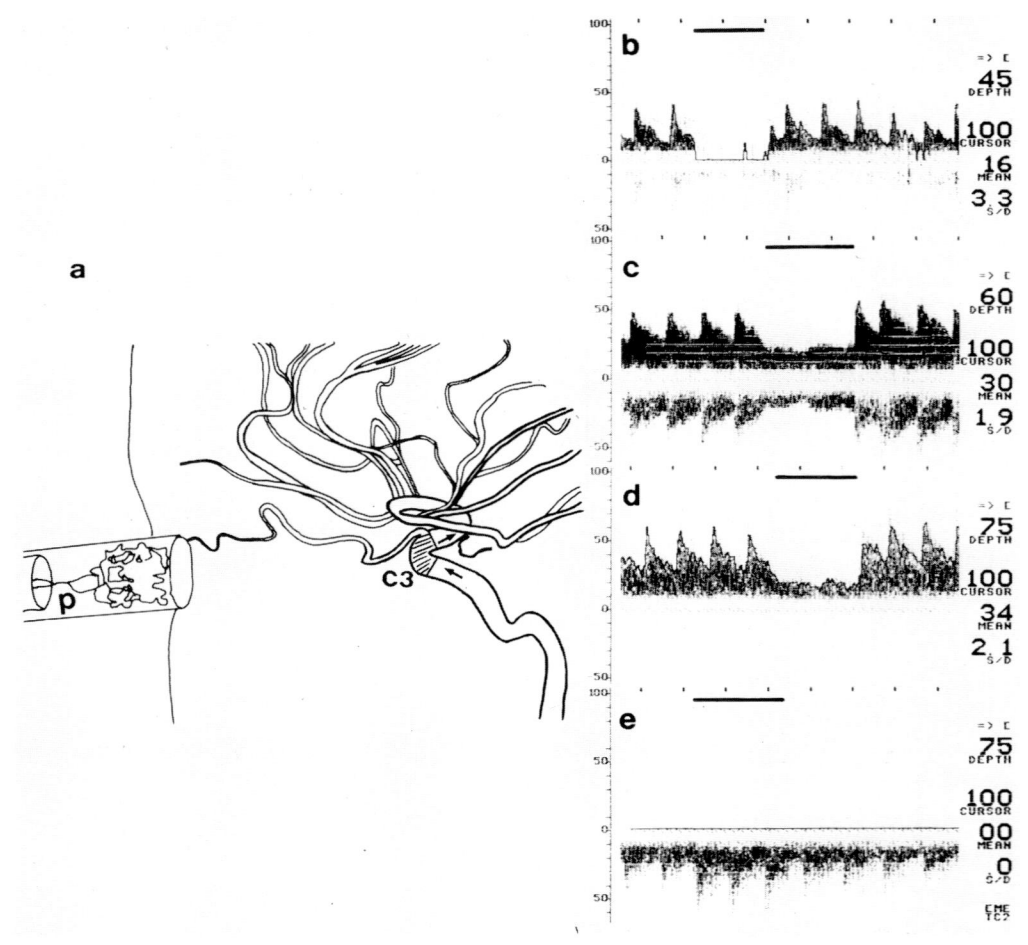

Figure 5–5. Transorbital insonation of the various segments of the carotid siphon. **a:** Drawing made from an angiogram with simultaneous transorbital insonation of the siphon. p, probe; C3, C3 segment of the carotid siphon. **b:** During insonation of the ophthalmic artery at 45 mm, flow is directed towards the probe. Compression of the common carotid artery (black bar) leads to complete stoppage of blood flow at this depth. **c:** Insonation of the C3 segment of the carotid siphon at 60/65 mm is indicated by a bidirectional flow signal, as flow at this site is directed both towards and away from the probe. **d,e:** At a greater depth, the C4 segment is insonated with flow directed towards the probe, while the C2 segment would show flow away from the probe. Compression of the ipsilateral (black bar in **d**) or contralateral common carotid artery (black bar in **e**) leads to decrease (**d**) or increase (**e**) of blood flow velocity.

flow. The latter is a phenomenologic description of what is displayed on the screen. Lack of any flow echo on the screen, however, does not necessarily indicate complete absence of flow within the vessel under study because a flow velocity of as low as 6 cm/sec or less can no longer be registered by the presently available devices.

In a series of 100 patients with angiographic visualization of the intracranial arteries, compression tests were performed and the type of response of various vessel segments was analyzed (Table 5.4). As is indicated, certain vessel segments most often revealed a uniform and thus typical reaction but can also respond less frequently in a different way. For example,

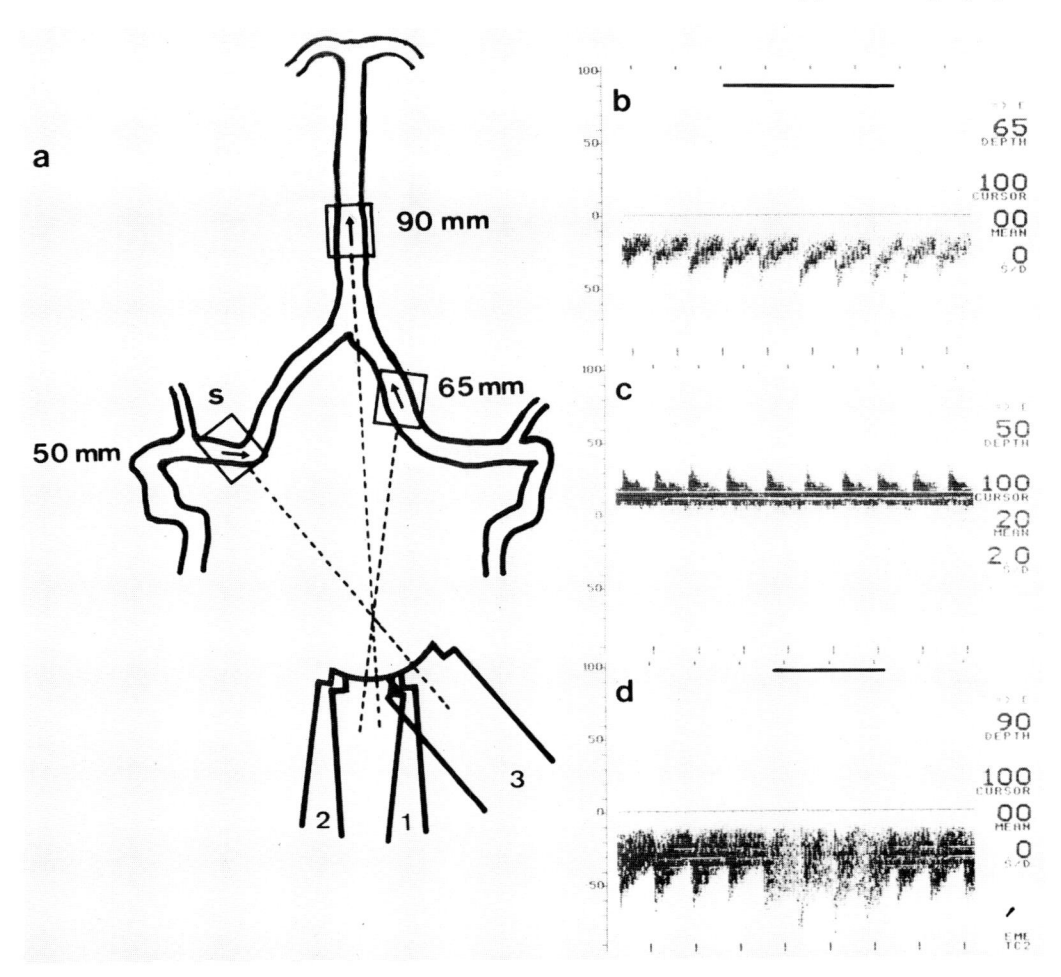

Figure 5–6. Insonation of the vertebrobasilar system from a suboccipital approach. **a:** Depending on the angulation of the probe (1, 2, 3), flow may be registered towards, or away from the probe. s, sample volume. **b:** At 65 mm insonation depth, the distal vertebral artery is insonated with flow away from the probe. **c:** At 50 mm insonation depth, a more proximal, extradural segment of the vertebral artery can be picked up, if the probe is angulated laterally. Flow is now directed towards the probe. **d:** At deeper insonation depths (90–125 mm) the basilar artery trunk can be found with flow away from the probe. Compression of the common carotid artery may lead to enhancement of antegrade basilar blood flow (black bar) if the posterior part of the circle of Willis is intact.

CCA compression did not affect contralateral MCA flow velocity in 82%, but led to a decrease in flow velocity in 11% of the cases. Flow velocity in the contralateral MCA may even increase in rare cases (1 of 79 patients), due to recruitment of leptomeningeal anastomoses, if both pericallosal arteries are exclusively supplied from one carotid system and the contralateral A1-segment is lacking. Certain theoretically expected types of response were not observed in the study so far (Table 5.4).

CLINICAL APPLICATIONS OF TCD

This overview focuses on a few major topics and does not refer in detail to each of the above-

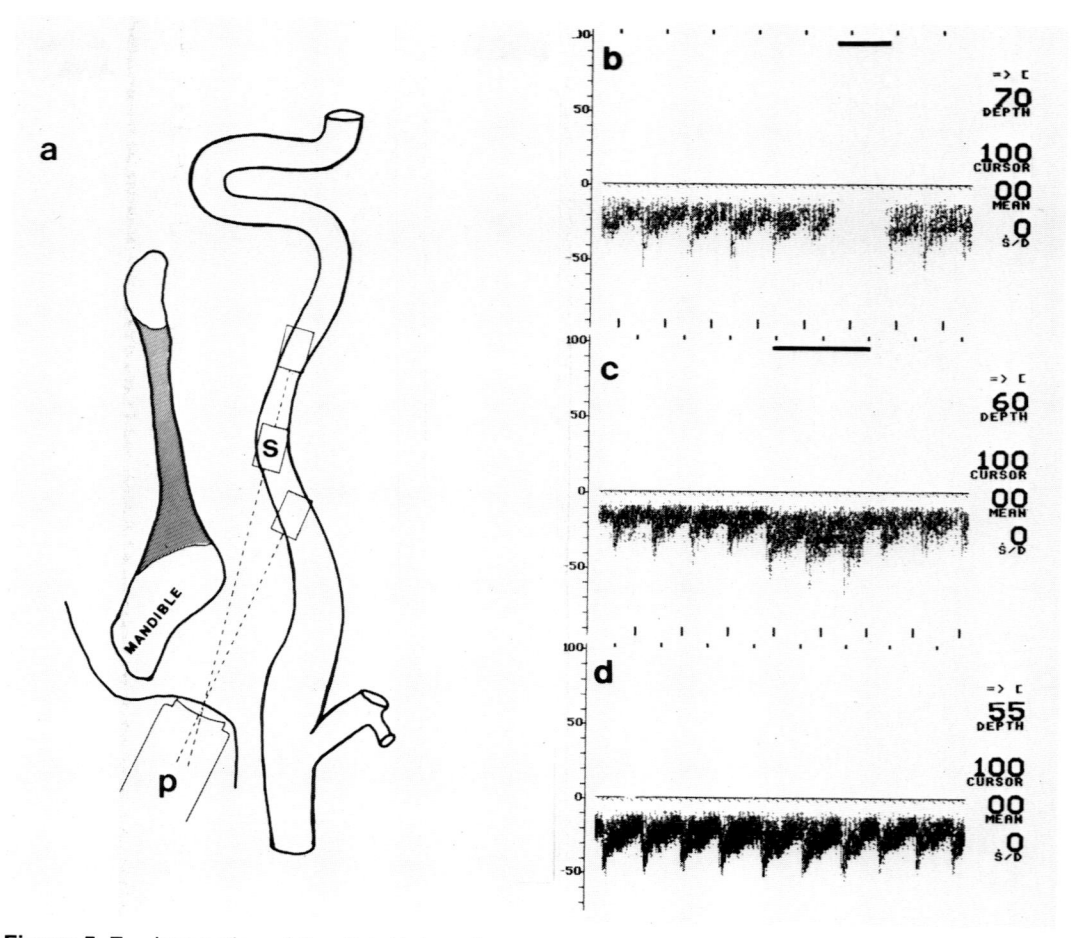

Figure 5–7. Insonation of the distal internal carotid artery from a submandibular approach. **a:** The probe should be placed medially from the mandible and should be angulated slightly medially and posteriorly to insonate the ICA. s, sample volume; p, probe. **b–d:** At various insonation depths, an ipsilateral common carotid artery compression test leads to stoppage of flow (b), whereas a contralateral common carotid artery compression test, as a rule, leads to increase of flow velocity (c). Compressions are indicated by black bar. The ICA can be tracked up to 80 (85) mm.

Figure 5–8. Temporal ultrasonic window of the skull. **a:** Standard (1), anterior (3), and posterior (2) window for placement of the probe. From my experience, position (1) is the most promising one. In position 2, the P2 segment of the PCA can easily be insonated for functional studies of the occipital lobe. **b,c:** Illumination of two different Caucasian skulls with a standardized light source indicates the broad variability in the configuration and extent of the so-called "temporal ultrasound window."

a

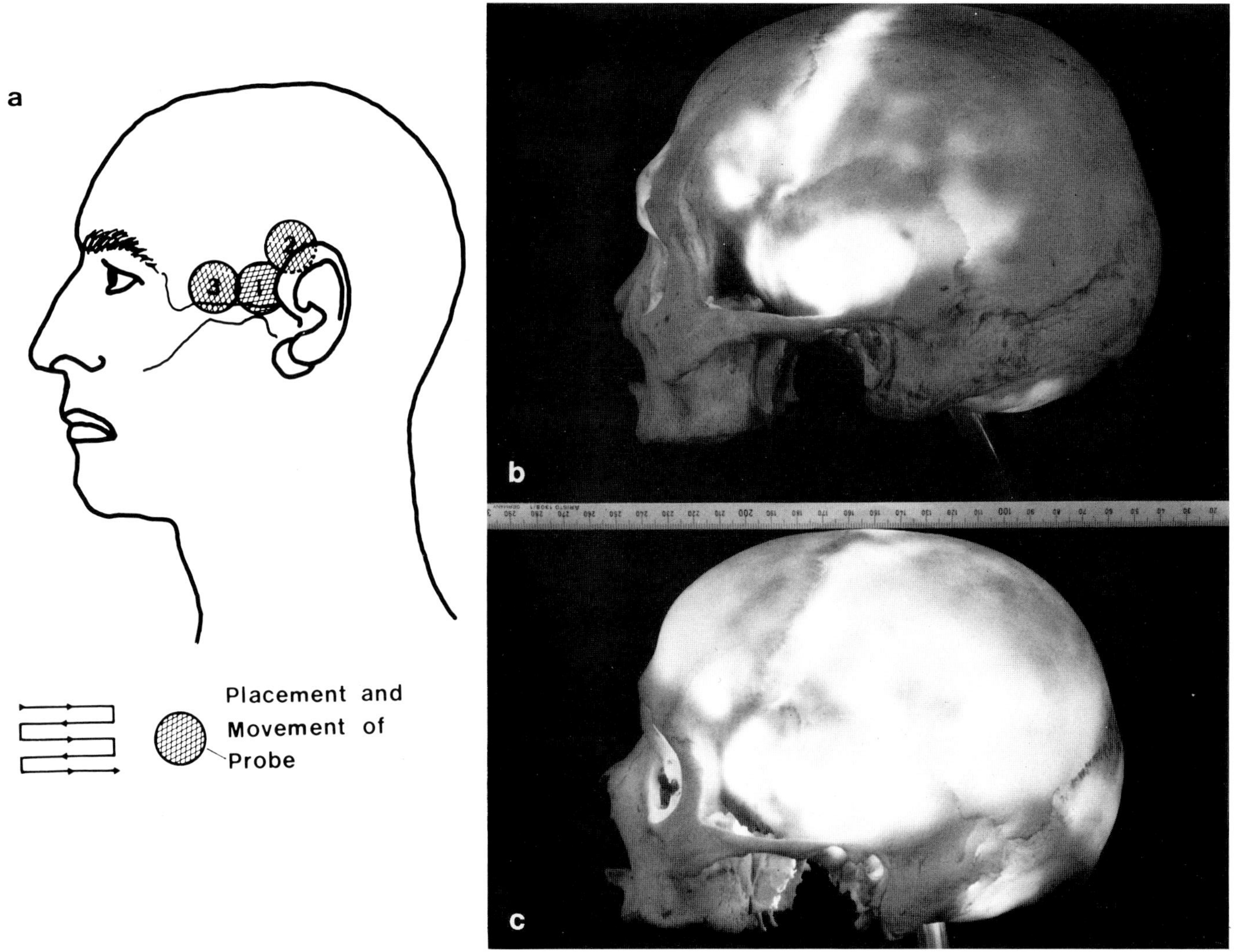

mentioned transcranial Doppler ultrasound applications.

Diagnosis of Cerebrovascular Disease

Clinically, the most obvious advantage of TCD application is the rapid screening of the acute stroke patient for intracranial high-grade stenoses or complete occlusions. Computerized tomography of the head and extracranial continuous-wave Doppler findings are also essential for an immediate diagnostic workup and, if reasonable, emergency echocardiography is additionally performed. The diagnostic categorization of the acute stroke patient can be done noninvasively and will lead to an etio-pathogenetically specified diagnosis in approximately 80% of the cases. This diagnosis should differentiate between 1) cerebral, small vessel disease; 2) intracranial, large vessel disease; 3) extracranial, large vessel disease; and 4) should further provide clues for a thrombotic, embolic, or hemodynamic mechanism of brain infarction [23,24]. If ultrasound and CT are not diagnostic, further analysis by means of repeat CT scanning and, finally, cerebral angiography may be necessary.

Distal cerebral artery branch occlusions are the major blind spot for TCD. This is also true for complete occlusions of the main branches of the MCA, but not for stenoses [25].

Normal TCD findings in an acute stroke patient have a considerable impact. They focus the clinical interest on the heart as the probable source of embolism, provided that an extracranial embolic source has been ruled out by sonographic studies, and intracerebral hemorrhage has been excluded by CT. In the elderly acute stroke patient, normal extra- and transcranial Doppler findings are frequently associated with signs of cerebral microangiopathy on CT (lacunar infarctions, periventricular translucencies, brain atrophy) [24].

The typical features of a circumscribed stenosis of a large basal cerebral artery are 1) acceleration of flow, i.e., increased flow velocity; 2) disturbed flow, as indicated by broadening of the frequency spectrum and enhancement of systolic low-frequency echo components; and 3) covibration phenomena of the vessel wall and surrounding soft tissue [25].

These covibrations can either present as a gruffing noise (visualized as symmetrically arranged, spindle-shaped, low-frequency enhancements of the spectrum during each systole with a maximum around zeroline) (compare Fig. 5-11) or as an abnormal tone with the features of a sea-gull-cry (also called "musical murmur" [2] and visualized during FFT frequency analysis as band-shaped enhancements of the spectrum symmetrically paralleling the zeroline) (compare Fig. 5-12b). Examples of typical TCD findings in intracranial stenoses at the siphon, middle cerebral, and vertebrobasilar arteries are shown in Figures 5-11–13.

Occlusion of the MCA can easily be assessed by lack of an MCA signal in spite of the presence of echos from the posterior and/or anterior cerebral arteries and/or the distal carotid siphon. Dislocation of the MCA due to intracerebral hematoma or tumor has to be excluded by CT because this may mimic absence of the MCA flow signal at the site where it is regularly expected to occur.

Occlusion of the proximal PCA or the A1 segment of the ACA cannot reliably be diagnosed by TCD. The reason is that aplasia or severe hypoplasia of these vessel segments is a not infrequent finding. On the contrary, stenoses at these sites, though very rare, are easily detected.

Spontaneous dissections of the internal carotid and vertebral arteries have been recognized as a relatively frequent etiologic entity underlying acute strokes in young and middle-age patients. This diagnosis should be considered, particularly if there is a history of whiplash trauma or excessive physical activity.

Figure 5–9. Demonstration of the various transorbital ultrasound approaches to the basal cerebral arteries. A human skull with an injection cast of the cerebral arteries in situ is shown. Three metal bars are inserted transorbitally via the inferior orbital fissure (**1**) for insonation of the knee (white arrow) of the carotid siphon, the superior orbital fissure (**2**) for insonation of the C1 segment of the carotid siphon, and via the optic canal (**3**) for insonation of the contralateral A1 segment (white arrow heads indicate ipsilateral A1 segment; black arrow indicates middle cerebral artery).

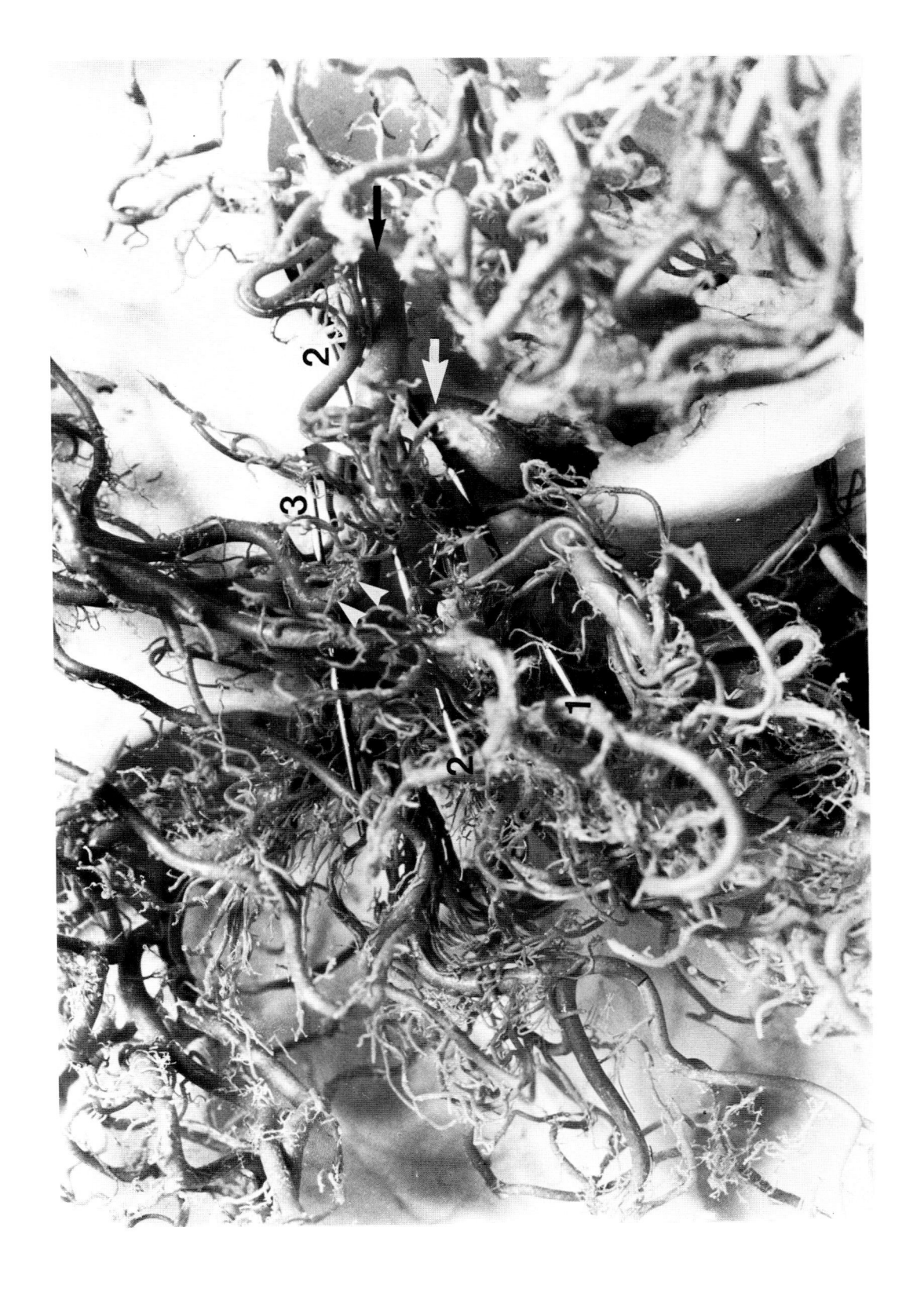

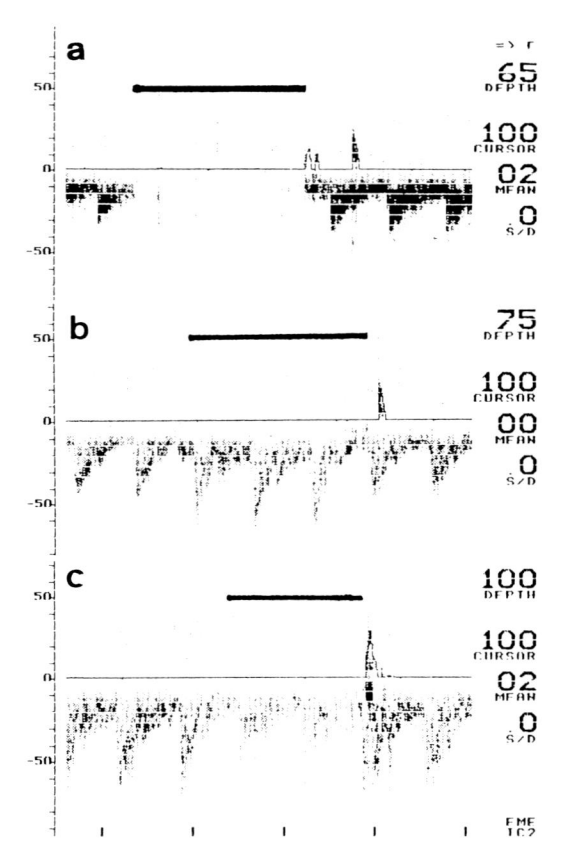

Figure 5–10. Effects of vertebral artery compression tests at the mastoid on intracranial vertebral artery and basilar artery blood flow velocity. **a:** The right vertebral artery is insonated with flow away from the probe (downward deflected curve) at an insonation depth of 65 mm. During compression of the vertebral artery at the mastoid process (black bar), stoppage of flow occurs (if insonation is performed distal to the origin of the posterior inferior cerebrellar artery, extracranial vertebral artery compression may lead to reversal of flow). **b:** During insonation of the left vertebral artery at 75 mm, extracranial compression of the right vertebral artery (black bar) leads to compensatory increase of flow velocity within the companion vessel. **c:** During insonation of the basilar artery at a depth of 100 mm, extracranial compression of the right vertebral artery (black bar) leads to reduction of flow velocity within the basilar trunk (upward deflected curve indicates movement artifact).

From a sonographer's point of view, the possibility of a dissecting aneurysm should always be presumed if 1) a proximal blind stump of the ICA can be detected by to-and-fro movement of the blood column during conventional Doppler techniques and 2) a stenosis seems to be present within the retromandibular part of the ICA, 2 to 3 cm distal to the carotid bifurcation. During the submandibular approach, TCD then regularly demonstrates a more distal extension of a high-grade "ICA-stenosis," sometimes far downstream, within the petrous part of the artery. In a few cases, I have also seen a valve mechanism of the dissected ICA, which means that the ICA is completely occluded during diastole but opens briefly during systole when there is maximal dilatation of the artery by the systolic pressure wave. Under these circumstances, a purely systolic, hissing flow signal could be registered in the carotid siphon. Insonation of the middle cerebral arteries in a series of ten patients with ICA dissections by Kapps et al. [26] revealed either stagnating or enhanced blood flow velocities reflecting hemodynamic significance of the dissecting aneurysm or reactive hyperemia within the MCA territory, respectively. Secondary embolization from the false ICA lumen to the MCA stem can also be detected by means of TCD (see above; MCA occlusion) and can be closely followed by daily reexaminations. Thus, spontaneous and therapeutically induced recanalization of the ICA/MCA pathway, or even progression of the occluding process, can be documented noninvasively. We have learned, that TCD findings in these patients may profoundly change from day to day. Spontaneous recanalization of the true lumen of the ICA is the rule. However, in some cases the artery progresses to complete occlusion in spite of therapeutic anticoagulation with heparin and never again reopens.

Reliability of TCD for the Diagnosis of Intracranial Cerebrovascular Disease

The reason why so little information is available concerning the sensitivity and specificity of TCD in the detection of intracranial lesions is at least fivefold. 1) It takes time to gather an adequate number of cases with both thorough TCD evaluation and closely time-related, high-quality intracerebral angiograms. Data on 72

Table 5.4
Effect of Common Carotid Artery Compression Test on Flow Characteristics of Intracranial Arteries

Vessel segment	II	IO	ID	OI	OO	OD	DI	DO	DD	SI	SO	SD	PI	PO	PD	RI	RO	RD	N
P1 bilateral	20	38	1		15	0													74
MCA							1	65	9		4	0							79
ICA							2	5		8	3						50		68
ACA A1							3	5		2	3					1	92		106
P2 unilateral		0	0		6	0		4	0		0								10
PCoA	0	0						0	0	0				0	0		4		4

[a]The type of response is indicated by a pair of symbols referring to the effects of both ipsilateral and contralateral CCA compression tests. Zero indicates types of response that were theoretically expected to occur but were never seen during this study. I = increase, D = decrease, 0 = no reaction, S = stoppage, R = reversal, P = pendulum-like flow, N = number of segments identified and tested.

such cases have recently been published by Ringelstein [4], indicating an overall 87.5% sensitivity and specificity of TCD when compared to highly selective intraarterial digital subtraction arteriography (i.a. DSA).

2) With improved experience, workers in this field realized increasing reliability of their diagnoses after an initial trial-and-error period. This made authors hesitate to publish their early findings. 3) A major problem is the strongly varying sensitivity and specificity of TCD from one vessel segment to another. This means that validity parameters have to be calculated separately for the carotid siphon; M1 and M2 segments of the middle cerebral artery; A1 segment, P1, and P2 segments of the anterior and posterior cerebral arteries, vertebral arteries, and basilar artery; and, additionally, have to be differentiated for the diagnosis of occlusion versus stenosis; the different degrees of stenosis have not yet been considered in this context. Such a thorough approach requires very large cohorts.

4) In internal carotid artery occlusions, the influx of blood from the PCOA working as a major collateral channel may mimic stenoses of the carotid siphon. For anatomic reasons, the insonation depths at which the PCOA may be hit during the transorbital approach can vary considerably between 65 and 80 mm. Once again, knowledge of extracranial CW Doppler findings is mandatory for correct interpretation of TCD findings. Common carotid artery compression tests may add important information to solve this diagnostic problem.

5) As soon as clinicians became aware of the obvious reliability of TCD in the diagnosis of intracranial stenoses they tended to avoid angiograms for confirmation of TCD findings, thus making data accumulation even more difficult.

Our recent findings in 133 patients subjected to both TCD evaluation of the intracranial arteries and subsequent high-quality arteriograms are summarized in Tables 5.4–7, referring to 632 visualized arterial segments. In summary, predictive values, overall accuracies, and sensitivity/specificity values of 90% or more have been obtained in the ICA-MCA system since 1984, with improving results due to thorough analysis of every false TCD diagnosis. By contrast, accuracy has been much lower in the vertebrobasilar system (Table 5-7).

The reason for the disturbing findings in the vertebrobasilar system are complex. 1) Course and site of the arteries are unpredictable in this distribution. Elongation and tortuosity of the basilar trunk may even mimic reversed flow. 2) The junction of the vertebral arteries cannot reliably be identified except in patients with subclavian steal mechanism [14] or in patients for whom bilateral vertebral artery compression tests are possible. 3) Absence of the VA flow signal on one side does not necessarily mean a pathologic condition but can be due to pronounced hypoplasia of the artery. 4) PICA

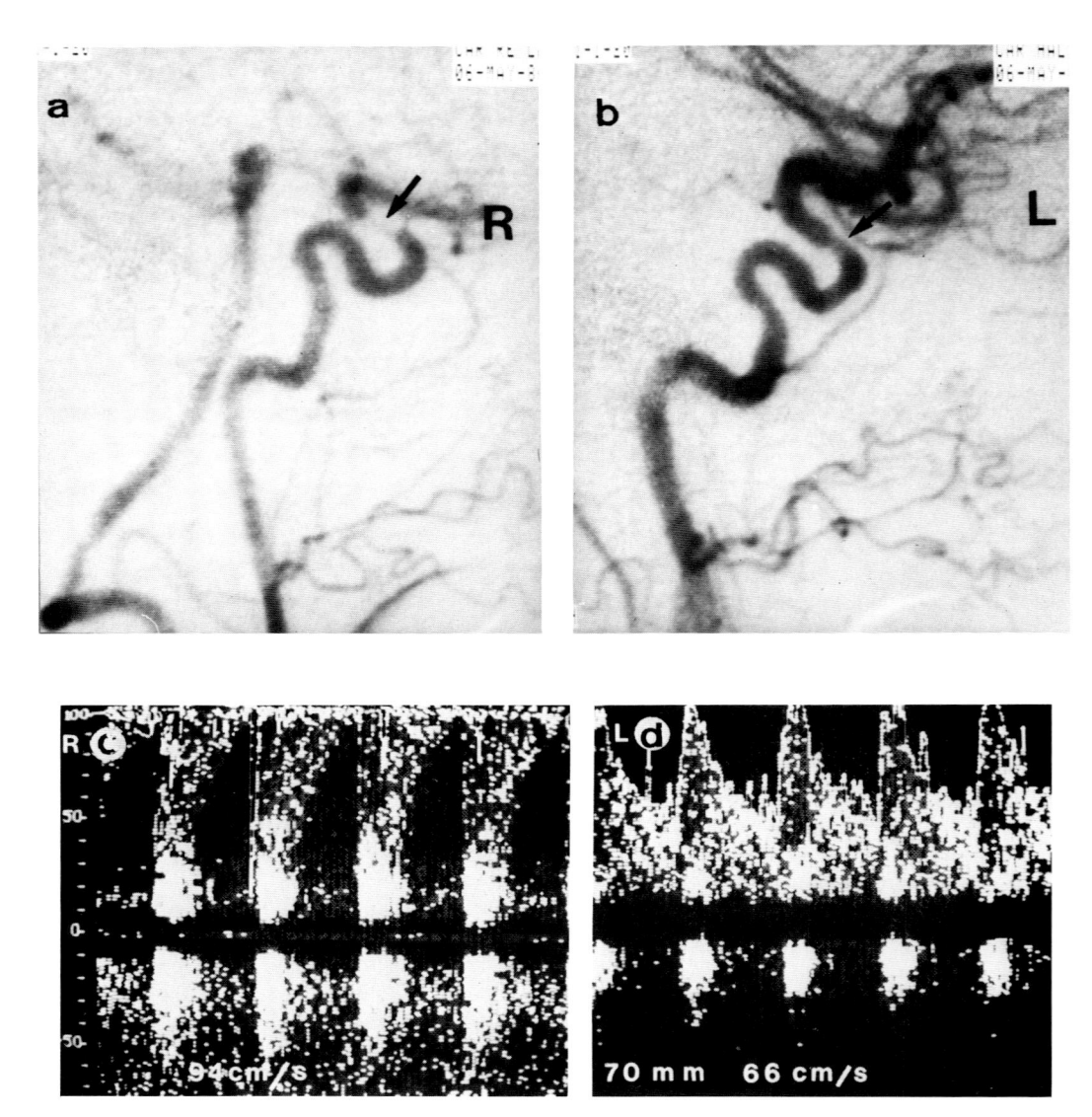

Figure 5–11. Bilateral siphon stenoses. **a:** A subtotal stenosis of the C2 segment of the carotid siphon is visible (arrow). **b:** Medium-grade siphon stenosis is also visible in the lower siphon on the left. **c,d:** The diagnosis was initially made by TCD showing abnormally increased flow velocities on both sides (94 cm/sec and 66 cm/sec). Insonation depth was 70 mm on both sides. The symmetrical systolic enhancement of low frequency noise (particularly in c) is an expression of severely disturbed flow. Due to very high frequency (> 3 kHz) some aliasing is also visible.

(posterior inferior cerebellar artery) -ending vertebral arteries also contribute to the examiner's confusion because occlusion of the very distal vertebral artery segment cannot be differentiated from a PICA-ending VA. 5) Occlusion of the extracranial vertebral artery(ies) does by no means predict intracranial flow abnormalities because the external occipital artery can easily provide sufficient support to the distal vertebral arteries. 6) Segmental oc-

**Table 5.5
Comparison of TCD and Angiographic Findings in the Carotid Siphon of 133 Patients**

Selective intra-arterial digital subtraction arteriography	TCD diagnosis			Total
	Normal	Stenosis	Occlusion	
Normal	111	4[a]	—	115
Stenosis	1	16	—	17
Occlusion	1	—	6	7
Total	113	20	6	139[b]

[a] In two cases, stenosis was mimicked by hyperdynamic PCOA flow.
[b] Number refers to perfectly visualized carotid siphons.

clusion of the basilar artery leads to prompt opening of anastomotic channels between cerebellar arteries that may give rise to misleading hyperdynamic flow phenomena, thus leading to the wrong diagnosis of basilar artery stenosis. 7) Reflux of blood in the distal basilar artery due to proximal occlusion may be so slow that flow velocity does not overcome the sensitivity threshold of the device (see above: 6 cm/sec). 8) A "top-of-basilar" occlusion does not necessarily lead to flow abnormalities in the patent proximal part of this artery because the cerebellar arteries are still regularly supplied and maintain a normal basilar flow velocity and flow profile. 9) With insonation depths of 90 mm or more, the signal-to-noise ratio becomes poor, and diagnostic decisions are even more difficult.

Some of the above-mentioned limitations and insecurities within the vertebrobasilar distribution can be overcome or ruled out by additional transtemporal insonation of the top-of-basilar bifurcation, particularly when combined with common carotid artery compression tests. There is not yet enough experience to judge the usefulness of the 3-dimensional color-flow-coded mapping system (Trans-Scan, EME, Überlingen, West Germany, or CME, King, NC, USA). Thus, I would like to make the following recommendations for a practical and reasonable TCD approach to the vertebrobasilar system.

1) The clinical findings (syndrome-like, progressive vertebrobasilar symptoms, stuttering course of vertebrobasilar stroke, CT/MRI imaging findings) must always be considered for the final "angiomorphologic" diagnosis.

2) Completely normal TCD findings during suboccipital TCD screening of the vertebrobasilar axis in conjunction with normal transtemporal findings at the top-of basilar reliably rule out significant large vessel disease in this distribution. In terms of strategic clinical decisions, this may be a very important and helpful finding in patients with coma of unknown origin. 3) Any vertebrobasilar abnormality during TCD in connection with clear-cut vertebrobasilar symptoms requires confirmation by angiography. When following this latter rule, our angiograms displayed severe vertebrobasilar large-vessel disease in more than two-thirds of these cases [22]. With respect to more aggressive antithrombotic (full heparin dosage) and thrombolytic (tPA, urokinase) regimens, precise definition of the underlying vascular disease is mandatory. In individual cases, dramatic improvement has been seen following thrombolytic treatment of vertebrobasilar occlusions [27].

In summary, when screening the intracranial arteries for occlusive lesions by TCD, typical sources of error are 1) misinterpretation of a hyperdynamic collateral channel as stenosis, 2) displacement of arteries due to space-occupying brain lesions, 3) misinterpretation of physiologic variabilities of the circle of Willis as a pathologic finding, 4) misdiagnosis of vasospasm as stenosis, 5) misinterpretation of reactive hyperemia as stenosis, and, last but not least, 6) poor false-negative angiograms producing seemingly false-positive TCD findings.

Concerning items 1–4, knowledge of both the clinical situation and CT findings is very helpful in avoiding errors. Contrary to the poor resolution of digital subtraction angiograms, conventional selective serial arteriography provides the best available data for validation of TCD findings, although even then it is questionable whether cerebral arteriography can serve as the true "gold standard" for ultrasound techniques.

With regard to confusion of vasospasm and stenosis, CT and/or lumbar tap findings immediately help to clarify the pathogenesis of flow abnormalities. In complicated migraine, typi-

Table 5.6
Comparison of TCD and Angiographic Findings in the Middle Cerebral Artery of 133 Patients

Selective intraarterial digital subtraction arteriography	TCD diagnosis Normal	Stenosis	Occlusion	Total
Normal	142	1[a]	1	144
Stenosis	2	12	—	14
Occlusion	—	1	10	11
Total	144	14	11	169[b]

[a]False-negative angiogram as demonstrated by repeat arteriography.
[b]Number refers to perfectly visualized middle cerebral arteries.

cal history, normal CT findings, and concomitant complaints will lead to the correct diagnosis. For sonographic differentiation of vasospasm and stenosis, it is helpful to consider that vasospasm 1) is usually less circumscribed than atherosclerotic disease, 2) often occurs bilaterally or in several arterial distributions, and 3) changes progressively or degressively over time. This means that daily TCD reexaminations are appropriate in such cases in order to correctly interpret ultrasound findings.

Diagnosis of AV Malformations and Fistulas

Both detection and identification of feeders of AV malformations, as well as abnormalities in their physiologic responsiveness to CO_2 stimuli or changes of systemic arterial blood pressure, respectively, have extensively been studied by Hassler [28]. An example from the Aachen clinic is given in Figure 5-14.

Arteries that exclusively or partially feed AV malformations can unequivocally be identified with TCD by means of their flow abnormalities (increased flow velocity, reduced pulsatility, reduced responsiveness to CO_2). This is only true, however, if the size of the angioma is large enough, i.e., greater than 2 cm^3. By means of transcranial Doppler sonographic criteria, it is of particular interest to define which of the basal cerebral arteries (MCA, ACA, PCA) are involved in the angioma and to what extent. According to Hassler [28], the following types of arteries should be differentiated with respect to their involvement in angiomatous disease. 1) Arteries exclusively supplying the angioma, with high systolic (> 180 cm/sec) and diastolic (> 140 cm/sec) flow velocities, severe reduction of pulsatility as indicated by a diastolic–systolic ratio of > 74% or low resistance index of < 0.27, and a striking interhemispheric difference of flow velocities during side-to-side comparisons. Flow velocities as high as 280 cm/sec can be measured in these feeders. Under CO_2 stimulation of the brain arteries, pure angioma feeders display either no changes in flow velocity or show only a slight increase of diastolic flow velocities during hypercapnia. These vessels are totally unresponsive to hypocapnia. Paradoxical phenomena due to steal mechanism may occur.

2) Arteries mainly supplying the angioma are characterized by still very high systolic (140–180 cm/sec) and diastolic flow velocities (120–140 cm/sec). The systolic-to-diastolic ve-

Figure 5–12. Transcranial Doppler flow mapping of the circle of Willis in a patient with right-sided MCA stenosis. **a:** At an insonation depth of 61 mm, increased flow velocity of 121 cm/sec and severely disturbed flow are registered immediately posterior to the stenotic channel (upper part). **Upper:** Large arrow, MCA stenosis; arrow heads, carotid siphon (AP view). **Lower:** small arrows, right P1 segment; double arrow, left P1 segment (axial view). **b:** At an insonation depth of 66 mm, musical murmurs occur, indicating the maximum stenosis. Note the red-colored, band-like, symmetrical, high-energy Doppler shift phenomena during each systole indicating harmonic covibrations of vessel tissue (i.e., musical murmurs). Flow direction and flow velocity are color-coded (yellow and red = towards the probe; blue and lilac = away from the probe). The size of the spots represents signal amplitude. (Reproduced in color on page 73.)

Transcranial Doppler Sonography 101

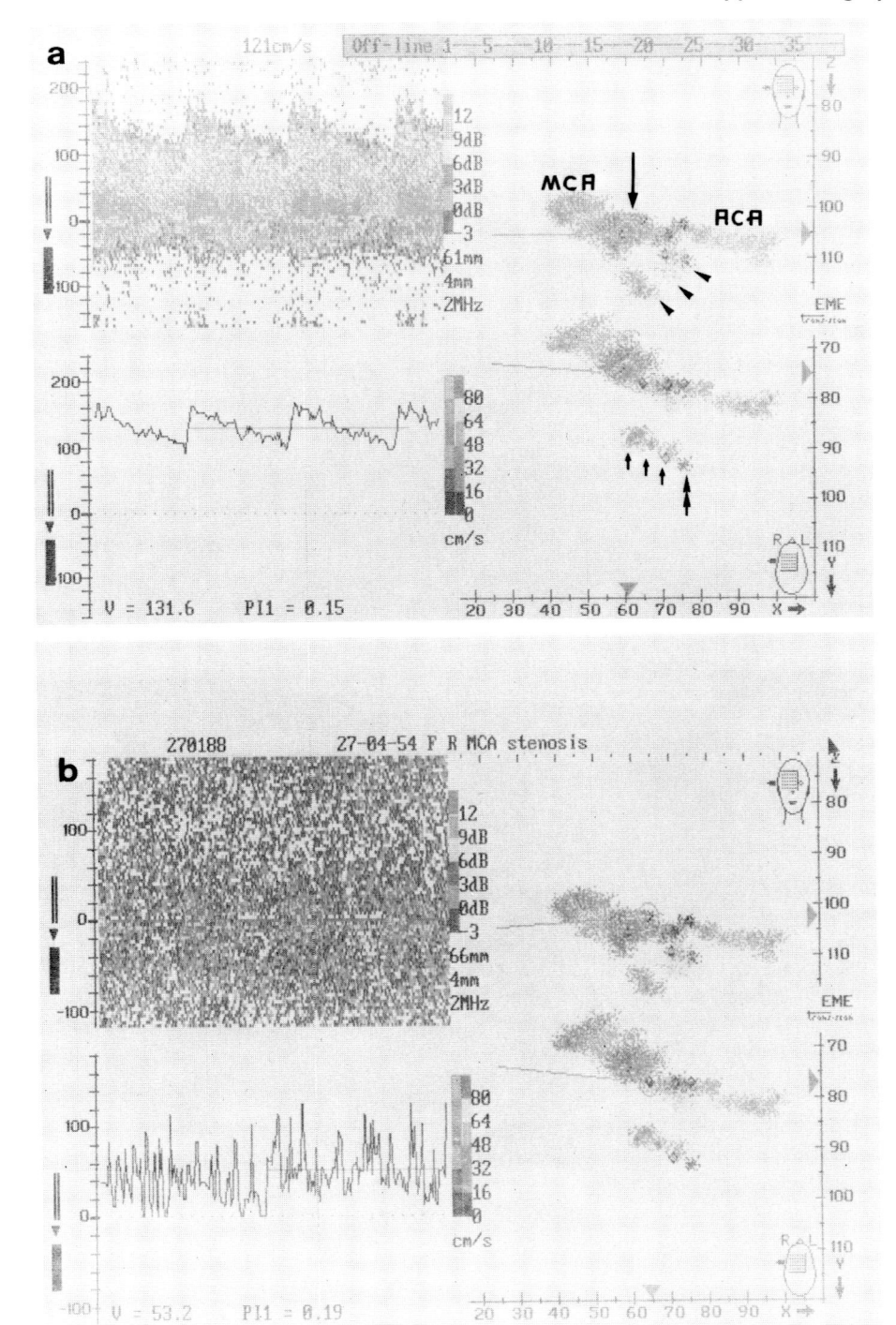

102 Ringelstein

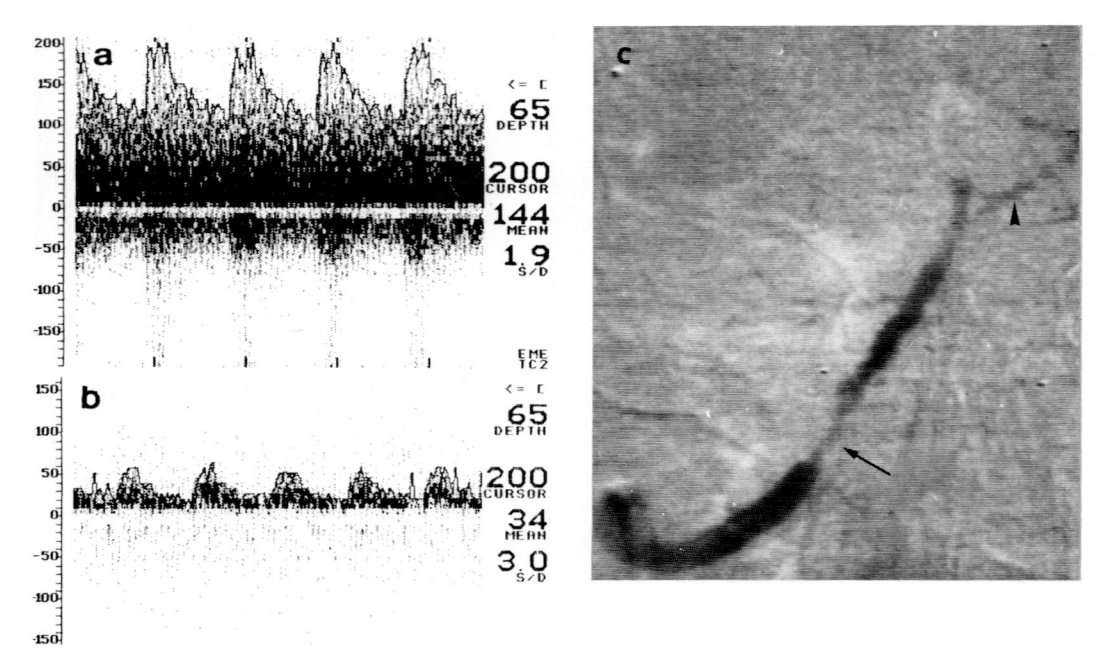

Figure 5–13. TCD findings in subtotal intracranial vertebrobasilar stenosis. **a:** At an insonation depth of 65 mm, a severely increased mean flow velocity (144 cm/sec) and turbulent blood flow were registered with the beam angulated slightly to the right. Poststenotic flow signal could not be picked up. Compression of the common carotid artery did not further increase flow velocity. **b:** When the beam was slightly angulated to the left, a low-flow signal was registered, attributable to the left intradural vertebral artery. This vessel, however, could not be tracked rostrally. Findings in a and b were interpreted as a high-grade vertebrobasilar stenosis on the right and hypoplasia of the vertebral artery on the left. Distal basilar artery thrombosis was also discussed. **c:** Angiography confirmed the diagnosis of vertebrobasilar stenosis, whereas the left, somewhat smaller vertebral artery turned out to be a PICA-ending vessel. The patient died from progressive brainstem stroke despite I.V. heparin treatment and fibrinolytic therapy with tissue plasminogen activator.

locity ratio is at least 70% with a low resistance index < 0.3. The interhemispheric difference is still > 40 cm/sec. Flow velocity changes during CO_2 application are small (40–80 cm/sec) with particularly poor responses during hypocapnia.

3) Tests of CO_2 reactivity allow for identification of arteries with only little contribution to the AV malformation, which may not be identified by velocity and pulsatility measurements during normocapnia alone. Again, it is the reduction of diastolic velocity due to hypocapnia that is less responsive than in normals.

4) Arteries not involved in the supply of the angioma are characterized by normal Doppler findings at rest (normal flow velocity, systolic diastolic velocity ratio < 50%, normal resistance index (0.53–0.56), and normal CO_2 responsiveness). The normal range of CO_2 reactivity approximates 100 cm/sec with a diastolic deceleration during hypocapnia down to 20/sec. However, in the vicinity of large angiomas, brain arteries show reduced responsiveness of the diastolic flow velocities to hypocapnia. This is due to maldistribution phenomena within the circle of Willis and subsequent reduced perfusion pressure within arteries not directly involved.

In angioma-feeding arteries, analysis of anatomic properties and their influence on flow characteristics revealed a linear relationship between mean flow velocity and length of feeder (negative), diameter of feeder (positive),

Table 5.7
Prevalence of Intracranial Arterial Lesions and Accuracy of TCD to Detect Them (n = 133 patients)

	Arterial segment			
	MCA	ICA siphon	ACA (A1)	PCA (P1)
No. of segments examined by TCD + angiogram	167 (one H2-segment)	139	142	52
Angiographically normal	142	115	141	51
Normality predicted by TCD	140	—	140	51
Angiographically stenosed	14	17	1	1
Stenosis predicted by TCD	12	—	—	1
Angiographically occluded	11	7	—	—
Occlusion predicted by TCD	10	7[a]	—	—
Angiographic prevalence of pathologic findings	25/167 (15%)	24/139 (17%)	<1%	~2%
Asymptomatic/symptomatic lesions	6/19	6/18	1/0	0/1
Normal findings in TCD	142	113	141	51
Angiographically confirmed (normal)	140	111	140	51
Stenoses in TCD	14	20	1	1
Angiographically confirmed stenoses	12[b]	16	—	1
Occlusions in TCD	11	6	—	—
Angiographically confirmed occlusions	10	6	—	—
TCD negative predictive value stenosis (%)	99	99		
TCD positive predictive value stenosis (%)	86	80		
TCD sensitivity stenosis (%)	86	94		
TCD specificity stenosis (%)	99	97		
TCD overall accuracy stenosis (%)	97	96		
TCD negative predictive value occlusion (%)	100	99		
TCD positive predictive value occlusion (%)	91	100		
TCD sensitivity occlusion (%)	100	86		
TCD specificity occlusion (%)	99	100		
TCD overall accuracy occlusion (%)	99	99		
TCD negative predictive value any lesion (%)	99	98		
TCD positive predictive value any lesion (%)	88	85		
TCD sensitivity any lesion (%)	92	92		
TCD specificity any lesion (%)	98	97		
TCD overall accuracy any lesion (%)	97	96		

[a]This diagnosis was made by means of extracranial CW Doppler sonography.
[b]One false-negative angiogram.

and volume of angioma (positive). Linear relationships could also be demonstrated between resistance index and length of feeder (positive), resistance index and volume of angioma (negative), and resistance index and the calculated flow rate of an AV feeder (negative) [28].

Angioma draining veins are characterized by a pulsatile flow that is most pronounced in close proximity to the angioma and a lack of flow changes during Valsalva maneuver.

Postoperatively, flow velocities in former feeders of angiomas drop dramatically below normal values (stoppage or near stoppage of the blood column during diastole) as an expression of the drastically increased peripheral resistance. On early postoperative angiograms, the ligated feeders can be identified as "stag-

104　Ringelstein

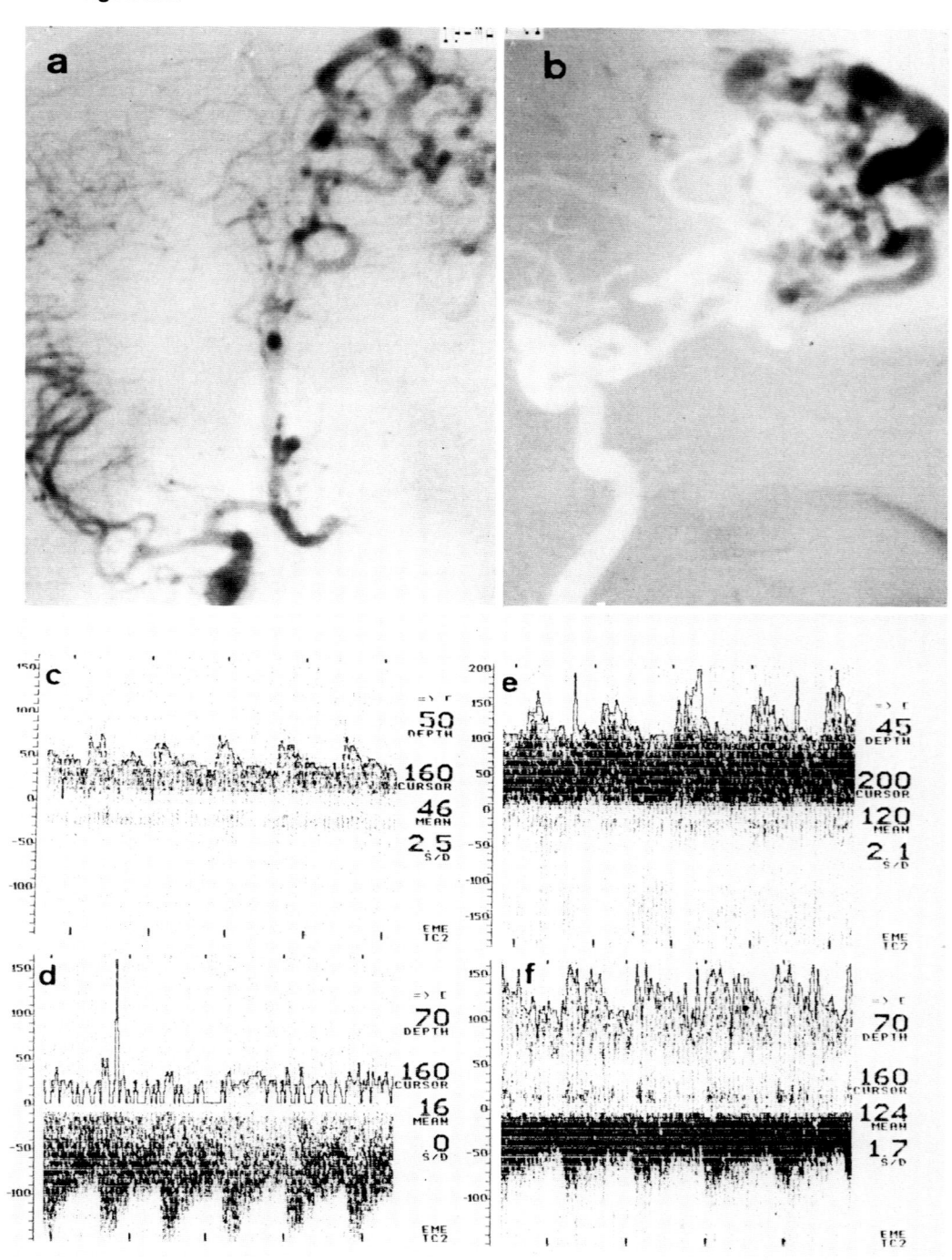

nating arteries." The vessels gradually readapt the flow characteristics of normal brain-supplying arteries. This may last up to 10 days, with faster readjustment in the arteries with less involvement in the angioma. Transcranial Doppler reexaminations after angioma surgery may be particularly helpful to detect feeders of residual angioma parts and identify other severe flow changes due to bleeding complications (e.g., pendulum-like reverberating flow in patients with life-threatening postoperative brain swelling). Hassler [28] has convincingly pointed out that TCD findings finally lead to concrete therapeutic consequences. Deeper insight into the complex pathophysiology of cerebral AV malformations caused rejection of Spetzler's "normal perfusion pressure breakthrough" theory for explanation of postoperative bleeding complications, and, simultaneously, improved both operation technique and postoperative results in angioma patients by more careful coagulation and ligation of thin-walled angioma vessels.

TCD also permits detection of other types of intracranial AV-shunts by demonstration of very high flow velocities and severly disturbed flow at the site of the lesion and of "arterialization" of the draining veins. This is particularly true for carotid siphon-cavernous sinus fistulas, either traumatic or spontaneous. Figure 5-15 shows the TCD findings during transorbital insonation of a young man with a small AV angioma at the frontal skull base, fed by the ophthalmic artery. It was extra- and intracranial Doppler ultrasound that detected the underlying etiology of the patient's throbbing pain and chronic congestion of the eye.

Intermittent Monitoring of Cerebral Vasospasm Following Subarachnoid Hemorrhage

The very first application of TCD by Aaslid et al. [1] was aimed at the detection and followup of vasospasm due to subarachnoid hemorrhage. Consequent reexamination of flow velocities within the basal arteries of patients with acute subarachnoid bleeding [1–3,29–31] could demonstrate a close correlation between increased flow velocities within the spastic basal arteries (MCA, PCA, ACA) and severity of the subarachnoid hemorrhage. This was true with respect to size and extent of the blood clot and the clinical state of the patients according to the Hunt and Hess Scale. Increased flow velocity also closely paralleled the angiographically documented severity of the spasm if Doppler shift was greater than 3 kHz or 120 cm/sec. The side with more severe flow changes during TCD screening corresponded to the predominant location of the blood clot and, also, the presumed site of the aneurysm. A steep increase in flow velocity within the first few days after the ictus was associated with a poor prognosis (> 20 cm/sec per day). Quite consistently, these authors were able to define prognostically relevant thresholds of increased flow velocities (or Doppler shifts) (Table 5.8), with the MCA flow velocity being critical at or above 3-kHz Doppler shift (corresponding to 120 cm/sec) and highly critical with ≥ 3.5 kHz corresponding to a velocity ≥ 140 cm/sec. These latter flow velocities indicated severe vasospasm and were frequently associated with subsequent brain infarction. All of Harder's patients who developed delayed ischemic symptoms were in the > 3 kHz group. Follow up of flow velocity in the basal cerebral arteries over time revealed a characteristic 4-week slope with an initial increase of flow velocity and a gradual decrease after an approximately 10-day plateau. Further, spasm-induced high flow velocities of the MCA were modulated in the expected direction by application of calcium channel blockers (decrease of flow velocity) and by performance of cerebral arteriogra-

Figure 5–14. TCD findings at the basal cerebral arteries in a 16-year-old woman with an arteriovenous angioma of the left hemisphere. **a:** During right carotid arteriography, it becomes obvious that the right ACA contributes to the angiomatous process. **b:** Left carotid angiogram. The main feeders are the left ICA, MCA, and also ACA. **c:** Low to normal MCA flow velocity on the right. **d:** Abnormally increased flow velocity (mean approximately 100 cm/sec) of the right ACA (A1 segment). **e:** Severely increased flow velocity of 120 cm/sec within the left MCA (main feeder of angioma). **f:** Extremely increased flow velocities within left distal carotid siphon (upward-deflected curve; 120 cm/sec) and moderately increased flow velocity within left A1 segment (downward-deflected curve; approximately 60 cm/sec).

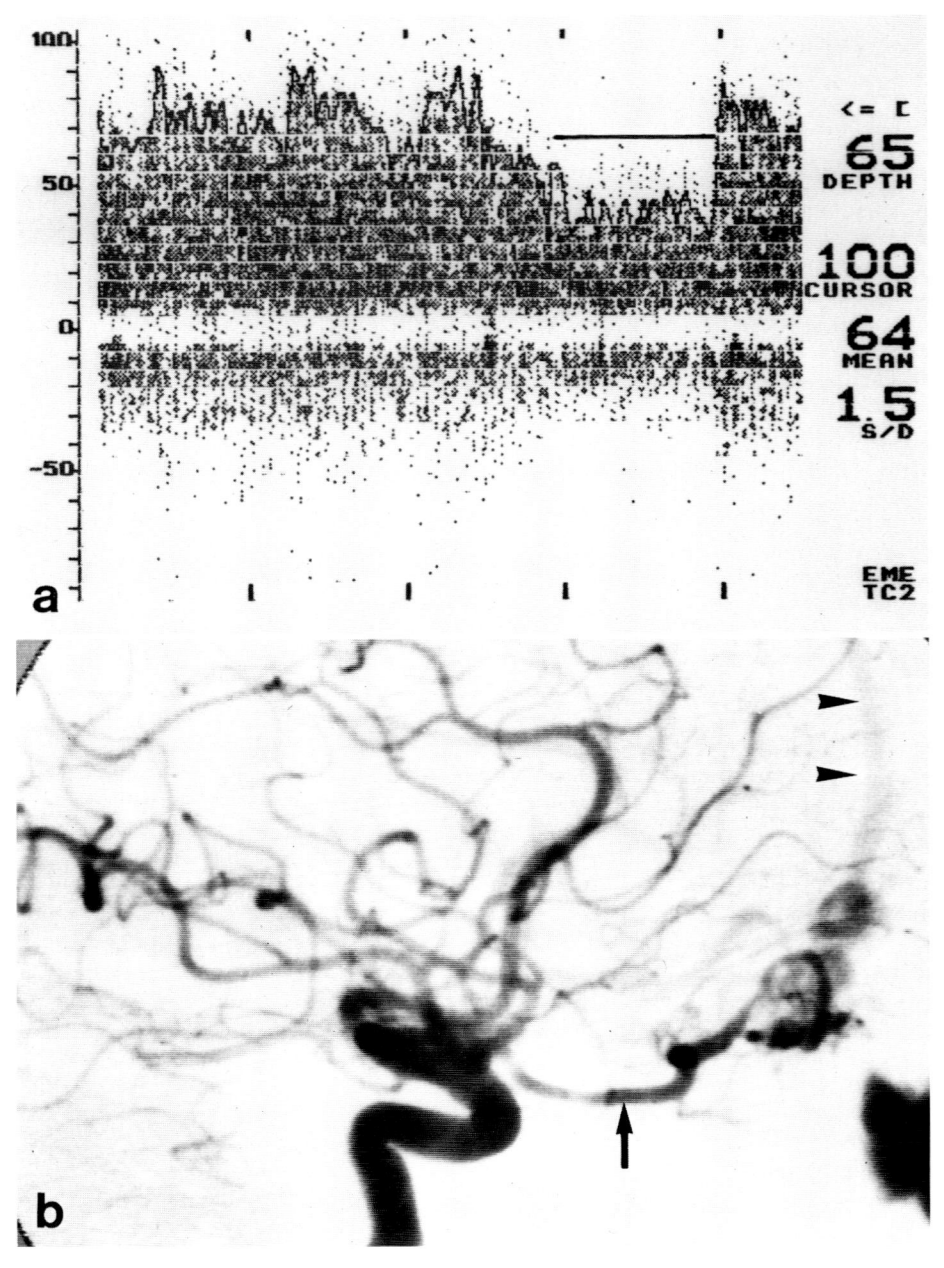

Figure 5–15. Detection of small AV malformation at the frontal lobe. **a:** Extremely elevated and turbulent flow velocity in the vicinity of the carotid siphon during transorbital insonation on the right (main flow direction away from probe). Compression of right CCA (black bar) reduced velocity to a nonpulsatile, residual, 40 cm/sec flow. Signal was attributed to arterialized vein, presumably cavernous sinus. Carotid cavernous fistula was presumed. Patient had throbbing pain and recurrent congestion of eye without trauma. **b:** Subsequent angiogram revealed small intradural AV malformation at frontal base of skull fed by ophthalmic artery (arrow). Arrowheads indicate early contrast enhancement of draining vein.

Table 5.8
TCD Diagnosis of Lesions Within the Intracranial Vertebrobasilar System

Segment	No. of patients examined by both TCD and Angiogram	Normal angiographic findings	Stenosis during TCD/ angiography	Occlusion TCD angiography[a]	Hypoplasia TCD/ angiography
Intradural vertebral artery	84	74	7[b]/6	3/3	0/1[b]
Basilar artery	48	39	6[c]/4	3[b]/5	—

[a]In conjunction with typical extracranial CW Doppler findings.
[b]Segmental hypolasia misdiagnosed as stenosis.
[c]Hyperdynamic flow in channels collateralizing basilar artery occlusion misdiagnosed as stenoses.

phy during the spasm phase (increase of flow velocity).

Spasm-induced brain infarction may lead to brain swelling and increased intracranial pressure, with the final consequence of circulatory arrest and brain death. If intracranial pressure overcomes perfusion pressure, a pendulum-like, reverberating (i.e., oscillating) flow occurs within the main cerebral arteries indicating complete stoppage of blood flow within the peripheral vascular network. Electrophysiologically, this is paralleled by progressive flattening of the EEG with burst suppression pattern and zeroline EEG, indicative of brain death [5]. The latter, however, should only be assumed if these abnormal flow findings are present for at least 1 hour because in individual cases complete reversibility of this alarming flow abnormality has been observed during acute peaks of intracranial pressure [28].

Effects of Extracranial Occlusive Disease on Intracranial Blood Flow Velocity

Evaluation of hemodynamic disturbances within the carotid artery-middle cerebral artery pathway is of particular interest in patients with subtotal ICA stenoses or both unilateral and bilateral occlusions. The predominant mechanism of stroke is thromboembolic rather than low-flow effect [32]. A small subgroup of patients, however, experience transient ischemic attacks, permanent stroke, and/or progressive ischemic eye disease due to critically reduced blood flow [33,34]. These patients may benefit from any kind of recanalizing vascular surgery including EC/IC bypass surgery. Identification of these individuals is based on the detection of an exhausted cerebrovascular reserve. The CO_2 responsiveness of the cerebral arteries has turned out to be a reliable indicator of the collateral reserve capacity in patients with severe carotid artery disease [35–38].

Transcranial Doppler sonographic evaluation of the flow velocity within the MCA can easily be used to measure the CO_2-induced cerebral vasomotor reactivity in the periphery [8,9,39]. As is shown in Figure 5-16, intraindividual flow changes within the MCA directly reflect the functional cerebral vasomotor state. This is only true, however, if the diameter of the middle cerebral artery stem is kept constant, irrespective of the concentration of CO_2 in the blood. Angiographic studies in the 1960s and 1970s have shown that this is obviously the case. With respect to the tremendous variability of normal flow velocities within individuals, absolute values should be transformed to relative values with the MCA-BVF at rest and breathing room air (normocapnia) being set 100%. Flow velocity changes during hyperventilation (hypocapnia) or during CO_2 inhalation (hypercapnia) were compared to this 100% value. At each steady state, the flow velocity value was plotted against the endtidal CO_2 value. As has been shown by Kirkham et al. [40], the end-tidal CO_2 volume percentage precisely reflects the true pCO_2 of the blood. During systematic measurements of the CO_2 reactivity in normals and in patients with unilateral or bilateral ICA occlusions, our group could consistently demonstrate a biasymptotic curve representing the MCA-BVF/pCO_2 rela-

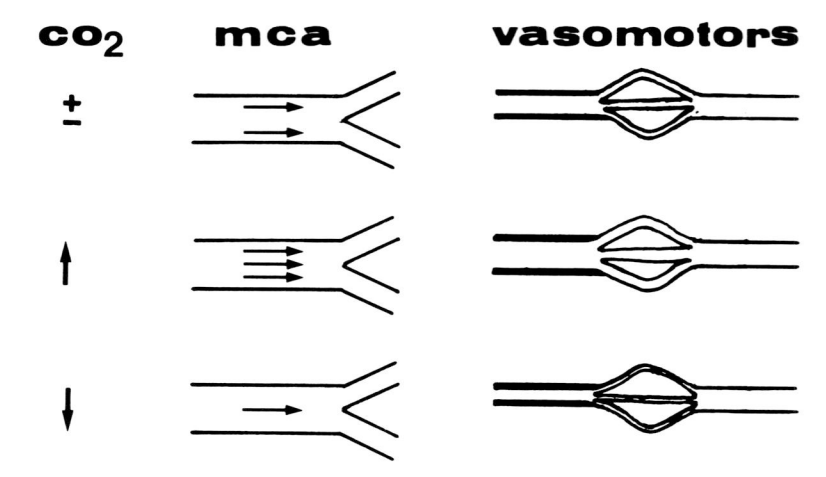

Figure 5–16. Dependency of vasomotor tone, and hence MCA flow velocity, on pCO$_2$. With normocapnia, MCA flow velocity (double arrow) and vasomotor tone are normal. Hypercapnia increases MCA flow velocity (triple arrow) due to peripheral vasodilation; hypocapnia does the contrary.

tionship (Fig. 5-17). The distance between the two asymptotes was defined to reflect the individual cerebral vasomotor reactivity (VMR). In a group of normals of different age and sex, we found a mean VMR of 85.6 ± 16%. Hassler [28] clearly demonstrated that this VMR span is age-dependent, with an approximately 30% reduction of the total reactivity range (maximal systolic to minimal diastolic flow velocity) at old age compared to young adults. If only mean flow velocities during hyper- and hypocapnia are considered, the reactivity span drops to about 10% in the later decades.

VMR was dramatically reduced in patients with unilateral or bilateral ICA occlusions, with a reduction to less than 34% being strongly associated with hemodynamically induced ischemic brain or eye symptoms, i.e., low-flow infarctions on CT, positional TIAs, and chronic ischemic eye disease. The VMR values also corresponded very nicely to the configuration of the circle of Willis, with the lower VMR values in patients with insufficient collateralizing capacities. As is shown in Figure 5-17c and d, the severity of the extracranial occlusive disease does not predict the hemodynamic relevance of extracranial lesions for the intracranial circulation in the individual case. Even in bilateral ICA occlusions, the vasomotor reactivity within the MCA territory may be normal on both sides. With application of CO$_2$, however, TCD flow velocity measurement permits individual quantification of cerebrovascular insufficiency and thus helps in the identification of candidates for beneficial EC/IC bypassing and other recanalizing surgery.

Subclavian steal mechanism (SSM) is the classic paradigm to study hemodynamic disturbances in the vertebrobasilar system in man. For the first time, workers in this field are now able to study and quantify rapid flow changes due to any kind of vertebral artery blood flow restriction directly within the basilar artery (Fig. 5-18).

SSM is a benign condition. Under resting conditions, blood flow within the basilar artery is rarely critically impaired, even if this steal is permanently operative due to complete subclavian artery occlusion. If the contralateral feeding vertebral artery is also diseased, basilar artery blood flow may become reduced in a few cases.

During hyperemia of the stealing arm, which can easily be induced by a 1- to 2-minute exercise during blockage of arterial blood flow with a cuff, the steal becomes dramatically enhanced and flow velocity and/or direction within the basilar trunk may become less or more affected. The latter case has been extensively studied by Ringelstein et al. [14] in 91 patients with subclavian steal mechanism of

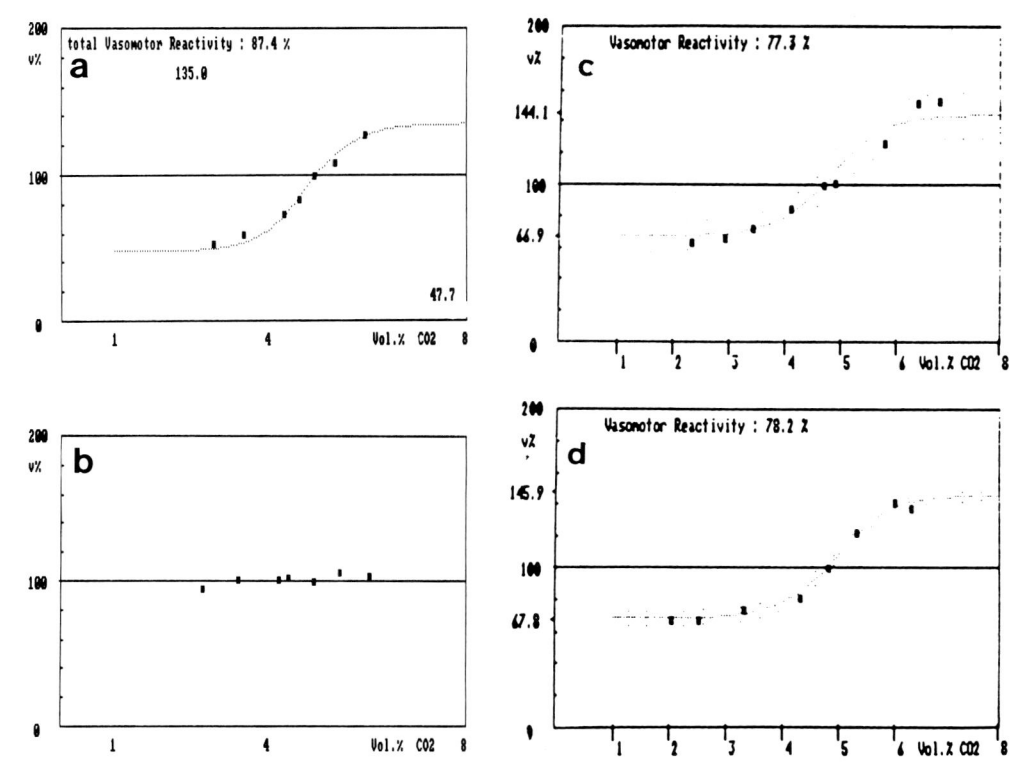

Figure 5-17. Vasomotor reactivity (VMR) in patients with unilateral and bilateral ICA occlusions. **a,b:** In a patient with unilateral ICA occlusion, VMR is normal on the patent side (upper curve), whereas complete loss of VMR was found on the occluded side (lower curve). This patient was symptomatic with ischemic ophthalmopathy and had a low-flow infarction on CT. **c,d:** In another patient with bilateral ICA occlusion, VMR was normal or nearly normal in both MCA territories due to excellent collateralization via the posterior communicating arteries. This case demonstrates that severity of extracranial occlusive disease does not always predict the hemodynamic impact on cerebral circulation. (For more details see Ringelstein et al. [8]).

varying severity. During this study it became obvious that patients with a latent (transient) steal mechanism did not show any reduction of basilar artery blood flow during hyperemia of the arm. (alternating flow, stoppage of flow, or flow reversal). This is also the case in patients with manifest subclavian steal unless the feeding vertebral artery or the contralateral subclavian are also severely affected (Table 5.9). In individual cases with severe multifocal occlusive disease of the extracranial arteries, major blood flow impairment within the basilar trunk may occur and may even be paralleled by transient vertebrobasilar symptoms or transient abnormalities of the acoustic evoked potentials [4,14,15]. In such cases, recanalizing procedures of the subclavian-vertebral axis (e.g., percutaneous transluminal angioplasty of the proximal subclavian and/or proximal vertebral artery) may be beneficial. But even in symptomatic patients, it should always be kept in mind that most of the vertebrobasilar symptoms are caused by cerebral microangiopathies and that PTA procedures, even if performed technically perfectly, do not make more than one-third of the patients symptom-free [41]. In the vertebrobasilar system, TCD has taught us that basilar artery blood flow is very resistant to any critical changes due to SSM. In rare cases, however, TCD has convincingly turned out to identify individuals for beneficial recanalizing intervention [4].

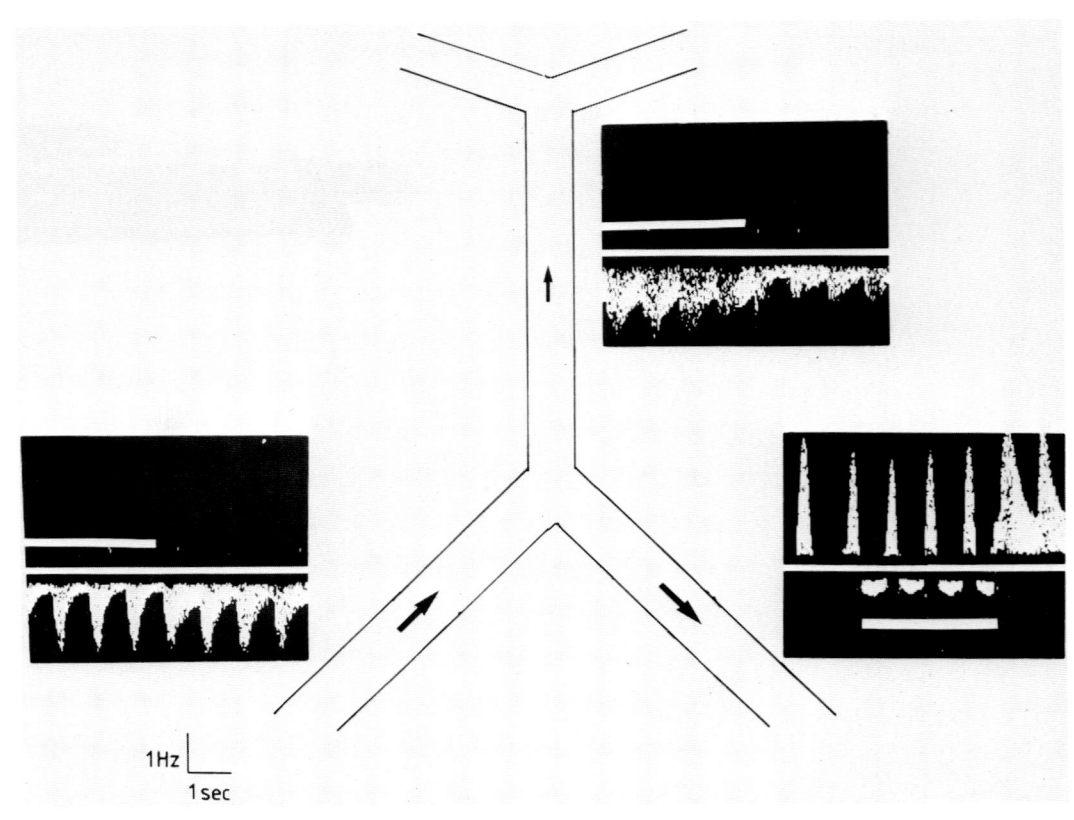

Figure 5–18. Transcranial Doppler evaluation of hemodynamic alteration of basilar artery blood flow velocity in manifest subclavian steal mechanism. **Left:** Flow within the feeding vertebral artery is directed cephalad (corresponding to downward-deflected curve). After release of compression (white bar) of the stealing left arm, hyperdynamic flow occurs. **Right:** In the stealing vertebral artery, flow at rest is constantly directed downward (manifest steal) but becomes slightly alternating during compression of the left arm (white bar). After cuff release, armward flow increases dramatically. **Top:** During insonation of the basilar trunk, flow is directed cephalad at rest. After cuff release, the steal mechanism is able to reduce basilar blood flow (modified from Busker et al., [15]).

Cerebral Blood Flow Monitoring by Means of Transcranial Doppler Sonography

The idea underlying the monitoring concept is the evaluation of nervous and/or circulatory functions of the brain in order to detect otherwise obscure alterations of the patient's condition. It is expected that monitoring delivers immediate information about potential hazards or the effectiveness of interventions and thus may lead to rapid modifications of therapy. Monitoring of representative parameters is of particular interest if the desired information cannot be acquired otherwise with more common methods, for instance, by clinical examination of the patient. Monitoring techniques are predominantly applied in noncooperative or comatous patients (e.g., in the operating room during intensive care and any kind of risky intervention and for evaluation of brain death).

As has already been pointed out, the unique advantage of TCD above other rCBF measurement techniques is the complete noninvasiveness of TCD, the ability to repeat the measurements as often as desired, and, above all, its potential to detect rapid alterations of blood supply in an on-line fashion. Although TCD

Table 5.9
Effects of Enhanced Subclavian Steal Mechanism on Basilar Artery Flow Velocity During Arm Hyperemia in 91 Patients*

	No. of cases	Arm hyperemia without effect on basilar flow velocity	Arm hyperemia with basilar FV reduction	Arm hyperemia with severe basilar flow disturbances[a]
Latent steal[b]	48	41	6	1
Manifest steal[b]	43	23	8	12[c]

*Modified from reference 14
[a]Severe means alternating flow or reversal of flow within basilar trunk.
[b]Latent steal means that blood flow in the stealing vertebral artery is decelerated or even reversed during early systole but antegrade during diastole with a net antegrade efflux, balanced flow, or slight net reserved flow. In manifest SSM, flow is permanently reversed both at rest and during hyperemia of the arm.
[c]All of these patients had contralateral disease of subclavian-vertebral axis.

only records the mean flow velocity of the blood column within the basal arteries, this parameter very closely reflects the true volume flow when measured both simultaneously and intraindividually [9]. Further advantages of the TCD technique for monitoring purposes are detailed elsewhere [5].

For monitoring purposes, the TCD device should be connected to a video-tape recorder or, at least, a commercial tape deck for analog storage of the signals. In the latter case, the flow signals can be displayed during playback in order to freeze and document the interesting phases of the procedure. So far, hand-held positioning of the probe is the method of choice. For more comfortable surveillance of intracranial blood flow velocity, several types of permanent temporal probes, mounted on the patient's head and fixed with bands or helmet-like constructions, have been developed. None of them has turned out to be truly without problems and to deliver artifact-free signals over a longer period of time. In most studies, the M1 segment of the MCA is insonated at an insonation depth of 55 mm. TCD monitoring can be performed either by repeat examinations in very short intervals (intermittent monitoring) or continuously over a longer period of time (continuous monitoring) (Table 5.10).

During open-heart surgery with cardiopulmonary bypass and extracorporeal oxygenation of the blood, TCD measurements have thrown considerable doubt on the theory that postoperative encephalopathy is caused by critical hypoperfusion [42]. On the contrary, accidental cerebral hyperperfusion may play a more decisive role with or without loss of cerebral autoregulation and/or showers of microbubbles from accidental air embolism [4].

Most experience with TCD monitoring has been accumulated during carotid endarterectomy [5,16,44,45,47,48]. The main finding was that during intraoperative clamping of the carotid artery, flow within the MCA is far less affected than was expected by vascular surgeons. The clinical consequence is, among others, that shunts are too often inserted, subjecting the patient to the intrinsic risks of shunting [46]. At least, two-thirds of the patients do not need a shunt; presumably the true percentage is over 90. In my experience, a residual MCA flow velocity of 30 cm/sec prevents the patient from any risk due to clamping-related ischemia. Preliminary recent experience with combined somatosensory evoked potential monitoring and TCD velocity monitoring of the MCA during carotid endarterectomy (Ringelstein and Schneider, unpublished data) have taught us that complete absence of any measurable MCA flow is necessary to rapidly and severely alter the somatosensory evoked cortical response (recall that the lower limit of TCD for registration of any blood flow velocity is at least 6 cm/sec). From a pathophysiologic point of view, these findings confirm our presumption that practically all of the postoperative neurologic deficits in these patients are

Table 5.10
Clinical Meaning of Increased MCA Flow Velocities After Subarachnoid Hemorrhage*

MCA flow velocity	Time-averaged peak velocity (mean; cm/sec)	Clinical consequences
Normal or unspecifically increased	≤ 80	Should be further observed
Subcritically accelerated	> 80–120	Moderate vasospasm, preventive therapy indicated
Critically accelerated	> 120–140	Severe vasospasm, consequent treatment necessary
Highly critical flow acceleration	> 140	Severe vasospasm, delayed ischemic deficit highly probable

*Modified from Reference 29.

brought about by acute thrombosis and/or operation-related embolism.

The effectiveness of removal of plaques and stenoses in the carotid bifurcation on MCA blood flow velocity can also be demonstrated by means of TCD (Fig. 5-14; Edelmann and Ringelstein, unpublished data). In retrospect, these data reconfirm that carotid endarterectomy is not predominantly aimed at improvement of perfusion pressure and intracranial hemodynamics but at removal of a source of embolism. The very few cases where carotid endarterectomy may improve critical impairment of hemispheric perfusion can easily be identified preoperatively by means of functional tests (see CO_2 stimulation above). The efficacy of the recanalizing procedure can objectively be measured during postoperative reexamination.

In a recent study of perioperative TCD findings in 40 carotid surgery patients, Schneider et al. [48] demonstrated a close linear correlation between stump pressure and the corresponding mean MCA flow velocity during cross-clamping (r = 0.81). They could further demonstrate that shunt placement restores both MCA flow velocity and pulsatility index to baseline levels. It has been demonstrated several times [5,45,48] that TCD monitoring immediately detects kinked or otherwise nonfunctioning shunts for rapid correction. Recruitment of intracranial collateral pathways via the circle of Willis with gradual increase of the degree of ICA stenoses could also be demonstrated during perioperative TCD measurements in CEA candidates, indicating that such compensatory mechanisms only occur if the degree of the ICA stenoses is more than 70%. Postoperatively, the previously recruited collateral pathways are no longer used and flow conditions normalize [47]. Preoperative evaluation of the collateralizing potentials of the circle of Willis in CEA patients revealed that those with well-developed collaterals had a significantly less pronounced drop in MCA flow velocity during carotid clamping and fewer EEG abnormalities of the compressed spectral array. EEG abnormalities seem to occur at higher residual MCA flow velocities when compared to SEPs (12 ± 10 cm/sec compared to nearly zero). Postoperative hyperperfusion for a few days was a common finding during TCD monitoring. The average MCA flow velocity was only slightly increased postoperatively when compared to preoperative values, again indicating that removal of the stenosis is only rarely of hemodynamic significance (Fig. 5-19). In conclusion, perioperative TCD monitoring immediately detects induced changes in the middle cerebral artery blood flow velocity, which correlates with systemic arterial pressure, depths of anesthesia, ICA stump pressure, and EEG or SEP changes. The ability to continuously examine the middle cerebral artery noninvasively provides a unique opportunity to rapidly respond to detected changes in MCA flow and may provide new insight regarding effects of carotid endarterectomy upon cerebral blood flow both during and after surgery (Table 5.11).

Mean flow [V]
at different Op situations

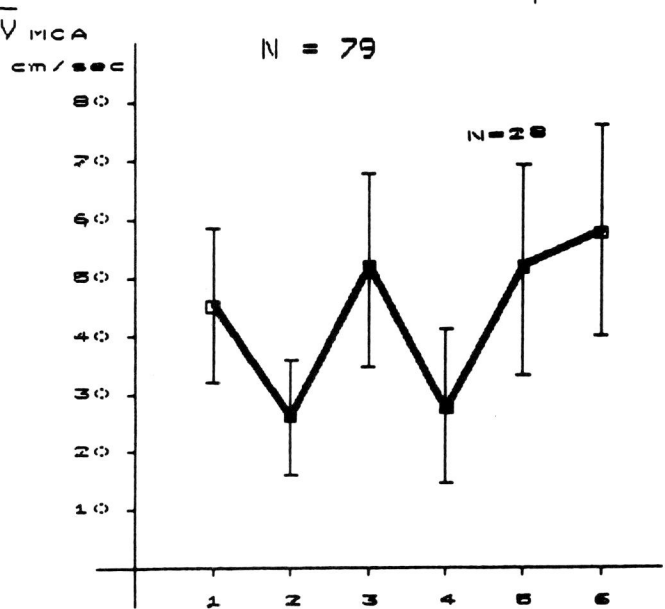

Figure 5–19. Mean flow velocities within the middle cerebral arteries before, during, and after carotid endarterectomy (n = 79). The mean flow velocities and the standard deviations are indicated at six different occasions (1, preoperative measurement at rest; 2, preoperative compression test at ipsilateral common carotid artery; 3, MCA flow velocity after beginning of anesthesia; 4, reduced flow velocity during intraoperative cross-clamping; 5, MCA flow velocity after insertion of shunt in subgroup of 28 patients; 6, mean flow velocity after flooding of recanalized carotid system. Note that the majority of cases shows residual MCA flow velocity during cross-clamping of more than 25 cm/sec. Note identity of flow velocity reduction during preoperative compression test (2) and intraoperative cross-clamping (4). Note restoration of preclamp MCA flow velocity by means of shunt insertion. Amazingly, shunt is not able to increase MCA flow velocity to higher values than those generated by the stenosed ICA itself. There is only slight increase of flow velocity after recanalization of the vessels, though percentage of high-grade lesions in this cohort was high (modified from Edelmann et al., [45]).

In the intensive care unit, TCD presumably will find a wider place in the future. This is particularly true for noninvasive assessment of increased intracranial pressure [49] for whatever reason. Any kind of cerebral low flow state can be assessed and analyzed with respect to yet unknown pathophysiologic phenomena. Studies for evaluation of the so-called "no reflow phenomenon" are under way (von Reutern, personal communication) and the same is true for daily or even hourly followup of embolic MCA occlusions with and without active fibrinolytic treatment.

Hyper- and hypoperfusion phenomena following blunt injury of the head are another exciting field for TCD monitoring, particularly with respect to the prognostic impact of these findings [5]. If continuous MCA flow velocity monitoring in conjunction with a complex registration of other extracranial circulatory parameters becomes accepted as an indicator of cerebral perfusion pressure, this would open completely a new field for controlled trials of anti-ICP substances in the large groups of intensive care patients with ICP elevation in neurosurgery, neurology, and anesthesiology.

Table 5.11
Effect of Intracranial Collateral Blood Flow on MCA Flow Velocity During Carotid Cross-Clamping*

Intraoperative procedure/findings	Presence of anterior communicating artery and/or ipsilateral posterior communicating artery (n = 22)	Collaterals impeded by proximal stenosis (n = 6)	No collaterals demonstrated preoperatively (n = 9)
MCA velocity during cross-clamp (cm/sec)	30.8 ± 11.4	16.2 ± 5.7[a]	5.5 ± 7.9[a]
Stump pressure (mmHg)	65.9 ± 15.9	41.7 ± 11.4[a]	38.7 ± 17.5[a]
Shunt placed	n = 2	n = 6	n = 8
Relative decrease of MCA flow velocity with cross clamp (%)	26.0 ± 23.5	56.3 ± 30.0[a]	76.2 ± 26.7[a]

*Modified from Reference 17.
[a]Significantly different when compared to group with well-developed collaterals.

MCA flow monitoring is a valuable ancillary method for the evaluation of the patient's cerebral circulation to assess cerebral circulatory arrest [5]. The characteristic and diagnostic phenomenon is an oscillating movement of the blood column within the intracranial arteries (reverberating flow, pendulum-like flow). Depending on the cardiac output, these flow profiles may be very sharp and pulsatile or, quite contrarily, may be sluggish or even absent. During critically increasing intracranial pressure, the flow profiles become pulsatile with loss of diastolic flow but reveal a clear-cut reflux during late systole. This reflux corresponds to the backward movement of the blood column due to the elastic properties of the arterial system. In patients with presumed circulatory arrest but where an intracranial flow signal cannot be detected within the basal arteries, probatory injection of 0.1 mg epinephrine leads to a short-lasting increase of heart ejection rate and systemic anterior pressure, thus bringing the hemodynamics to a level at which reverberatory blood flow may be registered (Fig. 5-20).

More recent monitoring applications of TCD were reported from orthostatic stress experiments in pilots, when vertical acceleration stress was simulated by seated lower body negative pressure. This is a setting in which TCD can be employed to test the effect of certain stresses on the cerebral circulation and the preventive effect of certain drugs [50]. Individuals at a higher risk of orthostatic intolerance may be identified in advance, and the pathogenetic mechanism of cerebral hypoperfusion can be defined. Another exciting application of TCD has been reported by Otis and coworkers [51] for better definition of the pathophysiology of acute mountain sickness at high altitude. Transcranial Doppler measurements of MCA flow velocity in conjunction with CO_2 stimulation of the cerebral vasomotor response indicated progressively increasing blood flow velocity and decreasing vasomotor reactivity values with increasing altitude. There was a clear association of low vasomotor reactivity with the development of clinical signs of acute mountain sickness, suggesting maximum arterial dilatation of the cortical resistance vessels in these individuals as a relevant pathogenetic factor for the development of high altitude illnesses.

Measurement and monitoring of flow velocities of the cerebral arteries before, during, and after attacks of common, classic, or complicated migraine are still under way, but have not yet led to conclusive results.

Functional Tests

Due to the excellent time resolution of TCD flow velocity measurements, this noninvasive technique is ideal for functional tests with rapid changes of cerebral perfusion. Such tests are predominantly aimed at the evaluation of the reserve mechanisms of the cerebral vasculature using various stimuli such as hypo- or hypercapnia, increased or reduced systemic arterial pressure, and hypoxia.

Reduced cerebral perfusion pressure due to extracranial occlusive disease or from other causes (migraine, hypoxia and high altitude, blunt head trauma, acute embolic stroke, etc.) induces vasodilation of the cortical resistant vessels in order to maintain constant cerebral blood flow and oxygen delivery or, as in head injury, because of vasomotor paralysis. The reason why CO_2 stimulation may deliver variable clinical information in patients with occlusive disease is the following: If the vasodilatatory perfusion reserve mechanism is curtailed or exhausted, other vasodilatatory stimuli, such as hypercarbia, cannot further dilate the brain arteries. Thus, the degree of vasomotor reactivity of the brain arteries during stimulation with CO_2 indicates the severity of low-flow states within the cerebral vasculature. As is shown in Fig. 5-16, flow velocity within the MCA directly reflects the functional cortical vasomotor state if measured intraindividually during different capnic states. Such measurements were systematically performed in normal volunteers of different age and sex, and in patients with unilateral or bilateral occlusions of the internal carotid arteries. Vasodilatatory stimuli were graded by stepwise inhalation of 6, 4, 3, and 2% CO_2 in air and, subsequently, by hyperventilation with increasing intensity. End-tidal CO_2 volume% values were measured as soon as steady states were reached and were correlated with the relative changes of mean blood flow velocity within the middle cerebral artery [8,9]. Curve-fitting revealed a biasymptotic line best described by a tangent hyperbolic function. The distance between the two asymptotes was defined as reflecting the individual vasomotor reactivity (VMR). In normals, VMR was 86 ± 16%, whereas in 40 patients with unilateral ICA occlusions, this value was significantly lower on both the occluded (45.2, median 50.4%) and on the nonoccluded side (67.7 ± 13%). Similar findings were seen in patients with bilateral ICA occlusions (VMR values 36.6 ± 16 and 44.9 ± 25%). The differences between symptomatic and asymptomatic ICA occlusions were significant. There was a clear association between VMR values of less than 34% and clinical signs of brain or eye ischemia such as hypostatic TIAs, infarctions of the low-flow type on CT and/or ischemic ophthalmopathy. Examples are given in Figure 5-17a–d. EC/IC bypass surgery in two patients with severely reduced VMR prompted cessation of hypostatic TIAs paralleled by improvement of the VMR during repeat measurement in the distribution of the bypass.

The usefulness of this technique to evaluate the hemodynamic impact of extracranial occlusive carotid disease could also be demonstrated in patients with severe ICA stenoses. Vasomotor reactivity in such patients with preoperative, severely reduced CO_2 response improved dramatically after removal of the lesion (n = 8; mean preoperative VMR = 34 ± 16, mean postoperative VMR = 75 ± 18%; $P < 0.01$; Ringelstein, unpublished data). This type of examination, obviously, detects a small, but definite subgroup of patients with severely impaired cerebral vasomotor reserve who will benefit from recanalizing procedures.

Further applications of CO_2 as a cerebrovascular stimulus have been shown to be of clinical and scientific usefulness in identifying conditions like acute mountain sickness, arteriovenous malformation, acute migraine attacks, acute and subacute strokes, and in general, any kind of alteration of the brain vasculature or brain injury where vasodilation may play a pathogenetic role. In rare cases, dissociation of the CO_2 response and the pressure-dependent cerebral perfusion reserve has to be considered before definite conclusions are drawn [8].

A recent attempt by Aaslid et al. to evaluate the true autoregulation of the brain vasculature by means of transcranial Doppler sonography has very elegantly demonstrated that such a measurement is indeed possible without subjecting the patient to any harm [52]. In the supine patient, cuffs are placed around the thighs of both legs, inflated to suprasystolic values, and left for 5 minutes. Both cuffs are then released abruptly and, simultaneously, the MCA flow velocity is monitored. The sudden drop in systemic arterial blood pressure leads

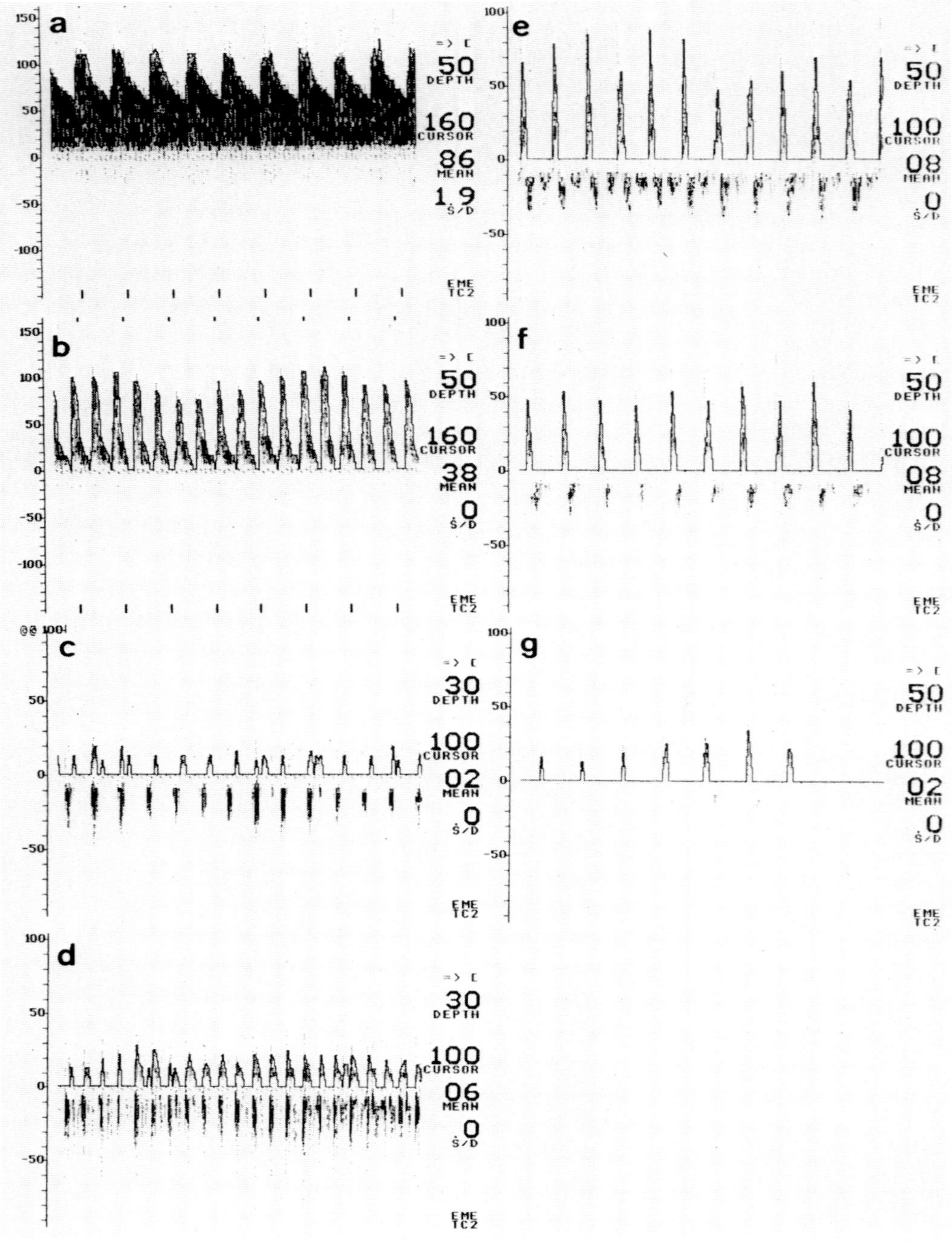
a
50
DEPTH
160
CURSOR
86
MEAN
1.9
S/D
EME
TC2
b
50
DEPTH
160
CURSOR
38
MEAN
0
S/D
EME
TC2
c
30
DEPTH
100
CURSOR
02
MEAN
0
S/D
EME
TC2
d
30
DEPTH
100
CURSOR
06
MEAN
0
S/D
EME
TC2
e
50
DEPTH
100
CURSOR
08
MEAN
0
S/D
EME
TC2
f
50
DEPTH
100
CURSOR
08
MEAN
0
S/D
EME
TC2
g
50
DEPTH
100
CURSOR
02
MEAN
0
S/D
EME
TC2

to an immediate reduction in MCA flow velocity, which is counterbalanced within a few seconds if cerebral autoregulation is intact (Fig. 5-20). The initial flow velocity should be restored after 10 seconds at the latest. Longer periods indicate impairment of cerebral autoregulation. So far, normal values in subjects of different age and sex have not been elaborated. The method, however, seems to be very promising, and the reset time in patients with reduced autoregulation seems to parallel loss of CO_2 reactivity (Ringelstein, unpublished data).

The efficacy and rapidity of autoregulation is clearly dependent on the degree of capnia, with a quicker reaction during hypocapnia, i.e., the response rate of the cerebral autoregulation in awake normal humans is profoundly pCO_2-dependent. The time course of the autoregulatory response to a step-wise blood pressure reduction is identical with a purely functional stimulus of the visual cortex [52]. These findings strongly support the hypothesis that the cerebral autoregulation relies on a metabolic and not on a nerve mechanism.

A principally different technique to study the physiologic changes in blood flow by TCD is to functionally stress the brain during experimental settings where performance tasks of various modalities (imagination of movements, reading, imaginative talking, visualization, etc.) are given (as has already been described in the rCBF literature) [53]. These performance tasks lead to enhancement in rCBF and/or metabolic parameters in certain brain areas corresponding to the type of task. Quite similar studies have now become possible by means of TCD concerning blood flow within the posterior cerebral artery to the visual cortex [13,51,54] and blood flow through the middle cerebral artery to the corresponding hemispheres (dominant versus nondominant during verbal versus spatial recognition tasks) [12]. Depending on the type of task, either the left hemisphere (verbal task) or both hemispheres (spatial tasks) were activated and showed characteristic changes and time profiles of MCA flow velocity (Fig. 5-21). During visual cortex stimulation, Klingelhöfer et al. found a clear dependency of posterior cerebral artery blood flow velocity on the complexity of the visual task [13].

FUTURE OF TCD

The first major step to make TCD a more comfortable, more reproducible, and more objective cerebrovascular examination technique was the development of a 3-dimensional scanning system by Aaslid [55]. I had the opportunity to use one of the devices of the first serial production. With updating of the program and probe technology, this system now is very precise in imaging the circle of Willis from both major approaches, the transtemporal and suboccipital. Two probes are mounted on a helmet-like holder that serves as a stable framework and provides the physical landmarks for the spatial arrangement of the vessels in a 3-dimensional system. The amount of data is immense, and it is necessary for the examiner to use both acoustic and visual color-coded input for reasonable processing of all this information (compare Figure 5–12). From my experience, 3-dimensional TC2 mapping is much more time-consuming than a rapid and

Figure 5–20. Extracranial and intracranial flow velocity findings during development of cerebral circulatory arrest and brain death. **a:** Patient was admitted with acute right-sided MCA territory and left-sided PCA territory infarctions. At this time, an elevated flow velocity with normal configuration of flow profiles was found in the left MCA. **b:** Thirty-six hours later, severe brain swelling had occurred, paralleled by a bulbar syndrome. The left MCA showed a dramatic increase in pulsatility of the signal with loss of diastolic blood flow due to increased peripheral resistance. Note fluctuations of flow velocity with respiration. **c:** Ten hours later, brain death was clinically diagnosed. At this time, not a single echo was available from intracranial arteries. By contrast, a weak flow signal was registered from the extracranial internal carotid artery showing reverberating flow during diastole. Note the different calibration of the ordinate, the shallow insonation depth, and that flow is mainly directed away from the probe. **d:** After administration of 0.1 mg epinephrine intravenously, pulse rate and stroke volume were enhanced (flow curves from left extracranial ICA). **e–g:** After epinephrine administration, a strong signal from the left MCA could be registered showing reverberatory flow, but gradually died out within a few minutes (f,g) with elimination of the epinephrine bolus. Findings are indicative of cerebral circulatory arrest.

118 Ringelstein

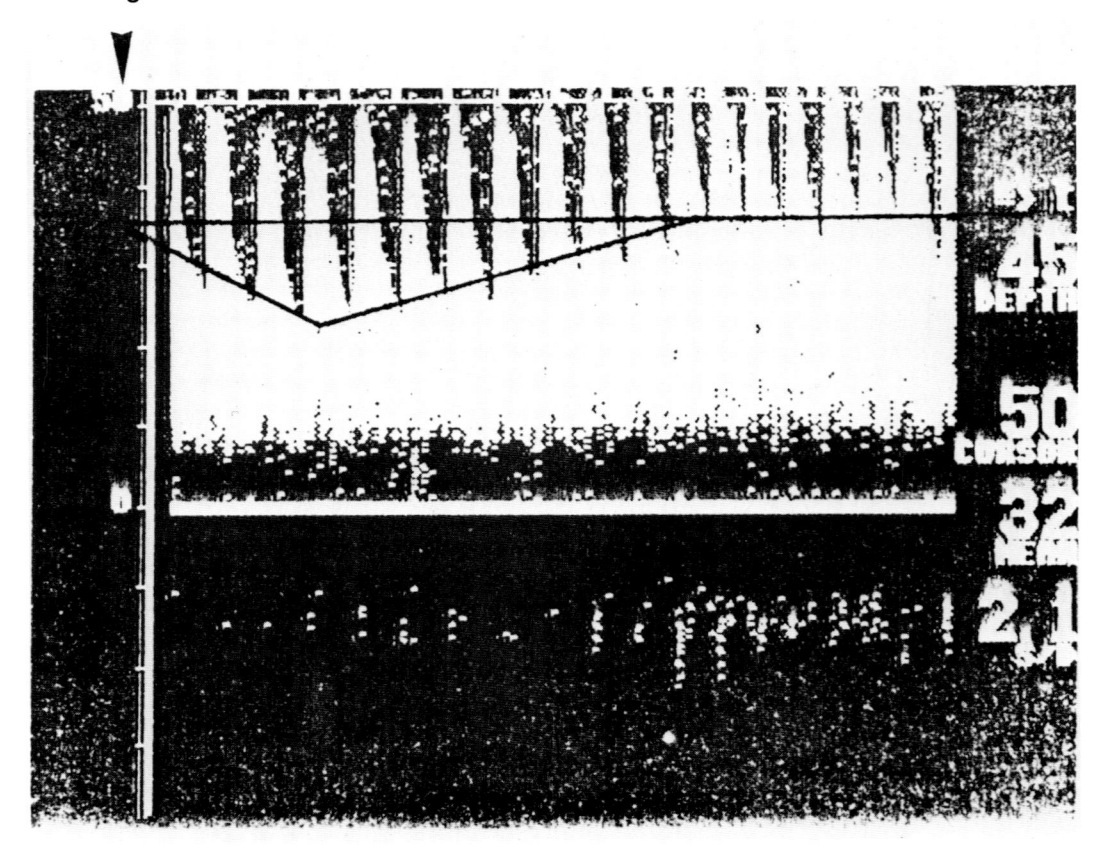

Figure 5–21. Measurement of MCA blood flow velocity during stepwise reduction of systemic arterial blood pressure. Cuffs at both legs were inflated and abruptly released. The resulting reduction of systemic arterial pressure led to a short-lasting decrease in MCA flow velocity. Black horizontal line indicates the normal diastolic flow velocity. Triangle indicates transient reduction of flow velocity and its restoration within approximately 7 sec. Arrowhead indicates release of cuff.

often more focused screening by means of the standard TCD-64 device. On the other hand, documentation of the findings is superb, and spatial orientation within the cerebral vasculature is facilitated, though this mapping system has its own sources of error. Further, the presently available mapping device did not turn out to make topographic orientation within the skull as easily as expected. The examiner has to have a precise idea of where to expect what, in order to make reasonable interpretation of the findings.

A possible step forward would be to automatize the whole device so that the probe is systematically shifted by a motor drive, and in each position the sample volume would be systematically moved forward and backward. The computer would then generate an image of the cerebral vasculature on its own. This idea will presumably be realized in subjects with normal or nearly normal anatomic conditions, but might fail to be informative for clinicians in more complex cerebrovascular disease. An example of imaging of a high-grade MCA stenosis is shown in Figure 5-12.

Another futuristic view is to use TCD as a completely noninvasive, but still reliable, monitoring system for evaluation of increased intracranial pressure. The continuously registered TCD data could be used for trend analysis and for automated application of pressure-reducing drugs. This development is still in its

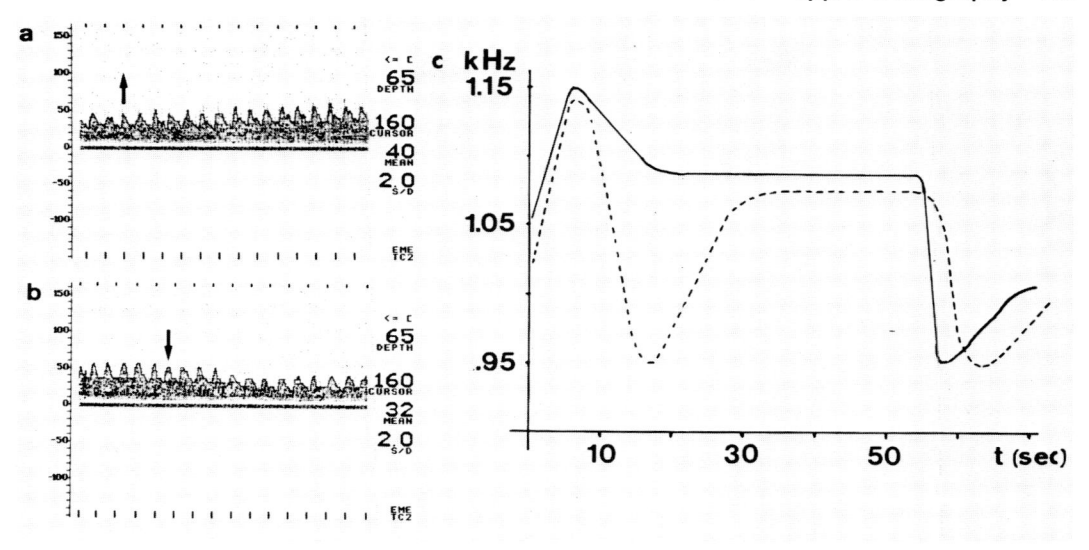

Figure 5–22. Changes of blood flow velocity within the feeding cerebral arteries during visual and mental stimulation of the cortex. **a,b:** Increase of blood flow velocity within the postcommunicating segment (P2) of the posterior cerebral artery when looking into a light. The identity of the vessel has previously been proven by a common carotid artery compression test (transtemporal supraauricular approach). Eye opening = upward arrow; eye closure = downward arrow. **c:** Influences of mental tasks on middle cerebral artery flow velocity (in kHz Doppler shift). Exposure to the task leads to a rapid peak of blood flow within the MCA (after approximately 7 sec). During the reading task (continuous line), MCA flow velocity of the dominant hemisphere rapidly reaches a plateau, the level of which is dependent on the loudness of reading. At the end of the task, flow velocity drops abruptly and then gradually gets up again. During the spatial imagination task (dotted line), the peak is always followed by a deep valley before reaching the plateau after 42 sec, at the latest (part C modified according to Harders and Droste [12]).

beginning stages. Its successful application would be of tremendous consequences for any kind of intensive care unit.

Functional tests of certain cortical areas have already been mentioned. This type of study seems to be very promising with improvement of probe technology. This would presumably allow one to pick up signals more distinctly from more distally placed brain arteries with a very circumscribed distribution. Very elegant functional tests of certain brain areas will be possible in the near future if the experimental setting is intelligent enough.

I should also mention the possibility of using TCD in experimental animals. I have personal experience with TCD measurements in baboons where ultrasound may help to make animal experiments more ethical and to make certain information less cost-intensive. Although the baboon's middle cerebral artery has a diameter of approximately 1 mm, the flow signal can easily be registered with a commercially available TC2-64 device and the echo provides a signal comparable to the human P1 or P2 echo. The topographic anatomy, however, is considerably different from human beings, with different sites of probe placement (more frontal window), posterior angulation of the probe during MCA insonation, and far more shallow insonation depths (e.g., M1 segment at 30 mm).

Diagnostic ultrasound has already been used in space. TCD now offers access to completely new types of experiments in space. Due to the perfect time resolution and extreme sensitivity to flow changes, TCD monitoring of blood flow velocities in the major brain arteries during gravity loss would provide information never before available.

References

1. Aaslid R, Markwalder TM, Nornes H (1982) Noninvasive transcranial Doppler ultrasound recording of

flow velocity in basal cerebral arteries. *J Neurosurg* 57:769–774.
2. Aaslid R, Nornes H (1984) Musical murmurs in human cerebral arteries after subarachnoid hemorrhage. *J Neurosurg* 60:32–36.
3. Aaslid R, Huber P, Nornes H (1984) Evaluation of cerebrovascular spasm with transcranial Doppler ultrasound. *J Neurosurg* 60:37–41.
4. Ringelstein EB (1987) Transcranial Doppler sonography. In Poeck K, Ringelstein EB, Hacke W (eds): *New Trends in Diagnosis and Management of Stroke*. Berlin: Springer pp 3–28.
5. Ringelstein EB (1986) Transcranial Doppler monitoring. In Aaslid R (ed): *Transcranial Doppler Sonography*. Wien: Springer, pp 147–163.
6. Ringelstein EB, Schneider PA, Edelmann M (1988) Multimodal monitoring during carotid endarterectomy by means of somatosensory evoked potentials and transcranial Doppler sonography. *J Vasc Surg* (submitted).
7. Grabielsen TO, Greitz T (1970) Normal size of the internal carotid, middle cerebral and anterior cerebral arteries. *Acta Radiol Diagn* 10:1–10.
8. Ringelstein EB, Sievers C, Ecker S, Schneider PA, Otis SM (1988) Non-invasive assessment of CO_2-induced cerebral vasomotor reactivity in normals and patients with internal carotid artery occlusions. *Stroke* 19: (in press).
9. Ringelstein EB, Otis SM, Schneider PA, (1988) Non-invasive assessment of CO_2-induced cerebral vasomotor reactivity. Comparison with rCBF-findings during 133-Xenon inhalation measurement. *J Cereb Blood Flow Metab* (submitted for publication).
10. Aaslid R (1987) Visually evoked dynamic blood flow response of the human cerebral circulation. *Stroke* 18:771–775.
11. Prohovnik I, Knudsen E, Risberg J (1983) Accuracy of models and algorithms for determination of fast-compartment flow by non-invasive 133-Xenon clearance. In Magistretti PL (ed): *Functional Radionuclide Imaging of the Brain*. New York: Raven Press, pp 87–115.
12. Harders A, Droste D (1988) Blood velocity changes in both middle cerebral arteries during rest and various mental activities. A transcranial Doppler study. In *2nd International Symposium on Intracranial Hemodynamics: Transcranial Doppler and Cerebral Blood Flow*. San Diego, California, February 16–18.
13. Klingenhöfer J, Konrad B, Frank B, Benecke R, Schneider M, Sander D (1988) Dynamics of local cerebral perfusion following different visual stimuli. In *2nd International Symposium on Intracranial Hemodynamics: Transcranial Doppler and Cerebral Blood Flow*. San Diego, California, February 16–18.
14. Ringelstein EB, Busker M, Buchner H (1988) Evaluation of hemodynamic effects of subclavian steal mechanism on basilar artery blood flow with the help of transcranial Doppler sonography. In Aaslid R, Fieschi C, Zanette EM, Eden A (eds): *Advances in Transcranial Doppler Sonography*. Wien: Springer (in press).
15. Busker M, Buchner H, Ringelstein EB (1987) Transkranielle Dopplersonographie beim Subclaviaanzapf-mechanismus: Anatomische Orientierungshilfen und Auswir-kungen auf den Basilariskreislauf. In Widder B, (ed): *Transkranielle Dopplersonographie bei zerebro-vaskulären Erkrankungen*. Springer, Heidelberg - New York, 46–49.
16. Edelmann M, Nielen C, Richert F, Skondras S, Ringelstein EB (1987) TCD monitoring of middle cerebral artery blood flow velocity during carotid endarterectomy: Further experiences. In Aaslid R, Fieschi C, Zanette EM, Eden A (eds): *Advances in Transcranial Doppler Sonography*. Wien: Springer (in press).
17. Schneider PA, Ringelstein EB, Rossman ME, Otis SM, Torem S, Dilley RB, Bernstein EF (1988) Perioperative evaluation of carotid surgery patients using transcranial Doppler sonography. In *2nd International Symposium on Intracranial Hemodynamics: Transcranial Doppler and Cerebral Blood Flow*. San Diego, California, February 16–18.
18. Arnolds DJ, von Reutern GM (1986) Transcranial Doppler sonography: Examination technique and normal reference values. *Ultrasound Med Biol* 12:115–123.
19. Ringelstein EB, Wulfinghoff F, Brückmann H, Hacke W, Zeumer H, Buchner H (1985) Transcranial Doppler sonography as a noninvasive guide for the transvascular treatment of an inoperable basilar artery aneurysm. *Neurol Res* 7:171–176.
20. Gilsbach J, Harders A (1986) Comparison of intraoperative and transcranial Doppler. In Aaslid R (ed): *Transcranial Doppler Sonography*. Wien: Springer, pp 106–117.
21. Spencer MP, Whisler D (1986) Transorbital Doppler diagnosis of intracranial arterial stenosis. *Stroke* 17:916–921.
22. Leonhardt G, Ringelstein EB (1988) Transcranial Doppler diagnosis of severe intracranial vertebrobasilar disease. *J Neurol* (submitted for publication).
23. Ringelstein EB (1988) Patterns of hemispheric brain infarctions. What can they tell us? In De Vleeschauwer PH, Horsch S (eds): *New Trends in Diagnostics and Clinical Experiences in Vascular Disease*. München: Zuckschwerdt (in press).
24. Zeumer H, Ringelstein EB (1987) Computed tomography patterns of brain infarctions as a pathogenetic key. In Poeck K, Ringelstein EB, Hacke W (eds): *New Trends in Diagnosis and Management of Stroke*. Berlin: Springer, pp 75–85.
25. Ringelstein EB, Zeumer H, Korbmacher G, Wulfinghoff F (1985) Transkranielle Dopplersonographie der hirnversorgenden Arterien: Atraumatische Diagnostik von Stenosen und Verschlüssen des Karotissiphn und der A. cerebri media. *Nervenarzt* 56:296–306.
26. Kapps M, Hornig C, Dorndorf W, Damian MS (1988) TCD follow-up studies in patients with cerebral ischemia due to spontaneous dissection of the internal carotid artery. In *2nd International Symposium on Intracranial Hemodynamics: Transcranial Doppler and Cerebral Blood Flow*. San Diego, California, February 16–18.
27. Zeumer H, Hacke W, Ringelstein EB (1983) Local intraarterial thrombolysis in vertebrobasilar thromboembolic disease. *Am J Neuroradiol* 4:401–404.

28. Hassler W (1986) Hemodynamic aspects of cerebral angiomas. Acta Neurochir (Suppl) 37:38–108.
29. Harders A (1986) *Neurosurgical Applications of Transcranial Doppler Sonography.* Wien: Springer, pp 35–71.
30. Seiler RW, Grolimund P, Aaslid R, Huber P, Nornes H (1986) Relation of cerebral vasospasm evaluated by transcranial Doppler ultrasound to clinical grade and CT-visualized subarachnoid hemorrhage. *J Neurosurg* 64:594–600.
31. Harders A (1986) Monitoring of hemodynamic changes related to vasospasm in the circle of Willis after aneurysm surgery. In Aaslid R (ed): *Transcranial Doppler Sonography.* Wien: Springer pp 132–146.
32. Ringelstein EB, Zeumer H, Angelou D (1983) The pathogenesis of strokes from internal carotid artery occlusion: Diagnostic and therapeutic implications. *Stroke* 14:867–875.
33. Caplan LR. Sergay S (1976) Positional cerebral ischemia. *J Neurol Neurosurg Psychiatry* 39:385–391.
34. Carter JE (1985) Chronic ocular ischemia and carotid vascular disease. *Stroke* 16:721–278.
35. Norrving B, Nilsson B, Risberg J (1982) rCBF in patients with carotid occlusion: Resting and hypercapnic flow related to collateral pattern. *Stroke* 13:155–162.
36. Gibbs JN, Wise RJS, Leenders KL, Jones T (1984) Evaluation of cerebral perfusion reserve in patients with carotid-artery occlusion. *Lancet* 1:310–314.
37. Bullock R, Mandelow AD, Bone I, Paterson J, Mcleod J, Allardice G (1985) Cerebral blood flow and CO_2 responsiveness as an indicator of collateral reserve capacity in patients with carotid arterial disease. *Br J Surg* 72:348–351.
38. Bishop CFR, Powell S, Insall M, Rutt D, Browse NL (1986) The effect of internal carotid artery occlusion on middle cerebral artery blood flow at rest and response to hypercapnia. *Lancet* 1:710–712.
39. Widder B, Paulat K, Hackspacher J, Mayr E (1986) Transcranial Doppler CO_2-test for the detection of hemodynamically critical carotid artery stenoses and occlusions. *Eur Arch Psychiatr Neurol Sci* 236:162–168.
40. Kirkham FJ, Padayachee TS, Parsons S, Seargeant LS, House FR, Gosling RG (1986) Transcranial measurement of blood velocities in the basal cerebral arteries using pulsed Doppler ultrasound: Velocity as an index of flow. *Ultrasound Med Biol* 12:15–21.
41. Brückman HJ, Ringelstein EB, Buchner H, Zeumer H (1987) Vascular recanalizing techniques in the hind brain circulation. *Neurosurg Rev* 10:197–199.
42. von Reutern GM, Hetzel A, Birnbaùm D, Schlosser V (1988) Transcranial Doppler ultrasonography during cardiopulmonary bypass in patients with severe carotid stenosis or occlusion. *Stroke* 19:674–680.
43. Ries F, Eicke M (1987) Auswirkungen der extrakorporalen Zirkulation auf die intrazerebrale Hämodynamik—Erklärung postoperativer neuropsychiatrischer Komplikationen. In Widder B (ed): *Transkranielle Dopplersonographie bei Zerebrovaskulären Erkrankungen.* Wien: Springer, pp 100–103.
44. Ringelstein EB, Richert F, Bardos S, Minale C, Alsukun M, Zeplin H, Schöndube F, Zeumer H, Messmer B (1985) Transkraniell-sonographisches Monitoring des Blutflusses der A. cerebri media während rekanalisierender Operationen an der extrakraniellen A. carotis interna. *Nervenarzt* 56:423–430.
45. Edelmann M, Ringelstein EB, Richert F (1986) Transcranial Doppler sonography for monitoring of the middle cerebral artery blood flow velocity during carotid endarterectomy. *Rev Bras Angiol Cli Vasc* 16:96–100.
46. Ferguson F (1982) Intra-operative monitoring and internal shunts: Are they necessary in carotid endarterectomy? *Stroke* 13:287–289.
47. Burmeister W, Fischer T, Maurer PC (1988) Transcranial Doppler investigations of collateralization capacity of basal cerebral arteries in patients with extracranial carotid stenoses before and after operative treatment. In *2nd International Symposium on Intracranial Hemodynamics: Transcranial Doppler and Cerebral Blood Flow.* San Diego, California, February 15–18.
48. Schneider PA, Ringelstein EB, Rossman ME, Otis SM, Torem S, Dilley RB, Bernstein EF (1988) Perioperative evaluation of carotid surgery patients using transcranial Doppler. In *2nd International Symposium on Intracranial Hemodynamics: Transcranial Doppler and Cerebral Blood Flow.* San Diego, California, February 15–18.
49. Aaslid R, Lindegaard KF (1986) Cerebral hemodynamics. In Aaslid A (ed): *Transcranial Doppler Sonography.* Wien: Springer, pp 60–85.
50. Sharma M, Teague SM, Saadatmanesh V, Voyles WF, Hordinsky J (1988) Middle cerebral blood flow monitoring during presyncope induced by orthostatic stress, hypoxia, and beta blockade. In *2nd International Symposium on Intracranial Hemodynamics: Transcranial Doppler and Cerebral Blood Flow.* San Diego, California, February 15–18.
51. Otis SM, Rossman ME, Schneider PA, Rush MP, Ringelstein EB (1988) Relationship of cerebral blood flow regulation to acute mountain sickness. *J Ultrasound Med* (in press).
52. Aaslid R, Lindegaard KF, Sorteberg W, Nornes H (1988) Cerebral autoregulation dynamics. In *2nd International Symposium on Intracranial Hemodynamics: Transcranial Doppler and Cerebral Blood Flow.* San Diego, California, February 16–18.
53. Phelps ME, Kuhl DE (1981) Metabolic mapping of the brain's response to visual stimulation: Studies in humans. *Science* 211:1445–1448.
54. Harders A, Seilacher E (1988) Blood flow velocity changes in both posterior cerebral arteries during visual cortex activities: A transcranial Doppler study. In *2nd International Symposium on Intracranial Hemodynamics: Transcranial Doppler and Cerebral Blood Flow.* San Diego, California, February 16–18.
55. Aaslid R (1986) Transcranial Doppler examination technique. In Aaslid R (ed): *Transcranial Doppler Sonography.* Wein: Springer, pp 39–59.

6

Magnetic Resonance Imaging (MRI) and Computerized Tomography (CT) in Cerebrovascular Disease

Gary Gerard, MD, Debra Shabas, MD, and Vidia Malhotra, MD

Department of Neurology, Winthrop-University Hospital, Mineola, New York 11501 (G.G.); Departments of Neurology (D.S.) and Neuroradiology (V.M.), Beth Israel Medical Center, New York, New York 10003

INTRODUCTION

The ability of magnetic resonance imaging (MRI) to detect changes in the ischemic brain was evident in the earliest investigative stages of this new technology. MRI is sensitive to physicochemical changes in brain tissues.

MRI images reflect the tissue state of hydration by mapping the characteristics of hydrogen (protons) in brain water. Increases in hydrogen density and proton physicochemical changes are reflected in prolongations of relaxation and resulting changes in image intensity.

The sensitivity of MRI in detecting ischemic changes is superior to that of other noninvestigational, noninvasive imaging modalities. The specificity of the MRI changes associated with ischemia is still low, as the intrinsic parameter changes (T_1 and T_2) are shared by numerous other pathologic processes.

It is probable that changes on positron emission tomography (PET), which reflect functional disturbances, will show abnormal changes more sensitively than MRI, but MRI as a noninvasive method provides important information.

The ability to do frequent and serial MR imaging will be applicable to monitoring the effects of drug regimens in clinical stroke studies and in this regard is complimentary to PET scanning.

Transient ischemic attacks (TIA) are by definition reversible clinical events, but there are permanent pathologic and MRI-detectable changes. It is now more clearly seen than ever that even when permanent tissue damage (infarction) occurs, there may be no apparent clinical manifestations.

MR contrast agents have not been rigorously tested in large-scale studies because conventional noncontrast-enhanced MR is so sensitive in detecting the changes associated with ischemia. It has been noted already that Gadolinium diethylenetriaminepentaacetic acid (Gd-DTPA), which has been approved for use by the Food and Drug Administration, is able to penetrate neural tissue, enhancing contrast when infarction impairs the integrity of the blood brain barrier. MR is a unique addition to our neuroimaging capabilities in the clinical approach to cerebral ischemia and provides an additional means to study characteristics of cerebral and extracranial blood flow.

CORTICAL INFARCTION

Numerous clinical studies have documented the superiority of MRI compared to CT scanning, in the detection of cerebral ischemic disease [1–6].

MRI is an entirely different imaging modality than CT. Proton MRI is based on the magnetic properties of the hydrogen nucleus. The brain contains a high concentration of hydrogen (protons) in water. In the earliest stages of ce-

---

We are indebted to Joan Nold for secretarial assistance.

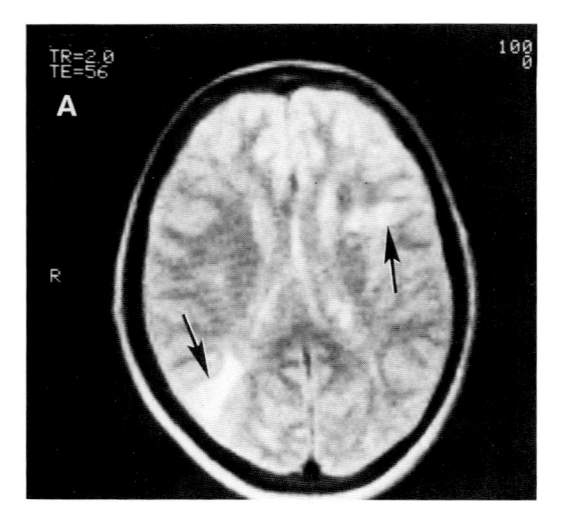

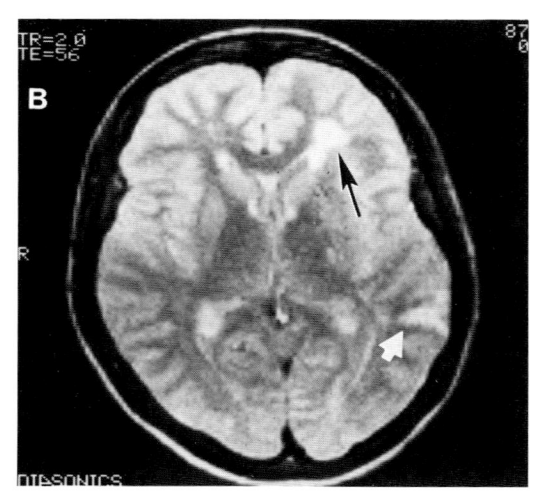

Figure 6–1. A: Bilateral acute cortical infarctions (arrows). **B:** Patient with lupus vasculitis. Cortical infarct, left (white arrow). Area of vasculitis (black arrow) that resolved with steroids.

is a unique tool in the evaluation of cerebral ischemia and infarction.

MRI can detect ischemic insults to the brain earlier than any other available method. MRI routinely demonstrates regions of abnormality before CT. Within the first 30 minutes of ischemia, there are already fluctuations in tissue water content resulting in cytotoxic edema. Studies have shown that ischemia can be detected on MRI within 30 minutes to 1 hour of onset and clearly seen within 3 hours of ischemic insult [4,8–10].

In a clinical study by Kertesz et al. [11], MRI was found to be significantly more sensitive than CT in detecting cerebral infarction within the first 48 hours of onset.

Ischemic brain infarction prolongs T_1 and T_2, with decreased signal intensity on T_1-weighted images, and increased signal intensity on T_2-weighted images. Images obtained with long TR and long TE, T_2-weighted images, have proven to be the most sensitive in acute infarction (Fig. 6-1). Also noted in the acute stage of infarction is the associated mass effect, which is reduced in subacute infarction [6]. Experimental data suggests that T_1 and T_2 prolongation is greatest in the earliest stage of ischemia. Later in the infarction, with destruction of the blood brain barrier, the influx of protein macromolecules into the area shortens the abnormally prolonged T_1 and T_2 [12] (Fig. 6-2). A more detailed description of the evolution of the appearances of acute and subacute infarction and their comparison to CT at each stage can be found in the literature [10].

Chronic infarction is usually well demarcated on MRI. The foci may show regions of focal cystic changes with marked prolongation of relaxation values or may show areas of focal encephalomalacia (Fig. 6-3).

The underlying structure is generally atrophic. Flannigan et al. [6] noted two types of MRI appearance of chronic infarction. Type I is described as having two distinct zones. They found one zone of the most severe tissue damage with a CSF-like intensity, representing macrocystic encephalomalacia, and a border zone of high intensity on T_2-weighted images, representing microcysts or gliosis (Fig. 6-4). Type II chronic infarction is described as an area of only CSF-like intensity and severe as-

rebral ischemia and infarction, there are changes in tissue water. These subtle alterations in water, to which MRI is exquisitely sensitive, does not significantly alter x-ray attenuation [7]. This forms the basis for the superiority of MRI over CT scanning in this setting. With the progression to infarction from prolonged ischemia, the changes in water content become more extensive. Due to the inherent sensitivity of MRI to water fluctuations, it

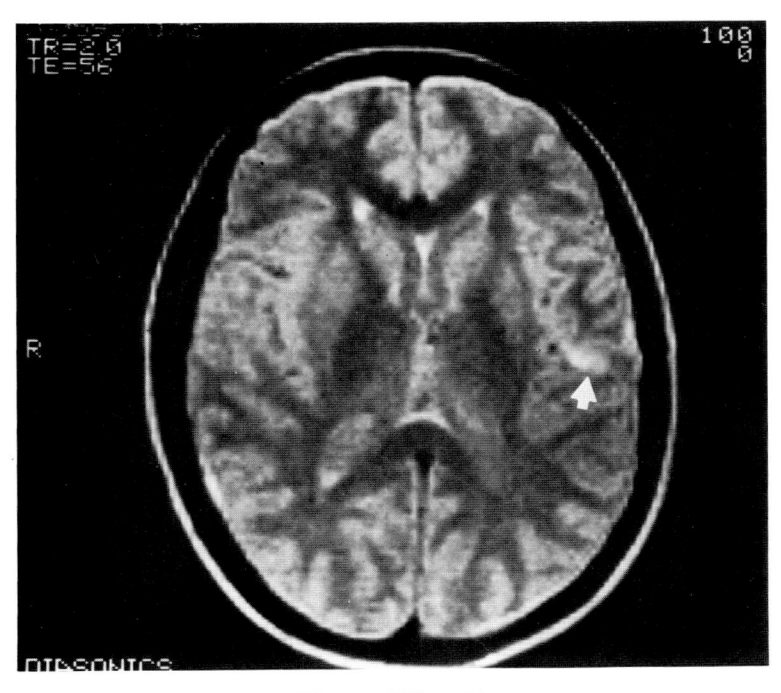

Figure 6–2. Subacute cortical infarct. TR = 2, TE = 56.

sociated atrophy, without the high intensity border zone (Fig. 6-5).

LACUNAR INFARCTS

Lacunar strokes are usually defined as small, deep infarcts resulting from a primary arteriopathy of small, penetrating branches of major cerebral arteries [13]. They are commonly associated with chronic hypertension and diabetes. Depending on their location, lacunes can be clinically silent or present with one of many well described clinical syndromes [85]. The focal area of ischemia is usually less than 1.5 mm in diameter (Fig. 6-6) and rarely exceeds 2 mm (Fig. 6-7) [14].

CT scanning often fails to demonstrate the lesion in patients with lacunar infarction. Small lacunes are beyond the resolution capacity of any type of CT. Demonstration of the larger lacunes by CT scanning depends on the resolution of the machine, the slice thickness, and the location of the lesion. However, even the smallest lacunes are seen on MRI. They appear as small, circular areas of prolonged T_1 and prolonged T_2 deep in the white matter

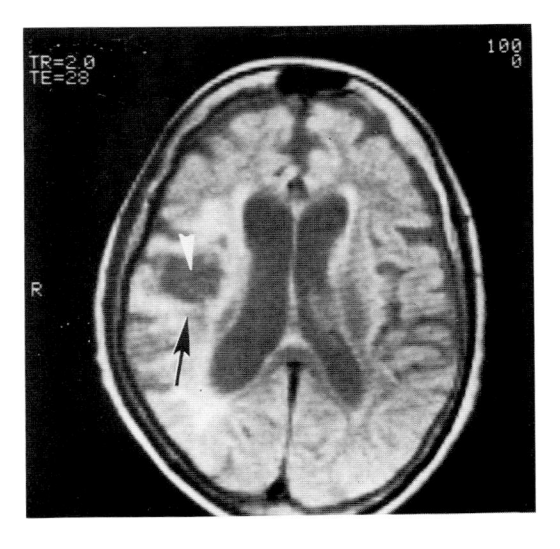

Figure 6–3. Large chronic cortical infarct with central cystic CSF density encephalomalacia (arrowhead) and high density peripheral gliosis (arrow).

126 Gerard et al.

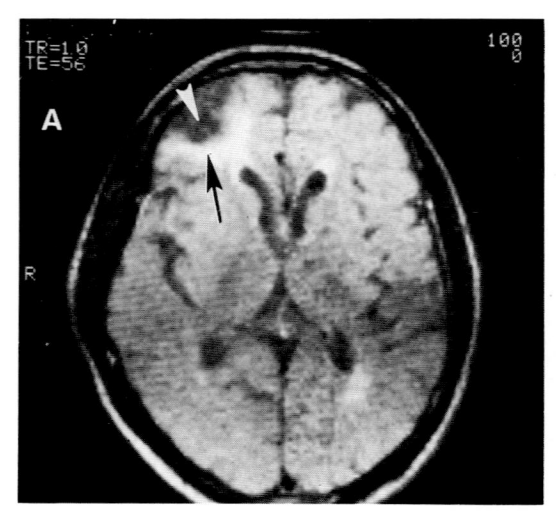

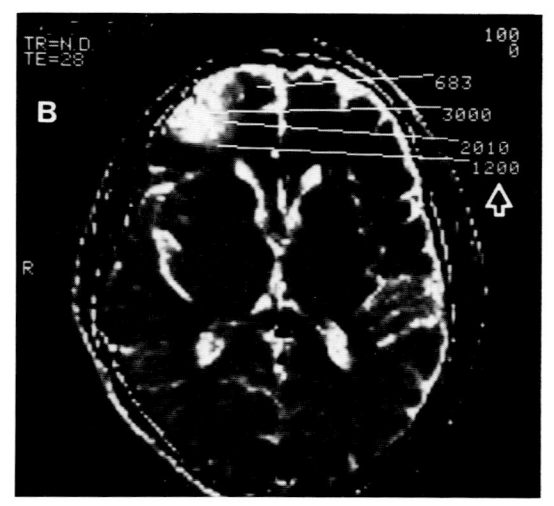

Figure 6–4. A: Chronic infarct: CSF density cystic change (arrowhead); high intensity periphery of gliosis (arrow). **B:** Calculated image. Arrow points to various relaxation times of calculations of different areas of chronic storke.

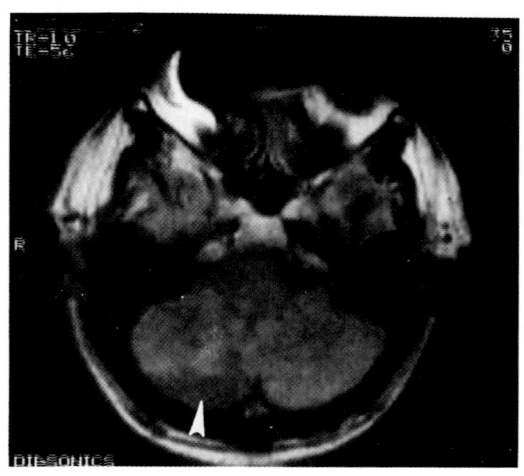

Figure 6–5. Cerebellar chronic infarct with CSF density cystic encephalomalacia (arrowhead).

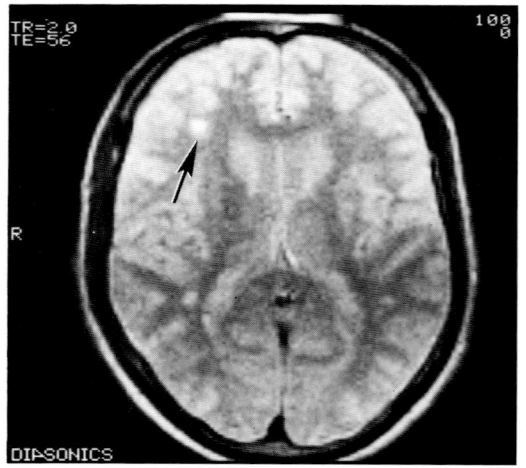

Figure 6–6. Small lacunar white matter infarct (arrow). TR = 2, TE = 56.

(Fig. 6-8). MRI is superior to CT scanning in identifying the small, deep lesions in patients with lacunar stroke [15].

POSTERIOR FOSSA INFARCTION

The diagnosis of small infarcts in the posterior fossa is facilitated by MRI. The visualization of posterior circulation infarcts by CT scanning is not as good as the demonstration of those in the anterior circulation. The CT evaluation of small brainstem lesions is usually poor or negative [16]. The small size of these infarcts, relative lack of edema, and degradation of images by bone streak artifacts all pose problems for their CT diagnosis [17].

As with other posterior fossa lesions, MRI has been found to be the best method to visualize infarctions in this location [18]. The su-

MRI and CT in Cerebrovascular Disease 127

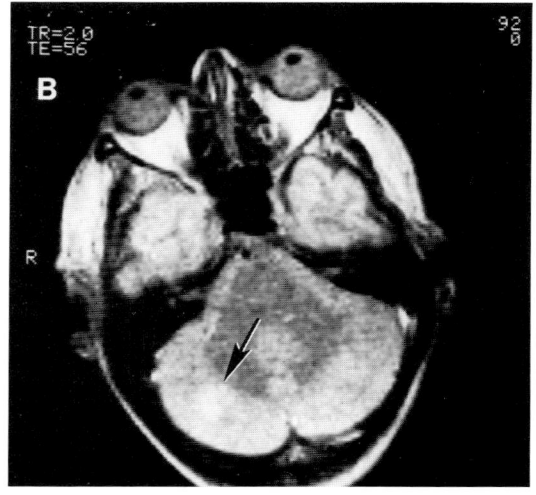

Figure 6–9. **A:** Oblique right parasagittal with subacute right cerebellar infarct (arrowhead). Acute deep white matter infarct (arrow). **B:** Axial view. Subacute right cerebellar infarct (arrow).

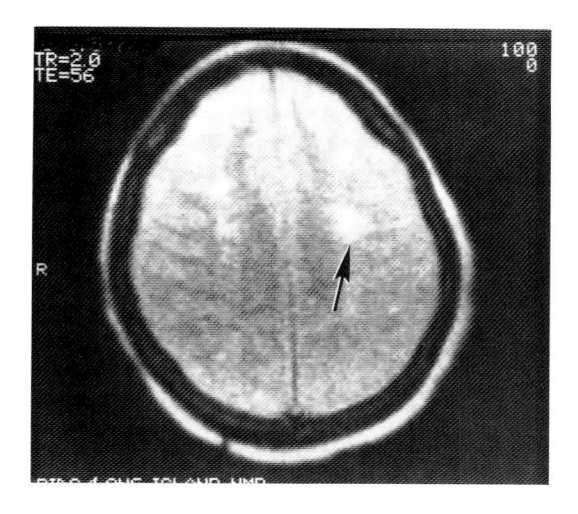

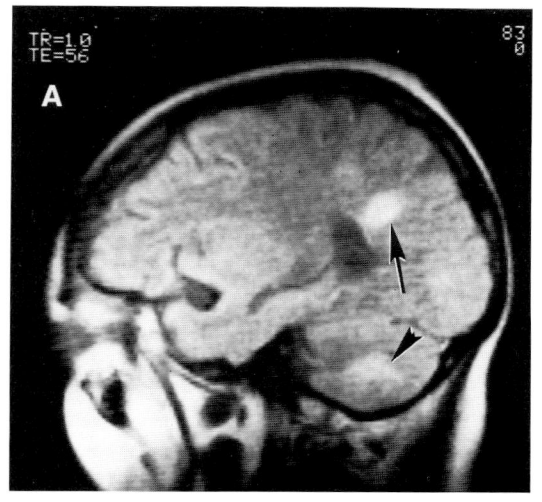

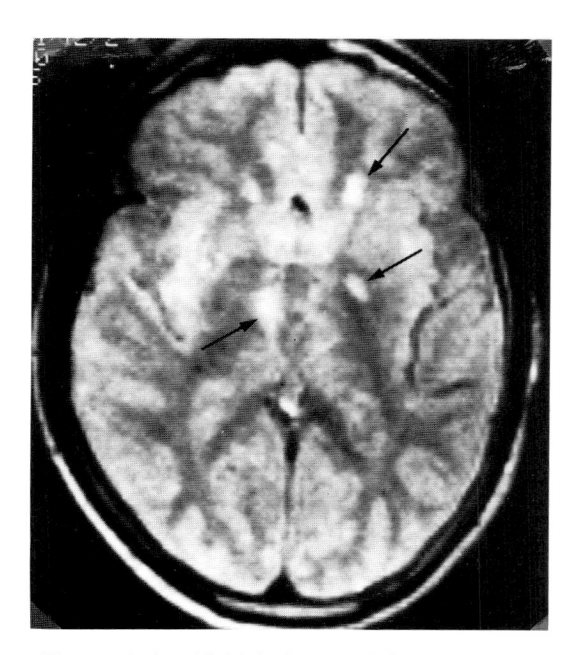

Figure 6–8. Multiple lacunar infarcts (arrows).

periority of MRI is due to its freedom from artifacts produced by cortical bone, the ability to obtain multiple imaging planes, and the high level of gray-white matter contrast resolution (Fig. 6-9). MRI is clearly the examination of choice in evaluating infarction in the posterior fossa [19].

In one study by Flannigan et al. [6], brainstem lesions of all ages were demonstrated on MR as increased intensity relative to normal brain on T_2-weighted images. Mass effect noted as displacement of the 4th ventricle was demonstrated on MR in severe acute infarcts. Acute and subacute brainstem infarcts had a higher signal intensity on the T_2-weighted images than old infarcts. These lesions were often missed by CT.

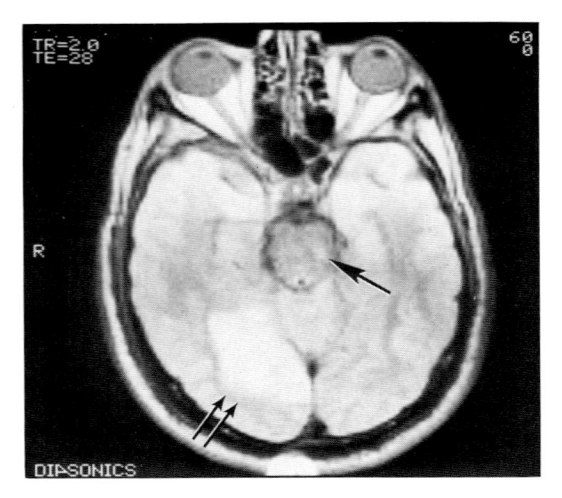

Figure 6–10. Pontine infarct, acute (arrow), and occipital infarct (double arrows).

Table 6.1
Various Names for Diffuse Cerebral Arteriosclerotic Vascular Disease

État crible (lacunes)
Encephalitis subcorticalis chronica progressiva [22]
État lacunaire (multiple lacunar state) [78]
Binswanger's disease [23]
Subcortical arteriosclerotic encephalopathy [79]
Periventricular atherosclerotic leukoencephalopathy [80]
Multiinfarct dementia [81]
Leukoaraiosis [82]

Table 6.2
Terms Used to Describe White Matter Radiographic Findings

CT Terminology
  Diffuse white matter hypodensities (DWMH) [42]
  Periventricular leukomalacia [83]
  Periventricular hypodensity (PVH)
MRI Terminology
  Patchy periventricular white matter lesions [29]
  Unidentified bright objects [61]
  Diffuse white matter hyperdensities
  Patchy subcortical foci of intensity [47]
  Periventricular hyperintensity (PVH) [31]
  Subcortical incidental lesions (ILs) [84]

In a study of patients with clinical pontine infarction, MRI was shown to be far superior in demonstrating the lesion than CT scanning (Fig. 6-10). The authors concluded that MRI was the imaging modality of choice for confirming pontine infarction [20].

A study of clinical medullary infarction similarly found MRI the modality of choice. Whereas three of five cases of clinical medullary infarction were documented by MRI, all the CT scans were obscured by artifacts through the lower stem [17]. Simmons et al. [21] found MRI a far more sensitive tool in the evaluation of cerebellar infarction as well.

DIFFUSE ARTERIOSCLEROTIC ISCHEMIC CEREBROVASCULAR DISEASE

Diffuse cerebral arteriolosclerotic vascular disease has been described by numerous terms (Table 6.1). With the advent of CT, neuroradiographic evidence of these syndromes was demonstrated as subcortical white matter hypodensities. With MRI, these white matter lesions were recognized with significantly increased frequency. The terms used to describe these findings are listed in Table 6-2; the first three terms relate to CT, the remainder relate to MRI.

Binswanger's disease (BD) has been infrequently diagnosed in the past. It was thought to be rare, and confusion exists as to the significance of asymptomatic patients with radiologic lesions only. Binswanger [22] first described patients with symptoms secondary to cerebral arteriosclerosis. Alzheimer [23] noted sparing of the cortex and atherosclerosis of the long penetrating vessels supplying the white matter. Caplan and Schoene [24] suggested the clinical features of subcortical arteriosclerotic encephalopathy and its relation to hypertension. In general Binswanger's disease or subcortical arteriosclerotic encephalopathy (SAE) is considered by most to be ischemic in origin, involving the periventricular white matter, sometimes causing dementia, and related to chronic arterial hypertension.

Recent reports suggest ischemic leukoencephalopathy is more common than historically assumed and is being recognized increasingly by MRI.

It is apparent that ischemic leukoencephalopathy exists in forms ranging from asymptomatic (only detectable radiologically) to advanced forms with severe dementia and focal deficits.

Whether SAE (Binswanger's disease) is a syndrome caused by different pathophysiologic mechanisms or is a distinct disease remains uncertain. It appears that clinical and radiographic features are characteristic enough to allow a diagnosis [25].

Numerous reports concerning the correlation of radiographic and clinical findings appear in the literature, and CT changes consistent with Binswanger's have been reported in normotensive, apparently healthy people [26,27].

Using MRI, patchy subcortical foci of abnormal signal intensity are seen frequently. Many investigators consider these incidental occult findings in neurologically intact elderly and consider it part of the aging process [28–32]. A physiologic explanation for periventricular hyperdensities in normal subjects other than ischemia has been proposed by Zimmerman [31] as a reflection of higher concentration of interstitial water at the ventricular lining.

Many authors are of the opinion that patchy periventricular hyperdensities are an early pathologic alteration and represent improved ability to detect preclinical cases [25,33–35].

Studies differ significantly in their use of the term, asymptomatic. Often the populations, extent of neurologic examinations, imaging techniques and criteria differ.

Sze [36] studied 56 normal patients and demonstrated punctate foci of high signal intensity anterior to the frontal horns in all patients. These increased densities were reported to be punctate, not larger than 1 centimeter, smooth, uniform, triangular in shape, with the base resting directly on the tips of the frontal horns immediately adjacent to the ependymal surface (Fig. 6-11). Pathologically, this region was found to have low myelin content, a loose network of axons, and increased water content.

In a study by Gerard and Weisberg [33] of 151 adults older than 50 years, the authors did not include punctate focal discrete round densities as abnormal if there were no other periventricular white matter lesions. Larger lesions that were dense and irregular were considered

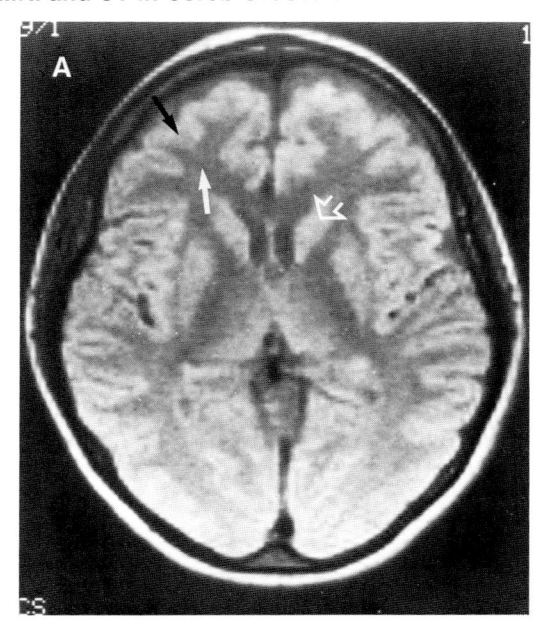

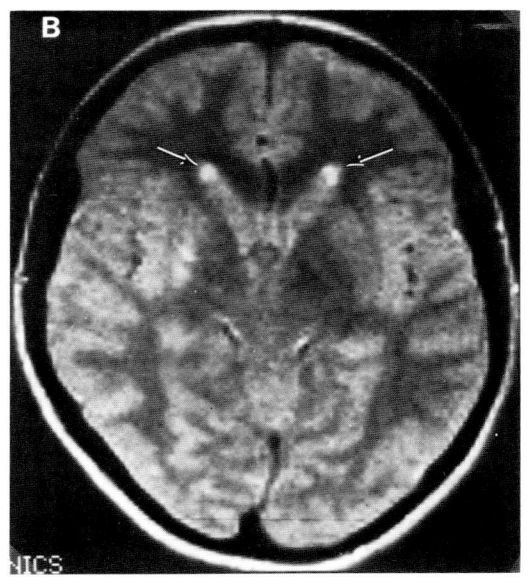

Figure 6–11. A: Normal image. Spin echo: TR = 2, TE = 28. Gray matter (black arrow), caudate nucleus (open white arrow), white matter (solid white arrow) are shown. B: Punctate density at tip of anterior frontal horns (arrows).

abnormal. The patients were categorized into three groups. Group 1 had symptoms of cerebrovascular disease (TIA, RIND, completed stroke). Group 2 had only risk factors for cerebrovascular disease (systemic arterial hypertension, cardiovascular disease, or diabetes mellitus). Group 3 had normal neurologic exams (not including neuropsychological testing), no symptoms or risk factors. Of the patients with no symptoms or risk factors, 7.8% had significant periventricular lesions. In group 2, 31% had lesions. With positive risk factors and positive symptoms (group 1), 78.5% had lesions. There was no relation to age except in group 1. It is probable that the aging process does not cause significant periventricular hyperdensities if cerebrovascular disease symptoms or risk factors are absent.

Awad [28] concluded that subcortical parenchymal lesions were frequent *incidental* findings on MRI and may be benign markers of normal physiologic processes, such as senescence, but may represent an index of chronic cerebrovascular disease. These lesions are incidental only in that they may not correlate with neurologic findings or may appear in asymptomatic patients. It is important to distinguish between normal healthy patients and those with subclinical disease, both groups being asymptomatic. This is an important distinction in a disease process such as SAE, which has a spectrum ranging from asymptomatic or minimally symptomatic patients with only radiographic findings to patients with severe diffuse and focal deficits.

Steingart [37] found significantly greater neuropsychologic deficits in a group of elderly volunteers with radiographic periventricular abnormalities when compared with matched controls without lesions.

Clinically, patients with SAE have a progressive dementia of slow onset and insidious progression [25]. Dougherty [38] found cognitive deficits in all patients confirmed by postmorten to have SAE. SAE is a subcortical dementia that fluctuates, frequently reaches a plateau, or even improves [39–41].

Abnormal neurologic findings are prominent in the advanced stages of SAE and include pseudobulbar palsy, gait difficulties, frontal lobe release signs, late onset seizures, and urinary incontinence.

Radiographic Features

CT findings of SAE (Binswanger's disease) were first reported by Caplan and Schoene in 1978 [24]. On CT, either diffuse or patchy low-density areas are seen, in the white matter of the centrum semiovale, frontal and occipital regions, with prominent involvement of the periventricular area. The changes occur bilaterally but not always in a symmetric pattern [42–44]. The incidence of CT findings suggesting SAE ranges from 0.5–8% of all CT scans, and there is a marked increased incidence in studies of patients older than age 60 years [26].

Information concerning CT changes in pathologically verified cases of SAE is limited [43,45,46]. Lotz [44] studied the brains of 202 patients who came to postmortem examination to determine the accuracy of CT in distinguishing SAE from other causes of low attenuation in the white matter and found the accuracy to be 90%.

It is apparent that there is a significant false-negative diagnosis rate in cases at the mild end of the SAE spectrum. Cases appearing to be mild on CT are often not so in terms of their clinical and pathologic evolution [44].

MRI is significantly more sensitive than CT in detecting early cases of SAE [29,31,33,47–50]. In many cases MRI shows extensive periventricular white matter involvement not seen at all on CT and is more accurate in determining the extent of involvement when seen on both.

As in chronic ischemic tissue seen in larger infarcts, there is decreased signal intensity on T_1-weighted images and increased signal on T_2-weighted images.

Several patterns of increasing extent are seen (Fig. 6-12), all which appear as periventricular high signal intensity areas (Table 6.3).

A grading system based on severity of involvement is presented in Table 6.4. The letters and numbers in Table 6.4 (grading system) correspond to the letters and numbers used to describe the various patterns of involvement in Table 6.3.

Lacunes are often not seen with early typical patterns of SAE until a continuous (diffuse) pattern of involvement is evident.

Uniform punctate foci of MRI signals (pseudolesions) directly anterior to the frontal horns, immediately adjacent to the ependymal surface, and triangular in shape, do not constitute pathology in and of themselves [36].

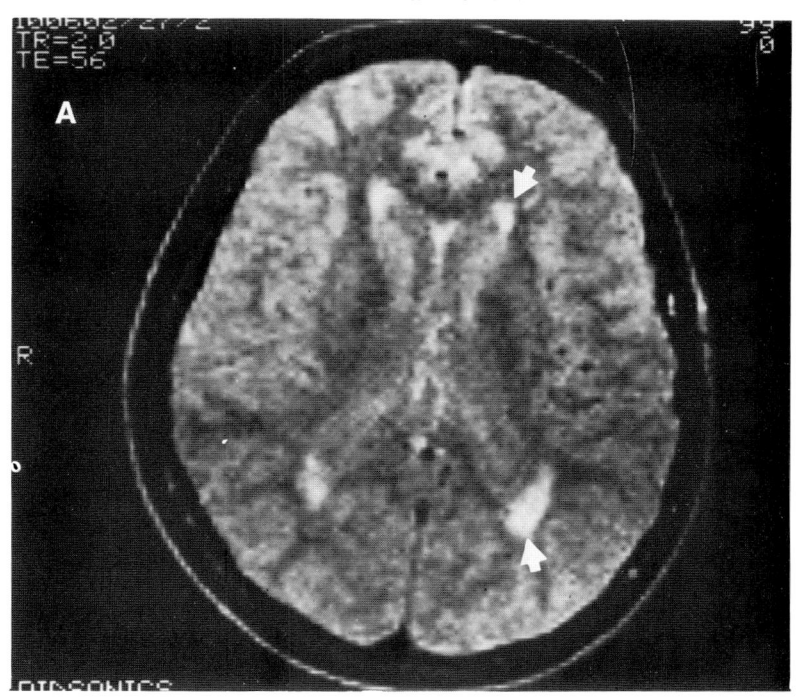

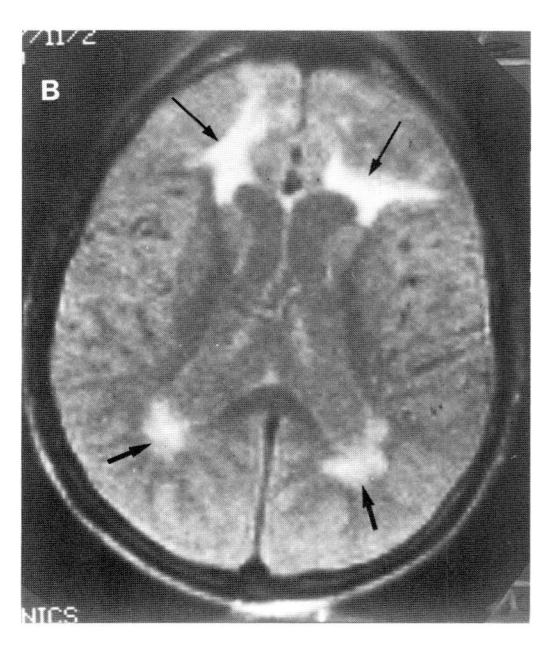

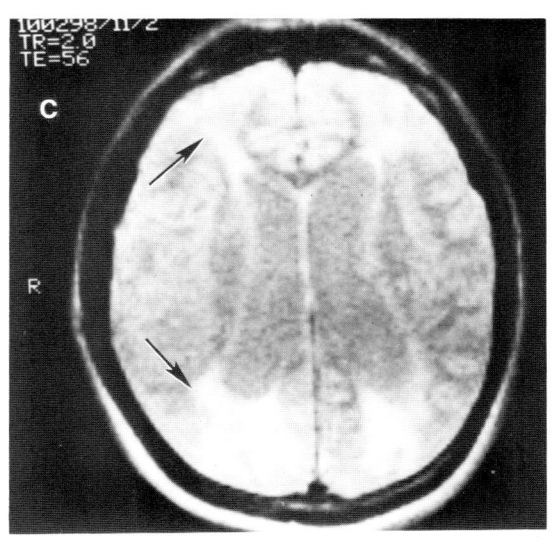

MRI and CT in Cerebrovascular Disease 131

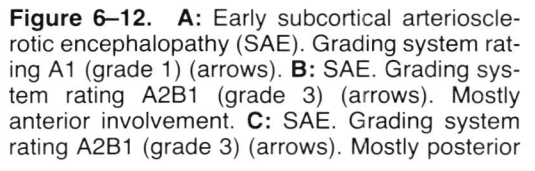

Figure 6–12. A: Early subcortical arteriosclerotic encephalopathy (SAE). Grading system rating A1 (grade 1) (arrows). **B:** SAE. Grading system rating A2B1 (grade 3) (arrows). Mostly anterior involvement. **C:** SAE. Grading system rating A2B1 (grade 3) (arrows). Mostly posterior involvement. **D:** SAE. Grading system rating A2B2 (grade 4) (arrows). **E:** SAE. Ischemic tissue (black arrows). Small lacunar infarcts (white arrows). Grading system rating A2B2 + C (grade 6). *(Continued on next page.)*

132   Gerard et al.

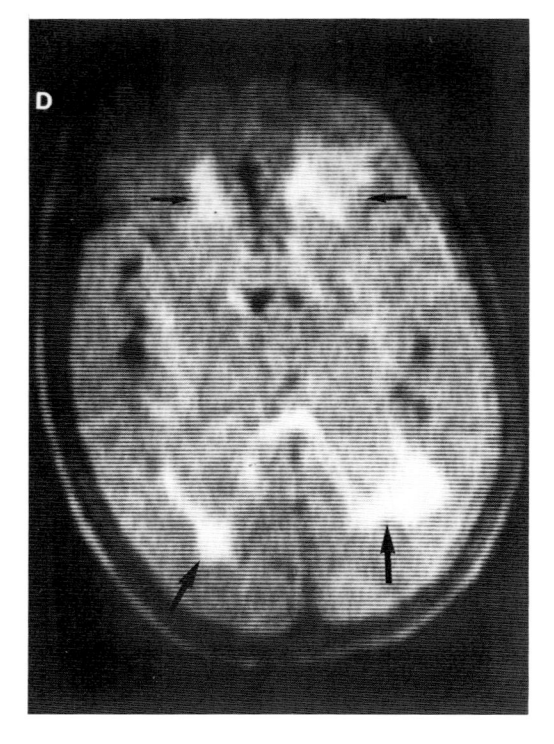

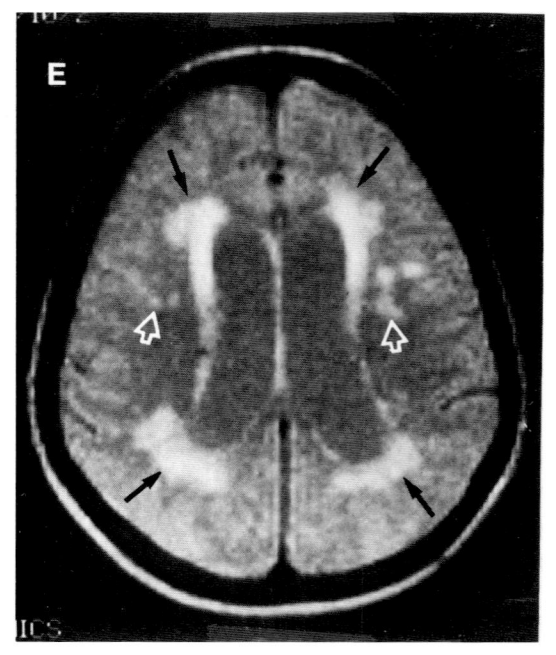

Figure 6-12   *(continued).*

Table 6.3
MRI Patterns of Periventricular Hyperdensity in Ischemic Leukoencephalopathy

A. Discontinuous
   1. Dense, thin, regular focal area adjacent to anterior frontal and occipital horns.
   2. Dense, thick, irregular (patchy) focal area adjacent to anterior and occipital horns.
B. Continuous (confluent)
   1. Thin, regular, band along the border of the lateral ventricles
   2. Thick, irregular, band of variable thickness confined to the borders of the lateral ventricles
   3. Thick, irregular, diffuse areas extending from the ventricular wall outward to the corticomedullary junction involving all or most of the white matter
C. Lacunes in the subcortical white matter outside the immediate periventricular area

Table 6.4
Grading System of Increasing Severity of Radiographic Involvement in SAE*

Grade 1 (mild)	A1
Grade 2	A2
Grade 3	A2B1
Grade 4	A2B2
Grade 5	A2B1 + C
Grade 6	A2B2 + C
Grade 7	A2B3
Grade 8 (severe)	A2B3 + C

*Letters and numbers correspond to descriptions in Table 6.3.

MRI and CT in Cerebrovascular Disease   133

Table 6.5
Adult Conditions With Diffuse Periventricular Involvement*

Multiple sclerosis
Subcortical arteriosclerotic encephalopathy (Binswanger's disease)
Hydrocephalus
Hypoxic leukoencephalopathy
Hypertensive encephalopathy
Vasculitis
Radiation-induced leukoencephalopathy
Muscular dystrophy
Carbon monoxide asphyxia
Acute necrotizing hemorrhagic encephalopathy
Bacterial meningitis
Head injury
Progressive multifocal leukoencephalopathy
Methotrexate-induced leukoencephalopathy
Cerebrotendinous xanthomatosis
Periventricular spread of tumor
Cytomegalovirus encephalitis
Polycystic lipomembranous osteodysplasia with sclerosing leukoencephalopathy
Creutzfeldt-Jakob disease (late stage)
Cerebral angioendotheliomatosis
Metachromatic leukodystrophy (adult onset)
Tuberous sclerosis
Acquired immunodeficiency syndrome (AIDS)

*From Reference 87.

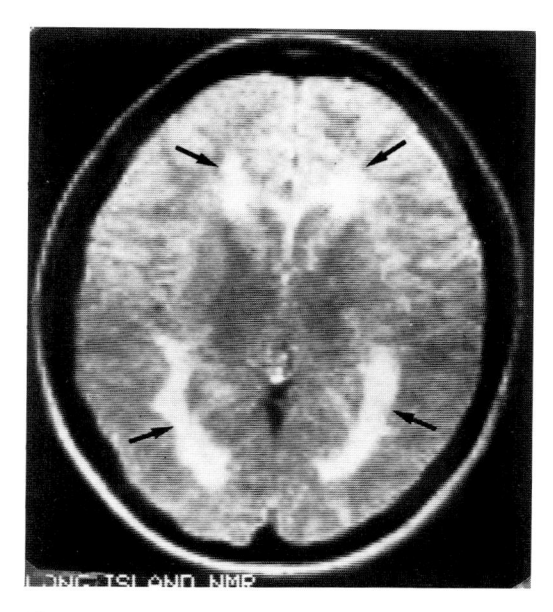

Figure 6–13. Chronic multiple sclerosis; confluent periventricular hyperintensity. Areas of patchy irregular demyelination (arrows).

Radiographic Differential Diagnosis

Diffuse white matter periventricular involvement may be found in a wide variety of pathologic processes (Table 6.5).

The two most important pathologic entities to consider in the differential diagnosis of SAE are multiple sclerosis (MS) and obstructive hydrocephalus, both the extraventricular (i.e., normal pressure hydrocephalus) and intraventricular types. Most other entities that resemble SAE radiographically can often be differentiated clinically.

Multiple sclerosis (Fig. 6-13) has a predilection for the white matter adjacent to the frontal and occipital horns and is seen in approximately 90% of cases [51]. In the advanced chronic stage of MS, diffuse irregular, confluent, relatively symmetric, periventricular involvement is typical. Differentiation should be possible based on, age, clinical history, ancillary electrodiagnostic tests, and CSF analysis.

In hydrocephalus, periventricular edema produces a halo of hyperintensity. In intraventricular obstructive hydrocephalus (IVOH), increased hydrostatic pressure causes a reversal of the direction of transependymal flow. In extraventricular obstructive hydrocephalus (EVOH), referred to as normal pressure hydrocephalus, periventricular edema produces a halo of hyperintensity, the mechanism of which has not yet been elucidated.

IVOH initially involves the anterior frontal and occipital horns (Fig. 6-14). Later, a halo of diffuse periventricular hyperdensity forms. The important differentiating feature is the smooth, thin width of the area of hyperintensity associated with enlargement of the ventricles and coincident loss of cortical sulci. Often the cause of the obstruction is demonstrated.

EVOH (normal pressure hydrocephalus) in its early stages initially involves the tips of the ventricular horns and is smooth (Fig. 6-15). It later progresses to diffusely involve the areas

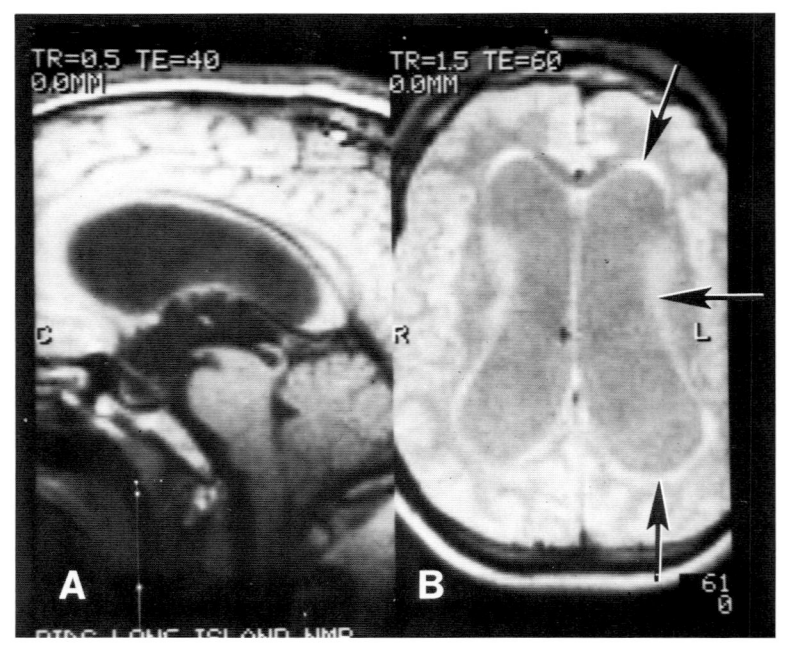

Figure 6–14. Intraventricular obstructive hydrocephalus (IVOH) with narrow aqueduct. Halo of thin diffuse hyperintensity of increased water content (arrows). **A:** Sagittal view, TR = 0.5, TE = 40. **B:** Axial view, TR = 1.5, TE = 60.

adjacent to the lateral ventricles. Most often, as in IVOH, the ventricles are enlarged, but there may be normal or enlarged sulci. In the late stages of EVOH, there may be a pattern indistinguishable from the grade 4 (A2B2) stage of SAE or advanced chronic MS. It is probable that long-standing periventricular interstitial edema eventually results in permanent demyelination of the areas involved. NPH occurs in the same age group as SAE and in its late stages is associated with dementia. It is at times radiographically and clinically indistinguishable from SAE. The presence of coincidental lacunes in the subcortical white matter outside the immediate periventricular area is somewhat more suggestive of SAE.

An MRI feature recently described by Bradley, a "signal void in the aqueduct," represents an alteration of cerebrospinal flow through the aqueduct [52]. This finding may prove useful in differentiating SAE from NPH.

Reports dealing with the MR appearance of Alzheimer's disease have been controversial and contradictory. Although most investiga-

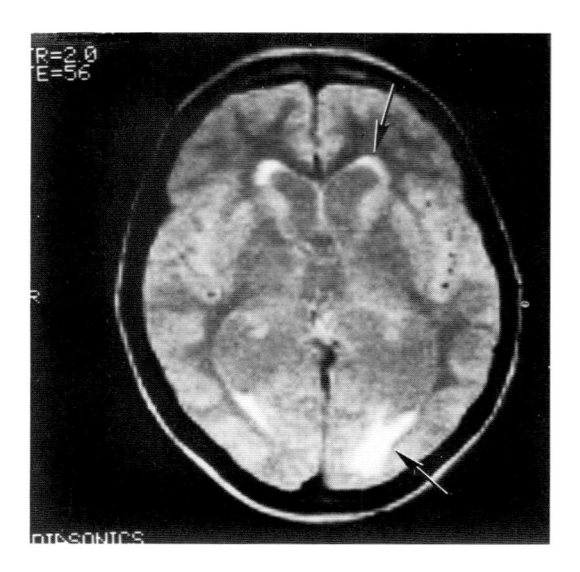

Figure 6–15. Extraventricular obstructive hydrocephalus (EVOH). Increased water content (arrows).

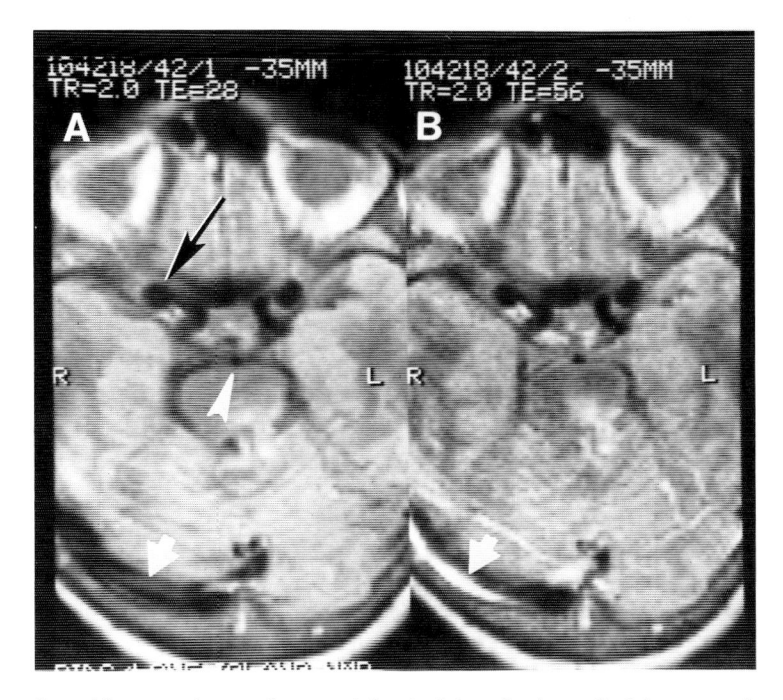

Figure 6–16. Carotid artery (normal) on axial view (black arrow). Basilar artery (normal) (arrowhead). Transverse sinus on right (normal) (white arrow). Note that arteries do not increase in intensity from first to second echo, whereas the sinus does change due to slower flow. **A:** TE = 28. **B:** TE = 56 (second echo).

tors have reported no signal abnormalities in Alzheimer's some have reported numerous periventricular white matter changes [53–55]. It has been suggested that MRI may be useful in differentiating vascular dementia from Alzheimer's disease, based on the presence or absence of periventricular white matter changes [50,56–58].

It is probable that white matter changes in patients with Alzheimer's disease are related to minor ischemic events [59,60]. It is probable that when ischemic leukoencephalopathy is present in association with Alzheimer's disease, there is a potentiating effect on the severity of the dementia [61].

Johnson found that dementia severity correlated with white matter periventricular abnormalities on both MRI and CT [50]. Hershey et al. found that enlargement of central CSF spaces was the only radiographic feature that was seen more commonly in demented than nondemented patients with ischemic cerebral vascular disease [57]. They found that periventricular white matter lesions were common in patients with known cerebral vascular disease (68% overall), but neither the presence nor the extent of white matter lesions distinguished demented and nondemented patients. This lack of relationship between the presence of dementia and the extent of white matter pathology in SAE has been previously described [62,63]. Kinkel et al. proposed broadening the term subacute arteriosclerotic encephalopathy to include individuals with characteristic periventricular lesions on MR scan even if they are not demented [49].

Zatz et al. reported decreased attentuation values of the white matter on CT in normal elderly people [64]. Authors have pointed out that small areas of long T_2 around the frontal horns might be considered normal in the elderly [36,65].

No study in which patients with cerebral vascular symptoms and risk factors were excluded has examined the type, frequency, and extent of MRI periventricular white matter signal abnormalities as they relate to normal aging. Our preliminary results suggest that in patients with cerebral vascular symptoms and risk factors, the frequency and extent of MRI white matter lesions increase with age, but there is no increase in white matter lesions in normal controls without symptoms or risk factors.

It is clear that additional studies are required before drawing definitive conclusions about the relation between periventricular high signal foci and normal aging as well as their correlation to dementia. Reports to date are conflicting and reflect the great sensitivity of MR in detecting tissue abnormalities but its low specificity in defining etiology. More extensive studies are necessary on the pathogenesis of SAE to define the role of cerebral small artery changes and the changes associated with the aging process.

MRI ANGIOGRAPHY

MR imaging may be used as a completely noninvasive angiography technique. No external contrast media is required. The high contrast difference between flowing blood and the vascular wall provides a means of assessing vascular patency and luminal irregularity. Rapid flow signal loss (flow void) permits the detection of extracranial and intracranial blood vessels, aneurysms, and arteriovenous malformations. Awareness of the mechanisms affecting signal intensity and analysis of vessel morphology provide a great deal of diagnostic information on routine MR images. Direction and magnitude of flow can be determined, and vascular stenoses and intraluminal thrombus can be detected.

Flowing blood can be bright or dark on MR images depending on its velocity. In general, rapidly flowing blood appears dark and slowly flowing blood is bright (Fig. 6-16). The appearance of flowing blood is markedly influenced by intrinsic factors such as velocity and turbulence as well as external factors such as pulse sequence and magnetic field strength.

The sensitivity of magnetic resonance to the movement of fluid was discovered in the mid 1940s and reported in the early 1950s [66,67]. The distinctive appearance of flowing blood was noted when the first human limb was imaged, and the possibility was recognized that MRI might provide an opportunity for circula-

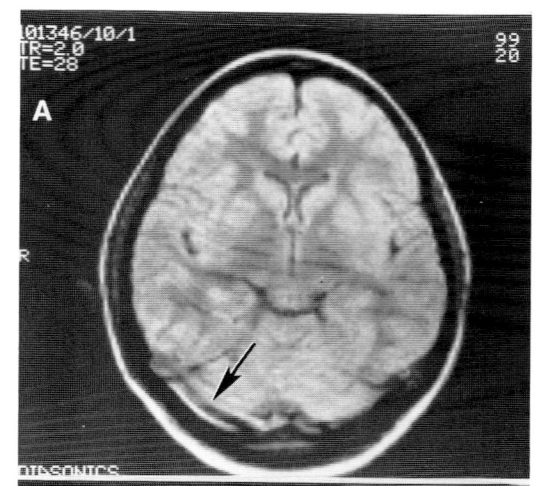

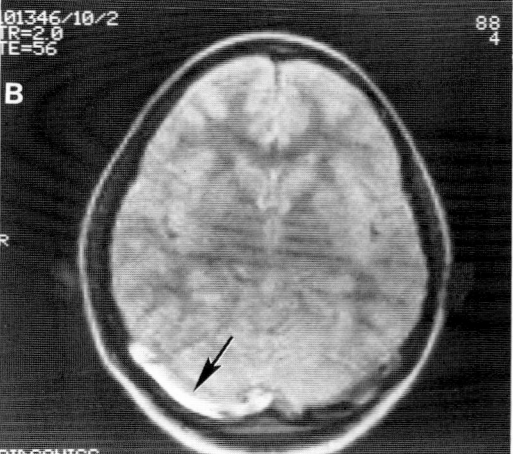

Figure 6–17. Transverse sinus (arrow). Rephasing phenomena due to slow flow. Increased on second echo. **A:** First echo TE = 28. **B:** Second echo TE = 56.

tory diagnosis [68,69]. Signal intensity depends on the position of the slice containing the vessel relative to the rest of the multislice imaging volume, the repetition time, echo delay time, echo number, and slice thickness [52].

The ability to distinguish slow-flowing blood from stationary blood depends on the signal intensity variations between the first and second echo delays when images are obtained with a single pulse sequence interval and two echo delays (Fig. 6-17).

Although MRI does not have the resolution

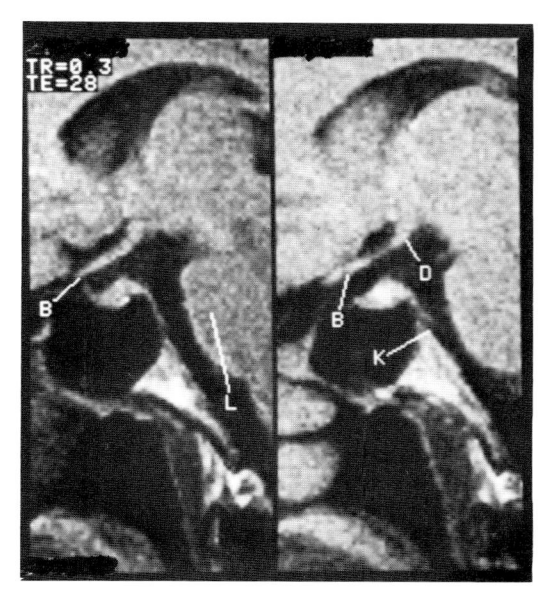

Figure 6–18. Inferior petrosal sinus anterior to brainstem on sagittal view (K). Right optic nerve (B). Right optic tract (D). Pons (L), (sagittal view).

of contrast angiography, when done properly, remarkable images are provided (Fig. 6-18). Studies are under way that are providing precise quantitative measures of circulatory function.

It is curious to note that when one considers flow, MRI may have more in common with Doppler ultrasound than with CT [70]. It is apparent that MRI angiography is useful as a qualitative means to demonstrate blood flow. MR angiography, although in its infancy, does measure and display blood velocity, not just vascular morphology. Despite practical and theoretical limitations, MR angiography provides dynamic images, and its clinical applications are expanding.

Distinguishing Between Arteries and Veins

In general rapidly flowing (arterial) blood appears dark and slower-flowing blood (venous) appears bright.

One specific factor affecting the signal intensity of flowing blood is the position in the multisection sequence. The first section of a sequence demonstrates the highest intensity for slowly flowing blood and the signal diminishes

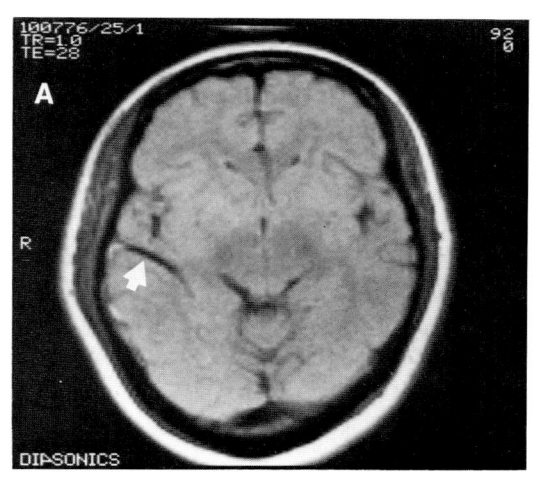

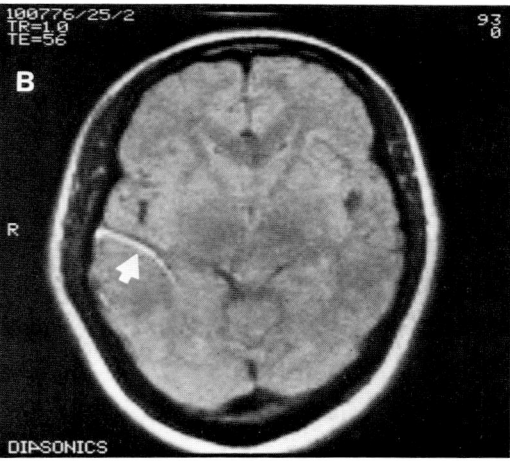

Figure 6–19. Second echo rephasing cortical vein. **A:** Dark on first echo, TE = 28. **B:** Brighter on second echo, TE = 56. Vein is identified by white arrow.

in subsequent images. This is an indicator of direction of flow and is helpful in distinguishing between arteries and veins. The enhancement of the MR signal is greatest in the sections first entered by the blood. A multisection sequence oriented with the most cephalad section first and the most caudad section last will demonstrate enhancement of arterial blood in the last caudad section for neck images. Venous blood will show the opposite pattern, with enhancement in the first cephalad section for neck images. This enhancement pattern reflects the

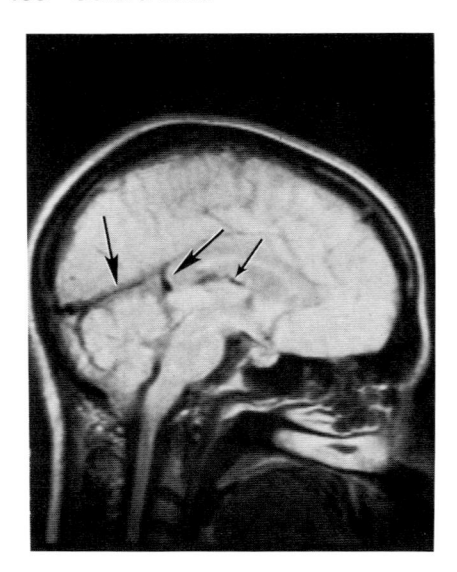

Figure 6–20. Deep cerebral veins (arrows). Sagittal view.

opposing directions of flow of arterial and venous blood.

On the usual MR image, cortical veins can be identified. On the first echo the cortical vessels are dark, whereas on the second echo the vessels are bright (Fig. 6-19). When the veins are dark on the image, they are difficult to distinguish from the cortical sulci containing cerebrospinal fluid. On the second echo these veins become bright and clearly identifiable. This increase in intensity should not be misdiagnosed as subarachnoid blood.

The deep cerebral veins, Galen's veins, and straight and sagittal sinuses can be identified (Figs. 6-20, 6-21). The basilar artery can be identified within the surrounding cerebrospinal fluid because of the signal void arteries create in relation to cerebrospinal fluid.

Changes in intensity seen in the transverse and sigmoid sinuses should not be confused with high intensity tumor (Fig. 6-22). By comparing the first and second echos and understanding the rephasing phenomenon, one should be able to identify structures as slow-flow vessels. When a high signal is seen on the MR image, the intensity on the first echo should be compared with the second echo, and if the lesion gains intensity it is likely to be a large, slow-flow vein. For a detailed explanation of the rephasing phenomenon, one can refer to an explanation by Waluch [86].

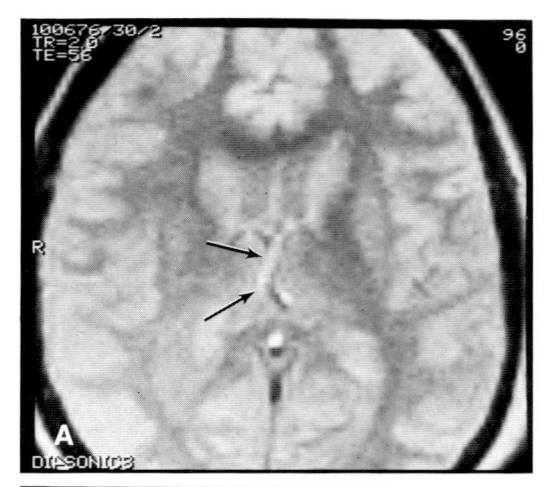

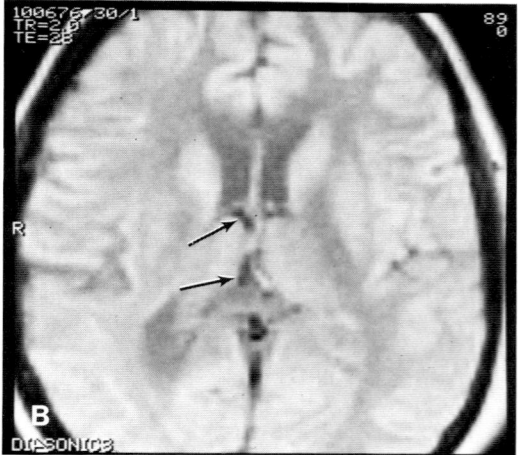

Figure 6–21. Internal cerebral vein. **A:** TE = 56. Second echo with increased intensity due to rephasing phenomena. **B:** TE = 28. First echo with lower intensity signal (arrows).

Vascular Occlusion

When even-echo rephasing is seen, it is usually evidence of flow. The relative signal increase on the second echo image is usually apparent merely by inspection of the two images.

High signal intensity results from stagnation of blood under various conditions. A technical factor that may cause high intraluminal signal is observed in arteries during diastole. This in-

MRI and CT in Cerebrovascular Disease   139

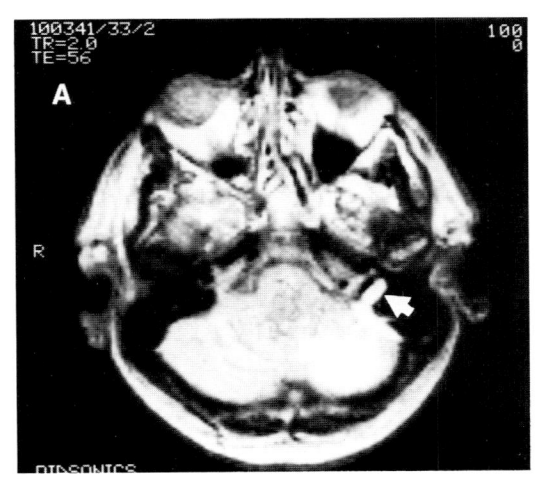

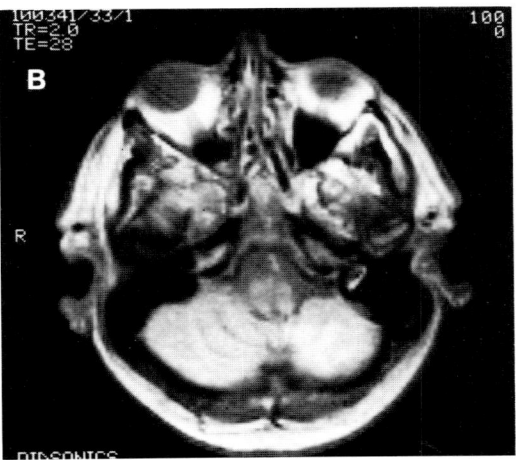

Figure 6–22. Sigmoid sinus jugular vein. High intensity area at first glance (**A**) looks like a lesion in the extraaxial cerebellar region, but the first echo image (**B**) at TE = 28 indicates this high intensity area (arrow) on the second echo at TE = 56 is due to slow flow.

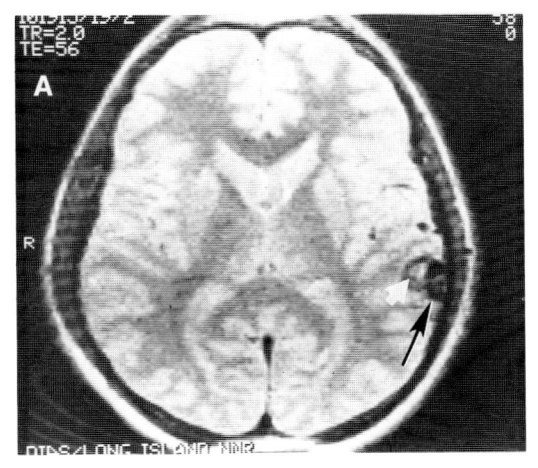

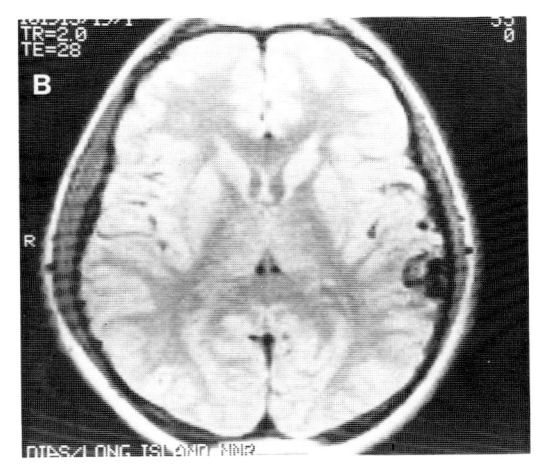

Figure 6–23. Arteriovenous malformation. **A:** Dark area corresponds to area of high flow (black arrow). **B:** Increased intensity corresponds to slow or stagnant flow, but lack of increased signal intensity from first to second echo suggests probable thrombus.

crease in signal occurring during diastole can be potentially mistaken for thrombus. It must be determined whether this high signal is a function of the cardiac cycle or a lesion is present. Various maneuvers are necessary to make this differentiation, and cardiac gaiting or repositioning of the patient may be necessary.

Vascular malformations may be partly clotted or totally clotted. Using angiography or CT one can only visualize the parts of a partially thrombosed AVM that fill with contrast. With MR one can visualize both the thrombosed and patent portions of the vascular malformation (Fig. 6-23).

Distinguishing slow flow from stationary blood depends on the signal intensity variations between the first and the second echo delays. Vascular occlusion or hemorrhage will result in a high intensity signal that diminishes or is unchanged between the first and second echo delays (Fig. 6-24). If the occlusion is not complete and slow flow is present, the signal

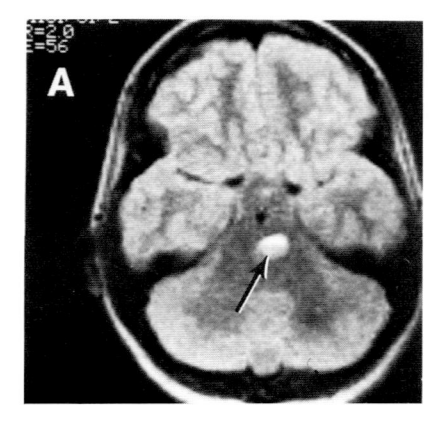

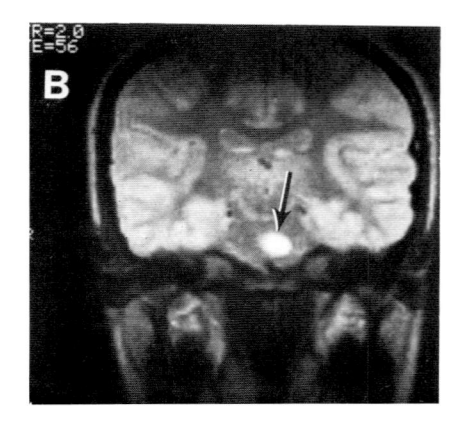

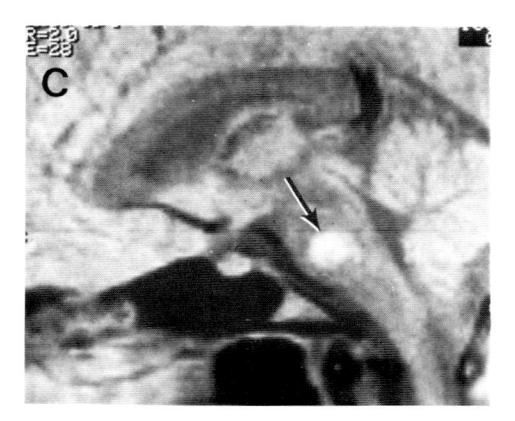

Figure 6–24. Subacute pontine hemorrhage in a patient with multiple arteriovenous malformations. **A:** Axial view. **B:** Coronal view. **C:** Sagittal view.

intensity will be equal or higher on the second echo compared to the first (Fig. 6-25).

Occlusion of the dural venous sinuses can be demonstrated by the absence of the usual flow phenomenon in the dural sinus with replacement by thrombus. The actual appearance depends on the age of the clot. The appearance in the late stages will depend on whether the sinus remains occluded or recanalizes. Only after normal flow effects are excluded can the diagnosis be made. Stationary blood gives rise to a signal intensity greater than rapidly flowing blood, but less than slow-flowing blood.

As a result of the signal intensity variability one can diagnose cartoid artery occlusion [71]. Intravascular thrombus results in an intravascular signal that, depending on age, composition, oxidation state of the hemoglobin, and the organization of the thrombus, shows a large variability in intensity [72–74].

A dark rim on the edge of a vessel containing signal, particularly if present on a first echo and total disappearance of signal or filling of the entire vessel with signal on second echo images, suggests that the observed signal comes from flowing blood rather than stationary tissue [75].

MRI has proved to be a useful, noninvasive means of detecting vascular occlusions. Cur-

MRI and CT in Cerebrovascular Disease   141

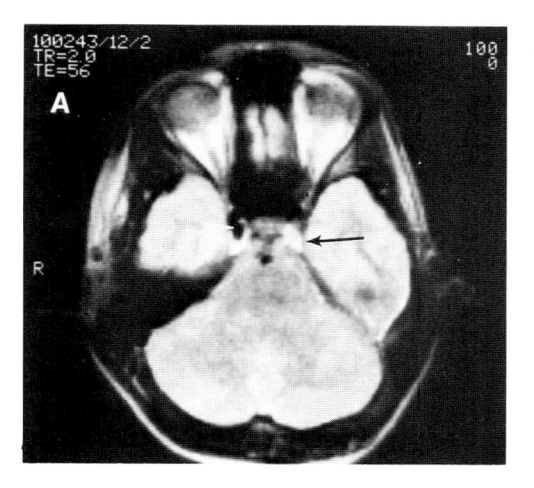

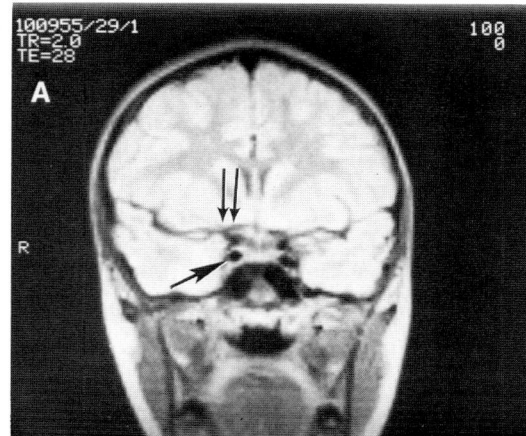

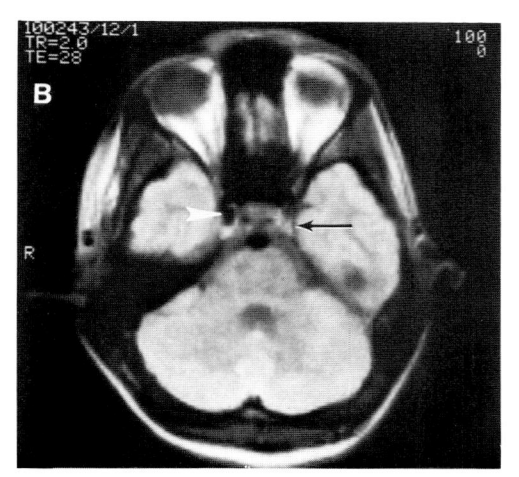

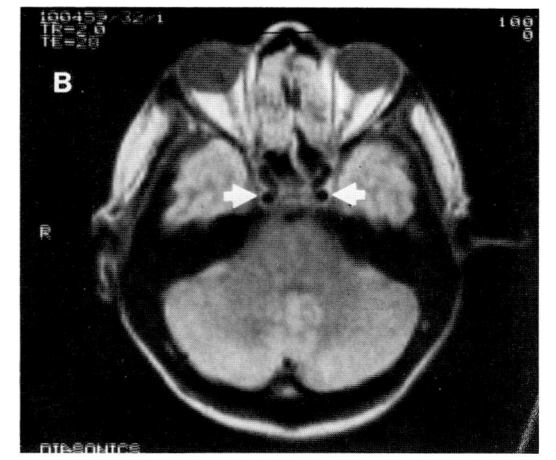

Figure 6–25. Carotid artery stenosis. **A:** On left (black arrow) increased signal intensity due to slow flow (second echo TE = 56). **B:** Atherosclerotic plaque can be seen narrowing the lumen of the left carotid artery (arrowhead) confirmed by angiography.

Figure 6–26. **A:** Coronal view of normal carotid artery siphon (arrow) and right middle cerebral artery (normal) (double arrows). **B:** Carotid siphon (normal) with dark fast-flowing blood (arrows). Axial view.

rently angiography is the best method of assessing vascular structures, but when vascular contrast agents cannot be used, MRI appears to offer promise as a means of detecting vascular occlusions.

Carotid MR Angiography

MR angiography has revealed the carotid arteries and anterior and middle cerebral arteries (Fig. 6-26). MR angiography does not remotely approach the resolution obtained with conventional film-based angiography, but MR angiography is hazard-free and may be useful in screening certain types of patients. Various techniques have been developed to image the carotid artery [76]. Imaging along an oblique angle has enabled investigators to directly examine the artery from the common carotid through the bifurcation to the internal and external carotid. Blood flow within the carotid is seen throughout the entire length of the vessel. Imaging in the oblique plane conforms to the spatial orientation of the carotid artery and al-

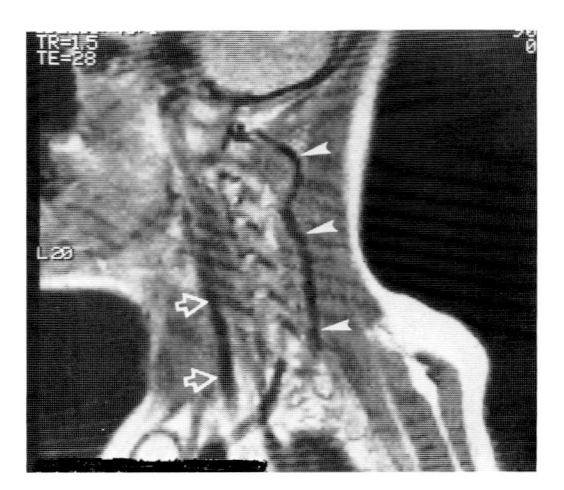

Figure 6–27. Extracranial arteries of the neck on oblique-parasagittal view. Common carotid (open arrows) and posterior vessel (arrowheads).

lows investigators to visualize the carotid artery in a single image without degradation of image quality or patient repositioning (Fig. 6-27).

Proton MRI has the potential to detect atherosclerotic disease of the arterial vasculature by depicting 1) physical distortion of the arterial lumen 2) anomolies in the intraarterial signal resulting from turbulence or variation in intraarterial velocity profile, and 3) gross MRI findings characteristic of plaque [77]. Direct depiction of the atherosclerotic involvement may also be possible. Protons of the aliphatic lipids are characterized by long T_2 values. Accordingly, signal intensity is increased in T_2 sensitive spin echo images and may allow visualization of early atherosclerotic plaque. Such information would be extremely useful in learning more about the natural history of atherosclerosis as well as in assessing the response of plaque to different kinds of therapy [77].

It is possible using chemical shift imaging to noninvasively characterize the composition of an atherosclerotic plaque.

Arteriovenous Malformations and Aneurysms

With an understanding of MRI flow phenomena one can determine the presence of

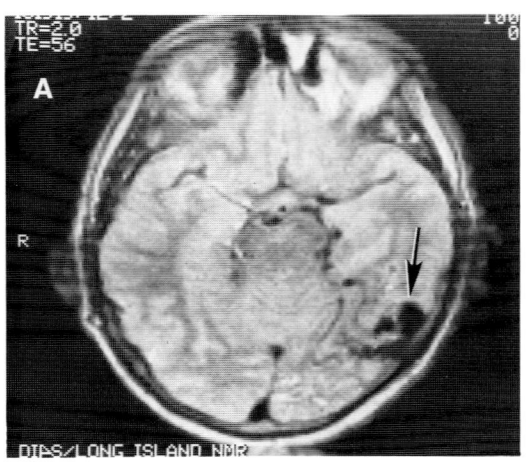

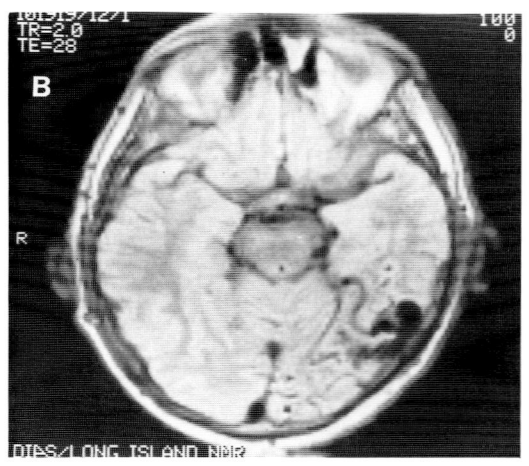

Figure 6–28. Arteriovenous malformation (arrow). Dark intensity on both first and second echoes indicates high flow vessels and no thrombus. **A:** TE = 56. **B:** TE = 28.

vascular malformations (Figs. 6-28, 6-29). One can usually conclude that a lesion is vascular in nature.

Flow in small venous angiomas may be below the resolution of some MR units, however, the presence of a draining vein may be seen in some cases.

Because flow is the only phenomenon known to increase intensity on the second echo, one can differentiate small vascular lesions from other high intensity lesions, such as multiple sclerosis plaques (Fig. 6-30).

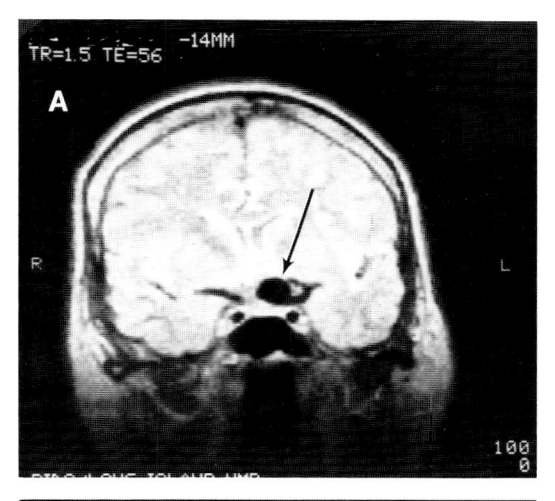

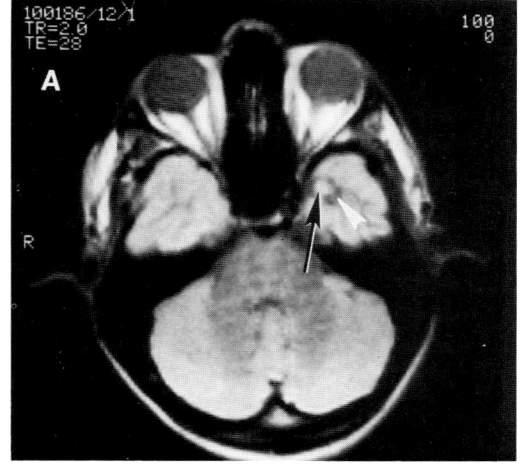

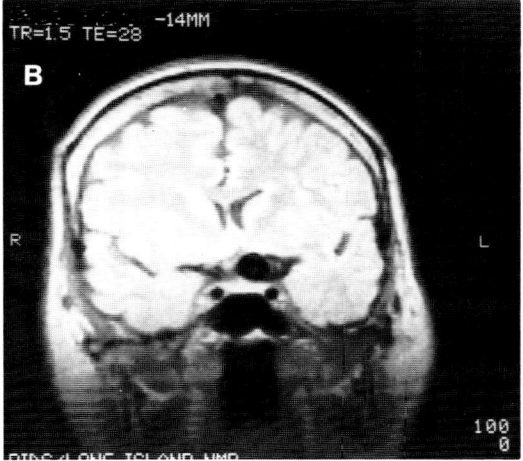

MRI and CT in Cerebrovascular Disease 143

Figure 6–29. Giant aneurysm, middle cerebral artery junction (arrow). Dark intensity indicates high flow. **A:** TE = 56. **B:** TE = 28.

Figure 6–30. AVM left temporal lobe. **A:** TE = 28. **B:** TE = 56. Note there is a fast flow (black arrow, dark area) and slow flow (bright intensity) seen on the second echo (white arrowhead).

CONCLUSIONS

Magnetic resonance imaging is clearly capable of identifying pathologic vascular lesions more accurately than computed tomography. It provides a better understanding of the pathophysiology of cerebral vascular diseases.

The major strength of MR imaging in evaluating cerebral ischemia is its sensitivity. This increased sensitivity in detecting the changes associated with ischemia will have a major impact on investigations of various forms of intervention in acute ischemia. Increased sensitivity may constitute an advance in the understanding of vascular dementia. If vascular dementia can be prevented or progression slowed, early diagnosis is essential.

MR imaging has undoubtedly expanded our knowledge of cerebral vascular disease. As with any new technologic advancement, many more questions have been posed concerning cerebral vascular disease than have been adequately answered, and many significant new findings are yet to be totally explained. The clinical and research applications of MR imaging as it applies to cerebral vascular disease have yet to reach their full potential.

References

1. Bryan RN, Willcott MR, Scheiders NJ, Ford JJ, Derman HS (1983) Nuclear magnetic resonance evaluation of stroke. A preliminary report. *Radiology* 149:189–192.
2. Sipponen JT, Kaste M, Ketonen L, Sepponen RE, Katevuo K, Sivula A (1983) Serial nuclear magnetic resonance (NMR) imaging in patients with cerebral infarction. *J Comput Assist Tomogr* 7:585–589.
3. Pykett IL, Buonanno FS, Brady TJ, Kistler JP (1983) True three-dimensional nuclear magnetic resonance neuroimaging in ischemic stroke; Correlation of NMR, x-ray CT and pathology. *Stroke* 14:173–177.
4. Kistler JP, Buonanno FS, DeWitt LD, David KR, Brady TJ, Fisher CM (1954) Vertebral-basilar posterior cerebral territory stroke: Delineation by proton nuclear magnetic resonance imaging. *Stroke* 15:417–426.
5. Brant-Zawadzki M, Solomon M, Newton TH, Weinstein P, Schmidley J, Norman D (1985) Basic principles of magnetic resonance imaging in cerebral ischemia and initial clinical experience. *Neuroradiology* 27:517–520.
6. Flannigan BD, Bradley WG, Kortman KE (1985) Evolution of cerebral infarction: MRI appearance with pathophysiological correlation. *Magn Reson Imaging* 3:174.
7. Brant-Zawadzki M, Kucharczyk W (1987) In Brant-Zawadzki M, Norman D (eds): Vascular Disease: Ischemia. In Magnetic Resonance Imaging of the Central Nervous System. New York: Raven Press, pp 221–234.
8. Naruse S, Horikawa Y, Tanaka C, Hirakawa K, Nishikawa H, Yoshizaki K (1982) Proton nuclear magnetic resonance studies on brain edema. *J Neurosurg* 56:747–752.
9. Brant-Zawadzki M, Pereira B, Weinstein P, Moore S, Kucharczyk W, Berry I, McNamara M, Derugin N (1986) MRI of acute experimental ischemia in rats. *AJNR* 7:7–11.
10. Kinkel WR (1986) Clinical value of magnetic resonance imaging for the evaluation of patients with stroke. In Lechner H, Meyer JS, Ott E (eds): *Cerebrovascular Disease: Research and Clinical Management*. Amsterdam: Elsevier, pp 319–324.
11. Kertesz A, Black SE, Nicholson L Carr T (1987) Sensitivity and specificity of MRI in stroke. *Neurology* 37:1580–1585.
12. Kucharczyk W, Brant-Zawadzki M (1987) Magnetic resonance imaging of cerebral ischemia and infarction. In Kressel HY(ed): *Magnetic Resonance Annual 1987*. New York: Raven Press, pp 49–69.
13. Mohr JP (1982) Lacunes. *Stroke* 13:3–11
14. Rothrock JF, Lyden PD, Hesselink JR, Brown JJ, Healy ME (1987) Brain magnetic resonance imaging in the evaluation of lacunar stroke. *Stroke* 18:781–786.
15. DeWitt LD (1986) Clinical use of nuclear magnetic resonance imaging in stroke. *Stroke* 17:328–331.
16. Bogousslavsky J, Fox AJ, Barnett HJ, Hachinski VC, Vinitski S, Carey LS (1986) Clinico-topographic correlation of small vertebrobasilar infarct using magnetic resonance imaging. *Stroke* 17:929–938.
17. Fox AJ, Bogousslavsky J, Carey LS, Barnett HJ, Vinitski S, et al. (1986) Magnetic resonance imaging of small medullary infarctions. *AJNR* 7:229–233.
18. Savdiardo M, Bracchi M, Passerini M (1987) The vascular territories in the cerebellum and brainstem: CT and MR study. *AJNR* 8: 199–209.
19. Kricheff II (1987) Arteriosclerotic ischemic cerebrovascular disease. *Radiology* 162:101–109.
20. Biller J, Adams HP Jr., Dunn V, et al. (1986) Dichotomy between clinical findings and MR abnormalities in pontine infarction. *JCAT* 10:379–385.
21. Simmons L, Biller J, Adams HP Jr, Dunn V, Jacoby CG (1986) Cerebellar infarction: Comparison of computed tomograph magnetic resonance imaging. *Ann Neurol* 19:291–293.
22. Binswanger O (1894) Die Abgrenzung des allgemeinen progressiven Paralysie. *Berl Klin Wochenscher* 31:1103–1105, 1137–1139, 1180–1186.
23. Alzheimer A (1902) Die Seelenstorungen auf arteriosclerotischer Grundlage. *Allgemeine Z Psychiatrie Psychisch-Gerichtliche Medicin* 59:695–711.
24. Caplan LR, Schoene WC (1978) Clinical features of subcortical arteriosclerotic encephalopathy (Binswanger disease). *Neurology* 18:1206–1215.
25. Babikian V, Ropper AH (1987) Binswanger's disease: A review. *Stroke* 18:2–12.
26. Pullicino C, Eskin T, Ketonen L (1983) Prevalence of Binswanger's disease. *Lancet* 1:939.
27. Rezek DL, Morris JC, Fulling KH, Gado MH (1986) Periventricular white matter lucencies in SDAT and healthy aging. *Neurology* 36(Suppl 1):263–264.
28. Awad IA, Johnson PC, Spetzler RF, et al. (1986) Incidental subcortical lesions noted on magnetic resonance imaging in the elderly. II. Postmortem pathological correlations. *Stroke* 17:1090–1097.
29. Bradley WG Jr, Waluch V, Brant-Zawadzki M, et al. (1984) Patchy periventricular white matter lesions in the elderly: A common observation during NMR imaging. *Noninvasive Med Imag* 1:35–41.
30. Salgado ED, Weinstein M, Furlan AJ, et al. (1986) Proton magnetic resonance imaging in ischemic cerebrovascular diseases. *Ann Neurol* 20:502–507.
31. Zimmerman RD, Fleming CA, Lee BCP, et al. (1986) Periventricular hyperintensity as seen by magnetic resonance: Prevalence and significance. *AJNR* 7:13–20.
32. George AE, de Leon MJ, Gentes CI, et al. (1986) Leukoencephalopathy in normal and pathologic aging: CT of brain lucencies. *AJNR* 7:561–566.
33. Gerard G, Weisberg LA (1986) MRI periventricular lesions in adults. *Neurology* 36:998–1001.
34. Bogousslavsky J, Regli F, Vske A (1987) Leukoencephalopathy in patients with ischemic stroke. *Stroke* 18:896–899.
35. Jacobs L, Kinkel W (1976) Computerized axial transverse tomography in normal pressure hydrocephalus. *Neurology* 26:501–507.

36. Sze G, DeArmond S, Brant-Zawadzki M (1985) "Abnormal" MRI foci anterior to the frontal horns: Pathologic correlates of an ubiquitous finding. AJNR 6:467–468.
37. Steingart A, Hachinski VC, Lau C, et al. (1987) Cognitive and neurologic findings in demented patients with diffuse white matter lucencies on computed tomographic scan (leukoaraiosis). Arch Neurol 44:36–39.
38. Dougherty JH, Simmonds JD, Parker J (1986) Subcortical ischemic disease: Clinical spectrum and MRI correlation. Stroke 17:146.
39. Cummings JL, Benson DF (1983) Dementia: A Clinical Approach. Stoneham, Mass.: Butterworths.
40. Roman GC (1987) Senile dementia of the Binswanger type. JAMA 258:1782–1788.
41. Whitehouse PJ (1986) The concept of subcortical and cortical dementia: Another look. Ann Neurol 19:1–6.
42. Rosenberg GA, Kornfeld M, Stovring J, et al. (1979) Subcortical arteriosclerotic encephalopathy (Binswanger): Computerized tomography. Neurology 29:1102–1106.
43. Zeumer H, Schonsky B, Sturn KW (1980) Predominant white matter involvement in subcortical arteriosclerotic encephalopathy (Binswanger disease). J Comput Assist Tomogr 4:14–19.
44. Lotz PR, Ballinger WE Jr, Quisling RG (1986) Subcortical arteriosclerotic encephalopathy: CT spectrum and pathologic correlation. AJNR 7:817–822.
45. Goto K, Ishii N, Fukasawa H (1981) Diffuse whitematter disease in the geriatric population: A clinical, neuropathological and CT study. Radiology 141:687–695.
46. Dupuis M, Brucher JM, Gonsette RE (1984) Observation anatomoclinique d'une encephalopathie souscorticale arteriosclercuse avec hypodensite de la substance blanche au scanner cerebral. Acta Neurol Belg 84:131–140.
47. Brant-Zawadzki M, Fein G, Van Dyke C, et al. (1985) MRI Imaging of the aging brain: Patchy white-matter lesions and dementia. AJNR 6:675–682.
48. Erkinjuntti T, Sipponen JT, Iivanainen M, et al. (1984) Cerebral NMR and CT imaging in dementia. J Comput Assist Tomogr 8:614–618.
49. Kinkel WR, Jacobs L, Polachini I, et al. (1985) Subcortical atherosclerotic encephalopathy (Binswanger's disease): Computerized tomography, nuclear magnetic resonance and clinical correlations. Arch Neurol 42:951–959.
50. Johnson K, Davis KR, Buonanno FS, Brady TJ, Rosen TJ, Growden JH (1987) Comparison of magnetic resonance and roentgen ray computed tomography in dementia. Arch Neurol 44:1075–1080.
51. Lumsden CE (1970) The neuropathology of multiple sclerosis. In Vinken PJ, Bruyn GW (eds): Handbook of Clinical Neurology. MS and Other Demyelinating Diseases. Vol. 9. New York: Elsevier, pp 217–309.
52. Bradley WG (1987) Sorting out the meaning of MRI flow phenomena. Diagn Imaging May 9:102–111.
53. Cherryman GR, Gemmell HG, Sharp PF, Besson JAO, Crawford J, Smith FW (1985) NMR demonstration of white matter changes in the watershed area of patients with dementia. Correlation with psychiatric evaluation and J-123-isopropylamphetamine cerebral blood flow imaging. Presented at the International Meeting of the Society of Magnetic Resonance in Medicine, London, Aug., 1985.
54. Fazekas F, Chawluk JB, Alavi A, et al. (1987) MR signal abnormalities at 1.5T in Alzheimer's dementia and normal aging. AJNR 8:421–426.
55. Besson JAO, Corrigan FM, Iljon Foreman E, et al. (1983) Differentiating senile dementia of Alzheimer type and multi-infarct dementia by proton NMR imaging. Lancet 2:789.
56. Erkinjuntti T, Ketonenl, Sulkava R, Sipponen J, Vuorialito M, Iivanainen M (1987) Do white matter changes on MRI and CT differentiate vascular dementia from Alzheimer's disease. J Neurol Neurosurg Psychiatry 50:37–42.
57. Hershey LA, Modic MT, Greenough G, et al. (1987) Magnetic resonance imaging in vascular dementia. Neurology 37:29–36.
58. Kinkel WR, Kinkel PR, Jacobs L, et al. (1985) Serial magnetic resonance imaging of the evolution of cerebral ischemia and infarction. Neurology 35(Suppl. 1):136.
59. Tomlinson BE, Blossed G, Roth M (1970) Observations on the brains of demented old people. J Neurol Sci 11:205–242.
60. Brun A, Englund E (1986) A white matter disorder in dementia of the Alzheimer type: A pathoanatomical study. Ann Neurol 19:253–262.
61. George AE (1987) Imaging techniques yield clues to memory disorders. Dia Imag Oct 9:122–126.
62. Huang K, Wu L, Luo Y (1985) Binswanger's disease: Progressive subcortical encephalopathy or multi-infarct dementia? Can J Neurol Sci 12:88–94.
63. Tomonoga M, Yamanovichi H, Toltgi H, et al. (1982) Clinicopathologic study of progressive subcortical vascular encephalopathy (Binswanger type) in the elderly. J Am Geriatr Soc 30:524–529.
64. Zatz LM, Jernigan TL, Ahumada AJ Jr (1982) White matter changes in cerebral computed tomography related to aging. J Comput Assist Tomogr 6:19–23.
65. Young IR, Randell CP, Kaplan PW, et al. (1983) Nuclear magnetic resonance (NMR) imaging in white matter disease of the brain using spin echo sequences. J Comput Assist Tomogr 7:290–294.
66. Hahn EL (1950) Spin echoes. Physiol Rev 80:580–594.
67. Suryan G (1951) Nuclear resonance in flowing liquids. Proc Indian Acad Sci (A) 33:107–111.
68. Lauterbur PC, Lai C-M (1977) Feasibility study of nuclear magnetic resonance zeugmatography for use in detecting atherosclerosis. In NHLBI, Division of Heart and Vascular Diseases, Devices and Technology Branch Contractors Meeting Proceedings. pp 205–206.
69. Hinshaw WS, Andrew ER, Bottomley PA, Holland GN, Moore WS, Worthington BS (1979) An in-vivo study of the forearm and hand using thin section NMR imaging. Br J Radiol 52:36–43.
70. Waluch V (1986) Magnetic resonance imaging of

blood flow. In Gerard G, Rossi DR (eds): *Seminars in Neurology*, vol. 6, pp. 65–71.

71. Alvarez O, Edwards JH, Hyman RA (1986) MR recognition of internal carotid artery occlusion. *AJNR* 47:359–360.

72. Gomori JM, Grossman RI, Goldberg HI, Zimmerman RA, Bilaniuk LT (1985) Intracranial hematomas: Imaging by high-field MR. *Radiology* 157:87–93.

73. Bradley WG, Schmidt PG (1985) Effect of methemoglobin formation on the MR appearance of subarachnoid hemorrhage. *Radiology* 156:99–103.

74. Swensen SJ, Keller PL, Berquist TH, et al. (1985) MRI hemorrhage. *AJR* 145:921–927.

75. Von Schulthess GK, Higgins CB (1985) Blood flow imaging with MR: Spin-phase phenomena. *Radiology* 157:687–695.

76. Ruszkowski JT, Damadian R, Giambolvo A, Gomes A, Hertz D, Lufkin R, Smith SD, Wortham D (1986) MRI angiography of the carotid artery. *Magn Reson Imaging* 4:497–502.

77. Jacobson HG (1988) Magnetic resonance imaging of the cardiovascular system. *JAMA* 259:2.

78. Marie P (1901) Des foyers lacunaires de desintegration et de differents autres etats cavitaires du cerveau. *Rev Med* 21:281–298.

79. Olszewski J (1962) Subcortical arteriosclerotic encephalopathy: Review of the literature on the so-called Binswanger's disease and presentation of two cases. *World Neurol* 8:359–375.

80. DeReuck J, Schaumburg HH (1972) Periventricular atherosclerotic leukoencephalopathy. *Neurology* 22:1094–1097.

81. Hachinski VC, Illiff LD, Zilkha E, et al. (1975) Cerebral blood flow in dementia. *Arch Neurol* 32:632–637.

82. Hachinski VC, Potter P, Merskey H (1987) Leukoaraiosis. *Arch Neurol* 44:21–23.

83. Kinkel WR, Jacobs L, Polachini I, et al. (1984) Late onset subcortical encephalopathy CT, NMR and clinical correlations. *Ann Neurol* 16:137–138.

84. Awad IA, Spetzler RF, Hodak JA, et al. (1987) Incidental lesions noted on magnetic resonance imaging of the brain: Prevalence and clinical significance in various age groups. *Neurosurgery* 20:222–227.

85. Fisher CM (1982) Lacunar strokes and infarcts: A review. *Neurology* 32:871.

86. Waluch V, Bradley WG (1984) NMR even echo rephasing in slow laminar flow. *J Comput Assist Tomogr* 8:594–598.

87. Gerard G, Weisberg LA (1986) Magnetic resonance imaging in adult white matter disorders and hydrocephalus. In Gerard G, Rossi DR (eds): *Seminars in Neurology*. Vol 6. pp 17–23.

7

SPECT Perfusion Imaging in Cerebrovascular Disease

B. Leonard Holman, MD, Jean-Luc Moretti, MD, PhD, and Thomas C. Hill, MD

Department of Radiology, Harvard Medical School, Brigham and Women's Hospital and New England Deaconess Hospital, Boston, Massachusetts 02115 (B.L.H., T.C.H.); Department de Biophysique et Medecine Nucleaire, Bobigny, Paris 13-93, France (J.-L.M.)

INTRODUCTION

A number of radiotracers have recently been developed that accumulate in the brain proportional to cerebral blood flow. These compounds are lipophilic, moving across the blood brain barrier with nearly complete extraction during a single passage through the cerebral circulation. Once inside the brain, they are either bound to nonspecific receptors or metabolized to nonlipophilic compounds. As a result, they maintain their distribution within the brain for some time after injection. The development of these commercially available tracers promises to bring to routine medical practice the remarkable diagnostic advances that have so far been limited to the small number of centers with positron emission tomography facilities.

RADIOPHARMACEUTICALS

Perfusion Agents

IMP

I-123 IMP N-isopropyl I-123 p-iodoamphetamine (IMP) is highly lipophilic, moving across the blood brain barrier with almost complete extraction during a single passage through the cerebral circulation [85,86]. The initial intracerebral distribution of IMP follows regional cerebral blood flow under normal physiologic conditions. However, when plasma pH is low, as in respiratory acidosis, metabolic acidosis, or ischemia, the IMP extraction is decreased [26]. The sequestration of basophilic amines by the brain and lung is a saturable process and is mediated by nonspecific mechanisms [59,60]. IMP is sequestered by binding to a high capacity cytoplasmic system, presumably a protein widely dispersed in organs and most abundant in the lung [67]. Trauble [74] has suggested that the saturability of amine transport may be due to mobile pores in the fluid membrane lipid and not due to carrier-mediated transport. Solubilization of the drug in brain lipids cannot be the only mechanism of uptake because there is no correlation between the lipid solubility of the drugs and their uptake in brain [60]. These amines have a low affinity for blood brain barrier transport sites, but the speed of uptake is very fast compared to glucose. Therefore, the capacity of the blood brain barrier lipophilic amine transport system is quite large. While less than 50% of IMP is unbound to proteins in blood in vitro, it is likely that dissociation from plasma proteins is enhanced in capillaries and that the concentration of unbound IMP is many times greater in vivo than in vitro [60].

Most brain tumors extract little IMP, probably because there is a deficiency in the lipophilic sequestration system [48]. Cerebral metastases from malignant melanoma [19] and oat cell tumors [72] do take up the tracer avidly, however, particularly if they are actively metabolizing amphetamine precursors. IMP uptake is decreased under anesthesia [29] perhaps because there is a decrease in the number

---

Noninvasive Imaging of Cerebrovascular
Disease, pages 147–162
© 1989 Alan R. Liss, Inc.

of perfused capillaries (about 50% of normal) under pentobarbital anesthesia.

In the monkey, IMP accumulates rapidly within the brain reaching 6–9 of the injected dose at 1 hour, with some evidence of washout by 4 hours [17]. By 24 hours, only 2% of the injected dose remains in the brain. The gray/white matter ratio is constant for the first hour, falling slightly by 4 hours and reversing by 24 hours.

IMP concentration in brain tissue immediately after an intravenous bolus injection is a reflection of blood flow. As the distribution of the tracer equilibrates between brain and blood over time, the brain concentration becomes a function of the partition coefficient. IMP washes out of the brain relatively slowly.

Rapin demonstrated that 3 minutes after injection of I-125 IMP in the rat, the ratio of gray to white matter was 10, and after 1 hour the ratio was 4.4 [63]. These findings suggest that either IMP is extracted from the blood by the gray matter before reaching white matter, IMP has a faster turnover in gray matter than in white matter, or that the coefficient of extraction of IMP is different in gray and white matter.

In the human, brain uptake of IMP is rapid, reaching 45% of the maximum brain activity by 2 minutes and 6–9% of the injected dose by 30 minutes [18]. The clearance of the tracer from the brain is balanced by slow release of IMP from the lungs. Thus, brain activity remains constant from 20 minutes to at least 60 minutes after injection. The gray/white matter activity ratio also remains constant during that time. By 24 hours, the gray/white matter activity ratio has reversed, and activity is higher in the white matter [18].

HIPDM

Kung and his colleagues have investigated a group of iodophenolic diamines that, like IMP, exhibit high uptake and long retention times in the brain [28]. Their most promising agent, N,N,N'-trimethyl-N'-(2 hydroxy-3-methyl-5-iodobenzyl)-1, 3-propanediamine (HIPDM), is extracted rapidly by the brain, rapid brain uptake reaching 4–5% of the injected dose in monkeys within 1 hour after injection.

HIPDM is taken up more rapidly by the brain than IMP, reaching 75% of maximum brain activity by 2 minutes [18]. The peak brain activity is significantly lower for HIPDM than for IMP, however. The lung clearance is slower for HIPDM than for IMP, and the amount of tracer reaching the liver is less [11].

Diamines take advantage of the pH gradient that exists between blood (pH 7.4) and brain (pH 7.0). As a result, nonspecific binding may account at least in part for brain retention of diamines as well as monoamines [27].

The activity distribution of IMP and HIPDM progressively changes from a flow dependence to a partition coefficient dependence. This effect is faster for IMP than for HIPDM [52]. Therefore, absolute quantitation of rCBF with these amines must take into account metabolites in the blood and diffusion of the tracers.

After the intravenous injection of IMP, only isopropyl iodoamphetamine (IMP) and iodoamphetamine are found in the brain [1,63]. These two compounds either equilibrate with the amines found in the blood at a rate determined by the partition coefficients of the blood and the brain, or the brain parenchyma releases hydrophilic metabolites into the blood at a rate determined by regional metabolism and turnover. Thus the temporal course of redistribution of the tracer from gray to white matter is either a function of the partition coefficient or results from the faster washout in cortex compared to the white matter with the rates determined by the rate of metabolism [62].

Data obtained with HIPDM helps us understand the process of amine redistribution [41]. Influx into brain is higher in gray matter (0.91) than in white matter (0.39). Washout is faster for gray cortex ($T_{\frac{1}{2}}$ = 33 minutes and 2.1%/minute) than for white matter ($T_{\frac{1}{2}}$ = 38.5/minutes and 1.8%/minute). Assuming a continuing amine influx from a lung reservoir of 2.1% to compensate for gray matter efflux, there is 0.3%/minute more influx than efflux in white cortex, leading to an additional 54% by 3 hours. White matter activity is 93%, of gray cortex activity by 3 hours. These data were obtained in rats, and the changes will be slower in humans.

Amines are cleared by the lung during their first pass through the pulmonary circulation and released slowly from the lung into the systemic circulation [73]. In humans, whole blood

IMP activity is less than 1.0% the injected dose by 1 minute after intravenous administration.

TL-201 DDC

Thallium-201 diethyldithiocarbamate (DDC) has recently been suggested as an alternative to I-123 IMP. The development of this imaging agent is based on the observation that treating patients for thallium intoxication with large doses of diethyldithiocarbamate causes increasing neurologic toxicity. In the human brain, uptake is complete after 90 seconds. There is almost complete extraction of the tracer during its first pass through the brain. Based on whole body distribution studies, the brain uptake is 4.3% of the injected dose. The Tl-201 DDC complex dissociates quickly in vivo and distributes as the Tl-201 ion. The DDC molecule probably serves as a lipophilic carrier for Tl-201 across the blood brain barrier [6].

Tl-201 DDC has a number of advantages over I-123 IMP: 1) no lung retention, 2) on-site preparation, 3) ease of preparation, and 4) considerable documentation of its distribution and toxicity. Tl-201 DDC has a number of disadvantages that will prevent its wide-scale application: 1) a photon energy that is too low for optimal imaging, 2) high radiation dose, 3) extracerebral uptake in the muscles surrounding the calvarium, and 4) instability in the vial before injection.

TC-99M DIAMINE DITHIOL (DADT)

N-piperidinyl ethyl DADT exhibits high initial uptake in mice brain (2.2% at 5 minutes) [39] but is cleared rapidly (0.5% of the injected dose at 30 minutes). Clearance of DADT Tc-99m from brain is also fast in monkeys ($T_{\frac{1}{2}}$ = 63 minutes) and baboons ($T_{\frac{1}{2}}$ = 5 minutes). These stable complexes are of great interest clinically because of the better imaging characteristics of Tc-99m, lower radiation dose, ready availability, and stability of the compound. Washout can be slowed by chemical or pharmacologic transformation. These compounds would be an attractive agent for perfusion imaging in humans.

TC-99M PAO

The macrocyclic amine, propyleneamine oxime (PnAO), has been labeled with technetium-99m [79]. This lipophilic compound crosses the blood brain barrier, but it has a very rapid clearance from the brain, precluding tomographic imaging with gamma cameras [16,75]. Significant improvements in brain residence time has been observed with new PnAO derivatives, however.

The d,l hexamethyl propylene amine-oxime (Tc-99m-HMPAO) stereisomer has a fairly high first-pass extraction through the cerebral circulation and has an initial cerebral distribution similar to IMP and HIPDM [54]. Unlike IMP, Tc-99m-HMPAO does not appear to redistribute within the brain for up to 8 hours after injection [68]. Unfortunately its blood clearance is slow, and its brain uptake is approximately 75% that of IMP, resulting in a degradation in image quality.

Tc-99m-HMPAO has significant advantages over either I-123 IMP or Tl-201 DDC: 1) onsight preparation, 2) lower radiation dose, 3) lower cost, 4) ideal physical characteristics, and 5) higher photon flux. But it is unstable in vitro by 30 to 60 minutes after preparation.

Diffuse Gas Tracers

Regional CBF can be measured quantitatively using the inert gas washout technique [30,31]. Advances in the technology have led to the replacement of Kr-85 with Xe-133 and to tomographic imaging systems [70]. Because this method requires special purpose equipment and is more difficult to perform than perfusion SPECT, Xe-133 SPECT has been limited to situations where absolute quantification of blood flow is necessary, where rapid serial studies are needed, and as a reference standard for the other soluble tracers such as IMP and Tc-99m HMPAO. When IMP and Xe-133 patterns are compared, they are similar as long as imaging with IMP is carried out within the first hour after injection [34].

Cerebral Blood Flow Volume Agents

SPECT can be performed following intravenous injection of Tc-99m-labeled red blood cells and plasma tracers such as Tc-99m albumin. Parametric images of the regional cerebral hematocrit are obtained from the regional ratios of red blood cell and plasma volumes [65]. Mean regional cerebral blood volume (CBV) averages 5 ml/100 g in the brain, and regional hematocrit averages 31%. During 5% CO_2 inhalation, CBV increases by 10% due to an increasing plasma volume and fall in hematocrit to 30% creating a physiologic hemidilution. During cerebral hypoperfusion, distal to internal carotid artery occlusion or severe stenosis, reduction in cerebral perfusion pressure, and central vasodilatation can be detected from parametric images of the ratio of perfusion (early IMP images) and CBV (labeled erythrocyte imaging).

INSTRUMENTATION

Single photon emission computed tomography (SPECT) of the brain can be performed using either multidetector or rotating gamma camera systems. Each imaging system has its advantages; the choice of equipment depends on the level of utilization and on the purposes for which the technique will be applied.

The high collection efficiency of the multidetector system makes rapid scanning (5–7.5 minutes) of an entire slice possible. The primary advantage of this system is its high sensitivity, resulting in high spatial resolution and rapid imaging. As a result, SPECT perfusion images of the brain can be obtained with a spatial resolution of 10 mm (full-width at half-maximum) in the plane of the slice. The multidetector system would, therefore, be the preferred instrument for studies requiring high spatial resolution, regional quantification, or rapid sequential imaging [45].

The rotating gamma camera approach is preferable for routine clinical imaging because of its availability and because it can be used for other types of tomographic and nontomographic imaging. The major constraint on rotating gamma camera tomography is sensitivity. The low sensitivity for each tomographic slice is compensated for by the fact that the gamma camera collects volumetric information as opposed to the single slice information obtained with the multidetector system. Improvements in camera designs [35], in collimator design (the slant-hole [61], long-bore [53], and fan-beam [76] collimators, for example), and in reconstruction algorithms have substantially improved the quality of SPECT perfusion images using the Anger-type gamma camera. Satisfactory tomographic imaging has been achieved with the rotating gamma camera using all of the perfusion agents described above.

RELATIVE QUANTIFICATION OF PERFUSION

The initial distribution of I-123 IMP is directly proportional to regional cerebral blood flow in normal brain. Quantifications of flow after intravenous injection in man is not an easy matter, however. There are both biologic constraints imposed by the mathematical model, and physical constraints imposed by the instrumentation.

A variation of the indicator fractionation technique of Sapirstein [66] has been proposed to measure regional blood flow using the tracer I-123 IMP [3]. This method requires a diffusible tracer and requires that 1) the tracer is delivered continuously to the brain, 2) the tracer is freely diffusible and completely removed on a single pass through the brain, 3) the tracer back diffuses slowly from the brain to the blood, and 4) the tracer can be distinguished from its polar metabolites. If these assumptions hold, flow can be calculated using the following formula:

$$\dot{C}_b = FC_a - kC_b$$

$$F \frac{C_b(T)}{C_a * e^{-kt}} = \frac{C_b(T)}{e^{-kt} \int_0^T C_a(t) e^{kt} dt},$$

where F is cerebral blood flow in ml/100 g/min, C_a is the arterial whole blood concentration of true tracer (mCi/ml), C_b is the brain activity concentration (mCi/100 g), $\dot{C}_b$ is the rate of change of C_b, k is the rate constant (per minute) for back diffusion, t is time, T is time of measurement, and * denotes the operation of convolution.

Measurement of regional cerebral blood flow is carried out after the intravenous injection of 5 mCi of IMP into an arm vein. Blood is withdrawn for 5 minutes from a small catheter placed in the radial artery using a Harvard pump at the rate of 0.9 ml/min. While scanning may continue for 1 hour after injection to obtain higher resolution images, quantitation of tissue activity is determined from the first 5 minutes of data collection. To use this technique with I-123 IMP, it is necessary to distinguish the tracer from its metabolites in the arterial blood sample by solvent or HPLC separation. There will be some washout of tracer from the brain during the initial 5-minute collection period, which will contaminate the arterial sample.

Using this method and attenuation compensation [5,25], it was determined that the normal value of whole brain CBF was 47 ± 5 ml/100 g/min, which is somewhat lower than the values obtained with xenon-133.

I-123 HIPDM does not appear to be suitable for quantification of regional cerebral blood flow using the indicator fractionation method because of rapid metabolism of the tracer, incomplete extraction of the tracer by brain tissue, and significant back flux of the tracer from the brain into the blood.

These techniques require accurate measurement of the absolute tracer activity within regions of the brain. Currently, only special purpose imaging devices comes close to meeting the specifications required for such a task. Photon attenuation and partial volume effects add to the difficulty.

It is probably more realistic and certainly simpler to limit quantitative schemes to the measurement of relative activities within brain regions. The ratio of activities between left and right regions can be used to evaluate asymmetries in focal diseases such as cerebral infarction, while the ratio of activities between the target region and ipsilateral normal regions can be used in bilaterally symmetric processes such as Alzheimer's disease.

Semiquantitative techniques have been developed to assess regional cerebral IMP activity [78]. Using the technique described by Moretti et al. [51], three symmetric regions of interest (ROI) are automatically defined for each transaxial slice from an external outline after manual exclusion of the parasagittal central region. The size of each automatic ROI is at least twice the spatial resolution of the reconstructed image (25 pixels). Differences between left and right ROI IMP activities are then determined for each region (six regions/patients).

A differential percentage of activity (DPA) is calculated for each transaxial slice. In control patients, the mean DPA obtained by automatic ROI quantification is 1.7 ± 4% (S.D.) (range 0–9.5%, n = 42). Therefore, areas are considered abnormal if the DPA is higher than 10%. The DPA on early (1 hour) images is called the *early index of hypoactivity* and the DPA on delayed (3–4 hours) IMP images is the *delayed index of hypoactivity* [50].

Partial redistribution will occur when tracer washin is slow due to marked reduction in perfusion. Redistribution will not be present on delayed images when there is absent perfusion because the initial IMP activity is absent or very low and because redistribution is due to slow washout in from ischemic zone. The redistribution amplitude (RA) is defined as:

$$RA = [(LHI - EHI)/EHI] \times 100.$$

Redistribution is complete if RA is greater than 90%, partial if 50% < RA < 90%, and absent if RA is less than 50%.

TECHNIQUE

Careful quality control is essential with SPECT. The relatively low photon flux from the target organ, the scattered radiation from the high energy gamma rays of I-123 and I-124, and the low photon energies associated with Tl-201 stretch the imaging process to its limits.

Between 3 and 5 mCi IMP is injected intravenously (3–4 mCi Tl-201 DDC [77] and 10–20 mCi if Tc-99m HMPAO [10]). Imaging begins 10 to 20 minutes after injection, with the patient supine and the head centered in the field of view. With IMP, imaging begins 20 minutes post injection and delayed image is obtained 3 hours later. The patient should be placed on a comfortable couch so that movement is reduced to a minimum during data acquisition.

A 64-frame, 360° study is acquired with the detector as close to the head as possible using a collimator optimized to the energies of the radionuclide. Each image takes from 20 to 40 seconds depending on the condition of the patient.

Reconstruction is performed after correcting the 64 frames with a 30–60 million count flood source image and after correcting for attenuation loss. Attenuation correction is more straightforward for imaging of the head than for imaging of the thorax or abdomen. Because the attenuation constant does not vary signifi-

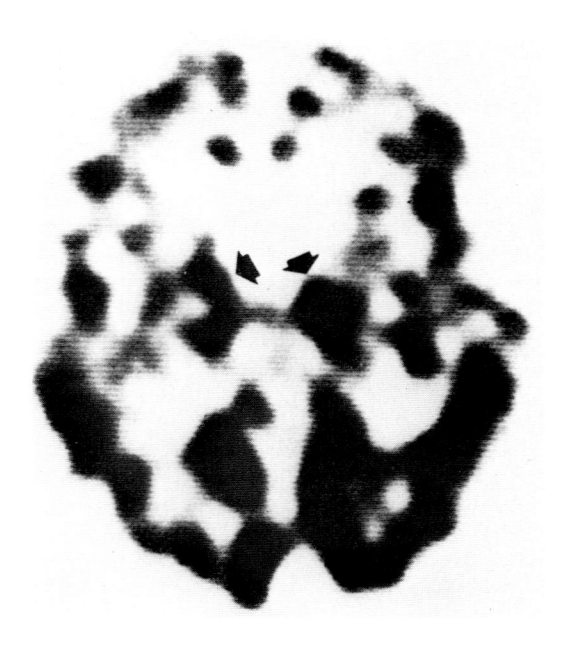

Figure 7–1. Normal I-123-IMP transaxial image. Cortical uptake appears to be related to gray matter blood flow, with good demarcation of the interlober fissure. In this tomographic slice taken 2 cm above the orbitomeatal line, the basal ganglia and thalamus are clearly defined (arrows) (reprinted from reference 14 with permission).

cantly throughout the brain, attenuation corrections such as those introduced by Sorensen or Chang are quite suitable for brain perfusion tomography.

Reconstruction is performed using a ramp filter. A three-dimensional Hanning filter is then applied to the reconstructed images to reduce the noise introduced from the out-of-slice planes as well as from the plane of the image. Reconstructions are performed along the plane parallel to the orbitomeatal line and in the coronal and sagittal planes.

CLINICAL APPLICATIONS
Normal Patterns

Patients without central nervous system disease and with normal x-ray CT examinations demonstrate bilaterally symmetric activity on the SPECT perfusion images (Fig. 7–1) [13]. Activity is greatest in a strip of cortex along the convexity of the frontal, temporal, parietal, and occipital lobes corresponding anatomically to cortical gray matter. Activity is also high in the region corresponding to the basal ganglia and thalamus. The regions between the basal ganglia and the convexity corresponding anatomically to cortical white matter and the ventricles have less activity.

Cerebrovascular Disease

ACUTE AND SUBACUTE INFARCTION

In patients with ischemic infarction, the brain usually appears normal on x-ray CT for several days after acute interruption of cerebral blood flow. Early changes in regional brain function have been observed using positron emission tomography (PET) well before transmission CT becomes abnormal. PET has limited potential for routine clinical applications because of its cost and lack of availability, however.

Perfusion SPECT accurately identifies acute infarction, using either the I-123 amines [9,37] or HMPAO Tc-99m [10]. With Tc-99m HMPAO, the intensity and extent of the perfusion defect remains fixed over time [40]. With IMP, the SPECT pattern changes over the course of time after injection especially in the ischemic focal lesion [64].

The decrease in IMP activity on early imaging is related to either an impairment in regional perfusion or to reduced IMP extraction [82]. In ischemic cortical tissue, IMP kinetics differ from normal cortex. This may be related to, 1) delayed uptake with redistribution of activity within the brain from normal cortical areas and the lung; 2) lower uptake due to metabolic acidosis associated with luxury perfusion or to a decrease number of functional binding sites; 3) slower metabolism due to reduced oxygen and enzyme activity, leading to impaired washout of metabolites and relative accumulation of activity; or 4) higher retention of IMP and its lipophilic metabolite, iodoamphetamine, resulting in a decrease in efflux back to the blood due to the acidic pH (lactate accumulation) [56].

The scintigraphic patterns of acute cerebral infarction correspond to the vascular anatomy of the brain. In patients with middle cerebral artery infarction, the perfusion defect involves the gray and white matter of the temporal lobe

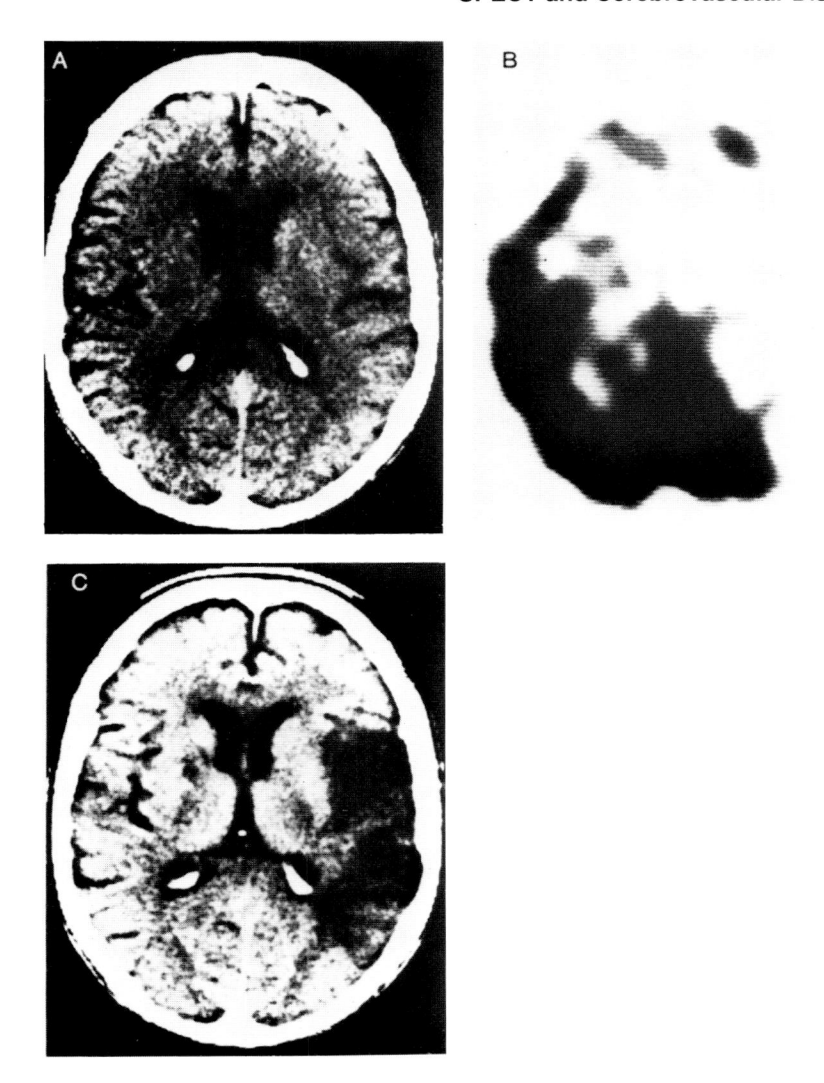

Figure 7–2. **A:** Initial x-ray CT scan obtained on the day of onset of right hemiparesis and aphasia is normal. **B:** I-123 IMP study shows absent uptake in the region of the left middle cerebral artery territory. **C:** Followup x-ray CT study 6 days after the acute event shows a low density area in the parietal lobe. Note that the resultant infarct is smaller than the ischemic tissue demonstrated on the IMP study (reprinted from reference 14 with permission.)

with variable extension into the frontal, parietal, and occipital lobes and the basal ganglia (Fig. 7–2). In patients with posterior cerebral infarction, the perfusion defects involve the occipital lobe and the visual associative areas. Acute anterior cerebral infarction involves a strip of the superior frontal cortex along the interhemispheric fissure. Infarction may be limited to the basal ganglia or the cerebellum. In the latter case, occlusion of the posteroinferior cerebellar artery may result in a perfusion defect involving the ipsilateral cerebellar hemisphere.

Emission computed tomography with I-123

IMP is more accurate than x-ray CT for the diagnosis of early cerebral infarction. In an evaluation of 25 patients with acute cerebral infarction, Hill et al. [15] found that 22 had perfusion defects on single slice emission tomography. Of the 22 abnormal IMP studies, six had normal transmission CT studies. In five of these six cases, the CT scan was obtained within 2 days of the onset of symptoms. In 16 patients with abnormal CT scans, only two of the patients had CT scans performed within the initial two days. In the three patients who had normal I-123 IMP studies, only one had an abnormal transmission CT study. More recent IMP studies with rotating gamma cameras suggest a sensitivity for detection of completed strokes close to 100% [2].

Not only does imaging with I-123 become abnormal sooner than computed tomography, but the extent of the perfusion defect may be substantially greater than the abnormality on CT. In eight of the 16 patients with abnormal CT scans studied by Hill et al. [15], the perfusion defect with I-123 IMP was much larger than the low density areas seen on the CT scan. This finding has been confirmed by other groups.

The discordance between CT and SPECT estimates of the size of the abnormality in patients with acute stroke is not surprising. The total extent of the ischemia is likely to be much larger than the extent of necrotic, irreversibly damaged tissue. Findings of persisting perfusion defects around the infarcted area on the CT image may indicate the occurrence of two phenomena: 1) an intracerebral neuronal diaschisis, 2) an incomplete infarction or 3) a diffuse selective neuronal cell loss [33,42]. Neuropathologic studies in animals who suffered either hypoxic insult show evidence of a reduction in neuronal density accompanied by microglia proliferation. Similar findings are present in zones surrounding the completed infarction [84]. Experimental studies have documented a correlation between cerebral blood flow and neuronal density using C-14 antipyrine [43].

Diaschisis is defined by (Von Monakow [44]) as a decrease in the functional capacity in a brain region caused by distant injury [22]. This phenomenom occurs when excitatory impulses through afferent fiber tracts are interrupted, reducing the functional status of the distal region. The observation that the countralateral cerebellar hemisphere has decreased blood flow and IMP uptake in many stroke patients in the absence of CT abnormalities in the cerebellum indicates that the flow asymmetry is due to diaschisis and not due to cerebellar infarction or atrophy. These disconnected regions have a coupled decrease in rCBF oxygen and glucose metabolism [58]. The incidence of cerebellar diaschisis is about 50% in stroke patients, and it is unrelated to clinical outcome [47].

Increased uptake of tracers [57,71] may be seen in areas of luxury perfusion [32]. This is a very unusual finding with I-123 IMP and is seen in less than 2% of patients with acute cerebral infarction. The area of increased uptake may appear in the border zone around the central infarct during the first 3 weeks after onset of symptoms and will usually disappear by 1 week. Luxury perfusion is not seen as commonly with I-123 IMP as with other radiotracers such as Tl-201 DDC and HMPAO [69].

Moretti et al. [49] have observed a major discrepancy between IMP and Tc-99m HMPAO distributions in stroke patients. During the subacute phase, uptake is decreased in the stroke area with IMP SPECT, while normal or hyperative areas may be present with HMPAO SPECT in 80% of middle cerebral artery stroke patients. IMP and HMPAO SPECT were similar by 3 months after onset of symptoms. When hyperemic infarcts are studied with PET, high oxygen uptake is never seen in those lesions [38], demonstrating that flow is in excess of the metabolic demand. The luxury perfusion syndrome is related to acute metabolic acidosis in damaged brain tissue [32], and is a rather frequent phenomenon, lasting several weeks in patients with strokes.

The mismatch between I-123 IMP and HMPAO Tc-99m suggests that IMP distribution is not only flow-limited but that its uptake in ischemic lesions may be dramatically decreased when focal arterial pH is low and binding capacity altered. In normal brain cells I-123 IMP follows CBF even in zones of increased blood flow because I-123 IMP uptake is high in focal epileptic seizures and brain stimulation [14,46].

Raynaud et al. [64] studied 17 patients with

chronic cerebral infarcts using early and delayed IMP I-123 SPECT (10 minutes, 2 hours, and 5 hours postinjection) and Xe-133 SPECT. Four of the 17 patients also had rCBF and $CMRO_2$ measured by PET. The central necrotic area seen on CT had a large decrease in activity with both IMP (34%) and xenon CBF (46%). The periinfarct area, which was normal on CT, had moderately decreased IMP activity (13%) and xenon CBF (19%). The peripheral areas were normal on delayed IMP SPECT. Peripheral hypoperfusion was found to persist with time.

Patients with the greatest neurologic deficits have the largest lesions on CT and I-123 IMP and have the greatest decrease in count density on SPECT. Neurologic deficit and psychological disability correlate well with the size of the peripheral abnormality but not with the central area of tissue necrosis [64]. Lee et al. [37] found that lesion size and uptake on early IMP SPECT images were not predictive of clinical outcome. By following clinical status for 3 months and performing early and delayed IMP SPECT images, Defer et al. [7] studied 21 ischemic patients including 16 with stroke, five with PRIND, and three with TIAs (Fig. 7-3). The redistribution amplitude averaged 44.5% in the group with poor clinical improvement, 83.7% in those patients with moderate improvement group, and 96% in patients with good improvement. Patients with PRIND and TIA had the least intense defects, whereas the stroke patients had the greatest reductions in tracer uptake. While there was some overlap among the groups, the method was sensitive enough for early evaluation of patient prognosis.

HEMODYNAMIC PATENCY

Cerebral blood flow may be reduced in patients with cerebrovascular disease due to either reduced metabolic demand in ischemic tissue or, less commonly, to vessel stenosis or narrowing. An arthromatous process must result in a stenosis of at least 50% to become hemodynamically significant and to result in a detectable reduction in internal carotid artery (ICA) blood flow.

Transient ischemic attacks (TIA) may either have a hemodynamic or embolic origin. A hemodynamic origin is assumed when postural changes provoke symptoms of short duration. This chronic hemodynamic insufficiency is due to the combination of severe ICA stenosis and a compromised collateral circulation. Patients with an inadequate collateral supply may drop their perfusion pressure below the lower limit of autoregulation.

Arteriolar vasodilation will be present in these patients at rest. Knapp et al. [24] using early IMP SPECT for perfusion imaging and Tc-99m red cell SPECT for CBV imaging showed that a focal decrease in I-123 IMP was accompanied by more than a 10% increase in Tc-99m red cell activity at the same site. The ratio of CBF/CBV was more sensitive in detecting hemodynamic risk in patients with carotid stenosis than perfusion imaging alone and may identify patients with a reduction in cerebral perfusion pressure even when ICA stenosis is less than 50%. CBF fails to change due to a compensatory drop in vascular resistance due to autoregulation, which is initiated by the release of vasodilator substances and reduced oxygen supply. When perfusion pressure distal to the arterial stenosis falls below the lower limit of autoregulation, CBF becomes pressure-dependent.

In the majority of patients with severe internal carotid artery stenosis, perfusion pressure is reduced only about 30%. An assessment of cerebrovascular flow capacity requires a vasodilating stimulus to enhance the hemodynamic effect of localized arteral disease. Hypercapnia has been used (5% CO_2 inhalation), but variability in flow response precludes accurate interpretation in individual cases [12,55]. A more uniform flow enhancement is obtained with acetazolamide (Diamox), a potent cerebral vasodilator [81,82]. Diamox (1 g IV) elicits an intracellular carbonic acidosis of brain tissue [23] and an additional hypoxic effect caused by inhibition of carbonic anhydrase in red cells due to the Bohr effect (less oxygen availability for tissues due to a lower pH). This second phenomenon seems to be of less importance because the consumption of oxygen ($CMRO_2$) is unchanged [36]. Cerebral vasodilation is rapid, and the maximum effect is achieved 20 to 30 minutes after acetazolamide injection. CBF increases more than 50% in normal controls and 33% in normal elderly [83].

Because reduced cerebral perfusion pressure

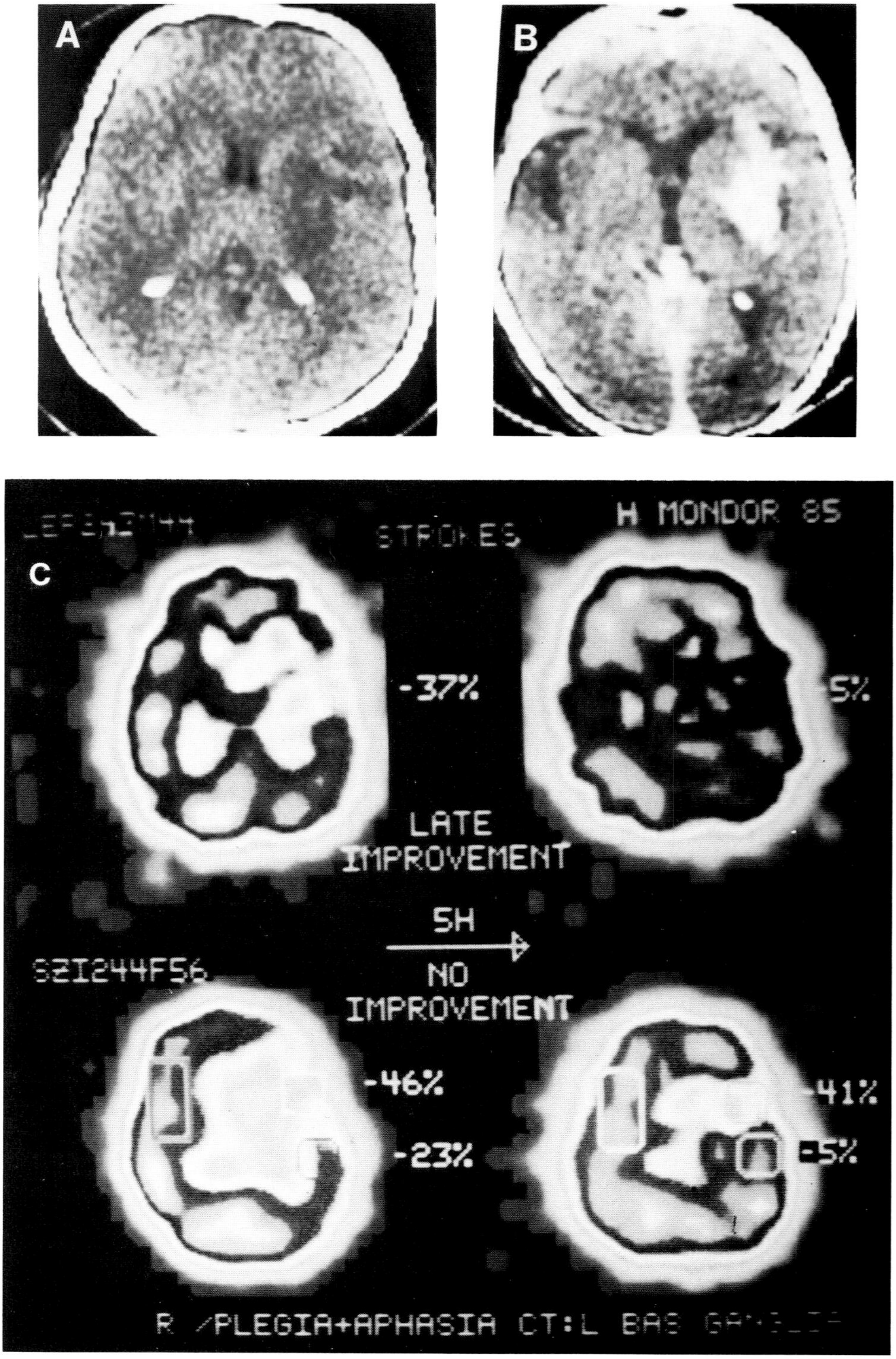
A
B
C
H MONDOR 85
STROKES
-37%
-5%
LATE
IMPROVEMENT
5H
NO
IMPROVEMENT
SZI244F56
-46%
-23%
-41%
-5%
R /PLEGIA+APHASIA CT:L BAS

accounts for about 10% of ischemic events, vasoreactivity can be used to identify patients with reduced cerebral flow capacity who are candidates for endarterectomy or extracranial-intracarnial arterial bypass (Fig. 7–4). Using Xe-133 SPECT, left-right asymmetries in cerebral blood flow asymmetries greater than 7% were found in 14 patients with a mean perfusion pressure of 50 mmHg versus 83 mmHg in 42 patients with asymmetries less than 7%. In the 14 patients with flow asymmetry, blood flow increased from 52 ml/min to 226 ml/min after surgery. CBF increased only from 103 ml/min to 170 ml/min in the other 42 patients.

In patients with minor strokes and/or transient ischemic attacks, Vorstrup et al. [82] showed that the permanent neurologic deficits remained unchanged following an extracranial-intracranial arterial bypass, surgery while almost all of the transient ischemic attacks stopped. Eighteen of 22 patients had no change in rCBF after surgery. In two of these patients, focal CBF improved on retesting 4 months after shunting; nine of 18 patients had significant flow asymmetries, while the other nine patients with a normal response had no increase in rCBF. These results underline the failure of extracranial-intracranial arterial bypass surgery to reduce the risk of ischemic stroke and complements the findings of others [8]. The only advantage of surgery was an increase in the regional vasodilatory capacity.

REVERSIBLE ISCHEMIA

The low sensitivity of CT in transient ischemia attacks is well documented [3]. Prolonged disturbances in cerebral blood flow are found, however, in patients with transient ischemic attacks and permanent regressive ischemic neurologic deficits (PRIND) using Xe-133 SPECT [13,80]. While Hill did not show IMP abnormalities in his early study, we found that the overall sensitivity of CT is 62% for PRIND, while the sensitivity of IMP SPECT is 87%. In the TIA group where CT was normal, the SPECT sensitivity is 56% when SPECT is carried out within 2 weeks of the onset of symptoms. Only 25% (3/4) of patients studied more than 3 months after the onset were abnormal, however. In five patients (35%) in the PRIND group, SPECT showed an additional ipsilateral cortical defect, while CT was abnormal only in the hypodense capsular lesions [4].

The intensity of the perfusion defect is much less in reversible ischemia than in completed stroke and redistribution is almost complete by 3 hours after injection in reversible ischemia. The high sensitivity of IMP SPECT in TIA and PRIND could be further improved by performing SPECT very soon after the onset of symptoms or by using acetazolamide enhancement.

DEMENTIAS

IMP SPECT has also been of value in differentiating multi-infarct dementia (Fig. 7–5) and Alzheimer's disease [20,21]. Patients with Alzheimer's disease have reductions in tracer uptake in the associative cortex, most profound in the posterior temporoparietal cortex. In patients with multiinfarct dementia, the defects are focal, heterogeneously distributed, and involve the primary cortex.

CONCLUSIONS

SPECT provides a functional evaluation of the cerebral parenchyma. The underlying phe-

---

Figure 7–3. Redistribution of I-123 IMP over 5 hours in two patients with similar neurologic status following their completed stroke but with different outcomes. **A:** CT without contrast 4 days after onset of symptoms with left middle cerebral artery distribution hypodensity. The patient had almost complete recovery of motor function but incomplete language recovery. **B:** CT with contrast 22 days after onset of symptoms in a patient with left middle cerebral artery infarct. This patient had no clinical recovery. **C:** I-123 IMP tomography in the two patients. The early image (upper left) in the patient whose CT scan is shown in A has hypoactivity in the area of the stroke (−37% compared to the opposite side) with redistribution at 5 hours (−5%) (upper right). Early image in the patient whose CT scan is shown in B (lower left) with two areas of hypoactivity in the left middle cerebral artery distribution (−46% and −23%). The most intense defect did not redistribute (−41%), while the activity in the second defect normalized (−5%) on delayed imaging (lower right).

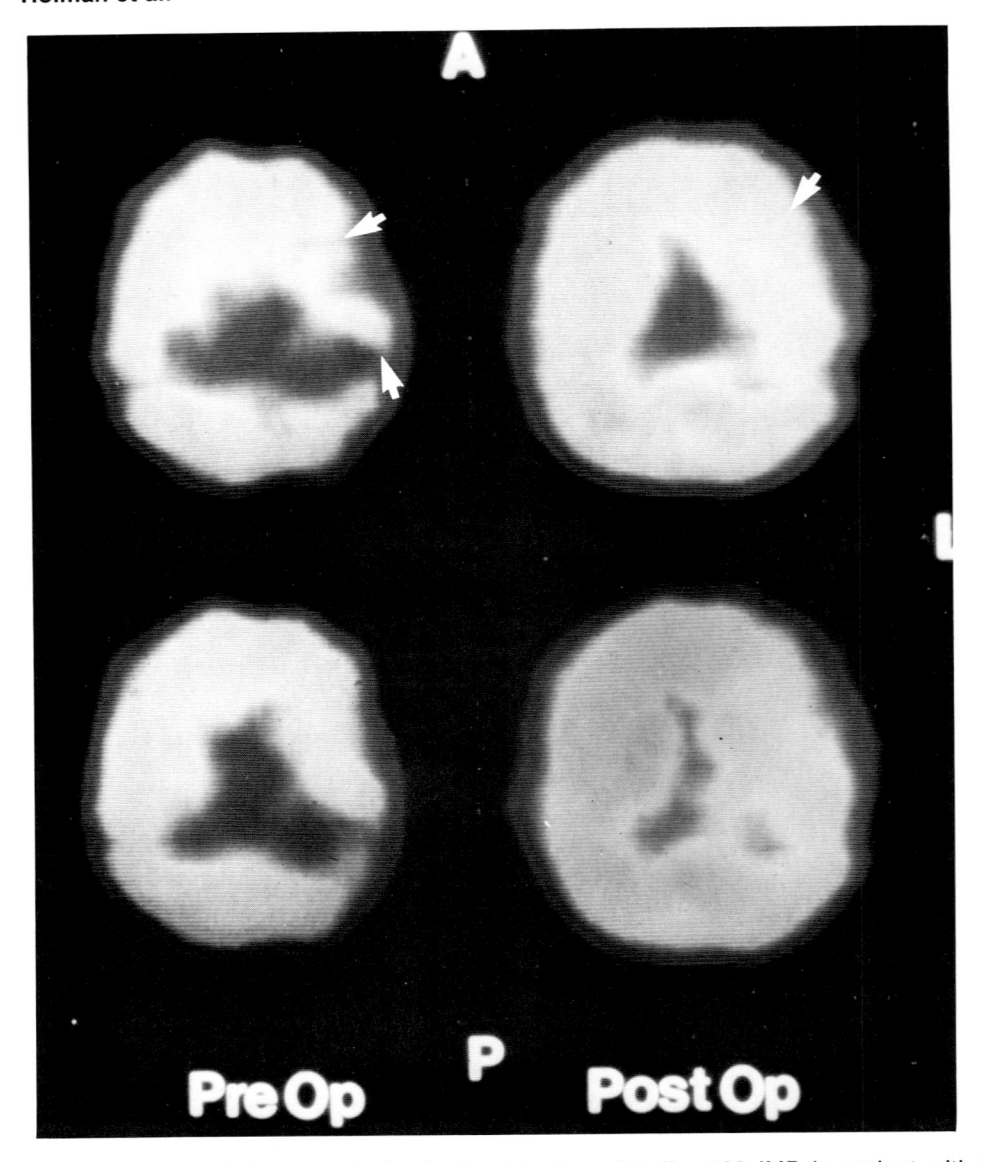

Figure 7-4. Transaxial images obtained after injection of iodine-123 IMP in patient with left internal carotid and middle cerebral artery stenoses. Left, extensive perfusion defect is noted in preoperative study (arrows). Right, after surgery, perfusion has improved to most of the hemisphere but with persistent perfusion defect at the site of surgery (arrow). Images were obtained with a rotating gamma camera. A indicates anterior; P, posterior. (Reproduced in color on page 74.)

nomena that occur in association with decreased tracer uptake involve either decreased blood flow, functional deactivation, metabolic impairment, or a combination of the three. As a result, identifying an ischemic area may be more difficult than defining the affected arterial territory.

SPECT imaging has a number of advantages in patients with cerebral ischemia. 1) It may be used as a guide in following the evolution of

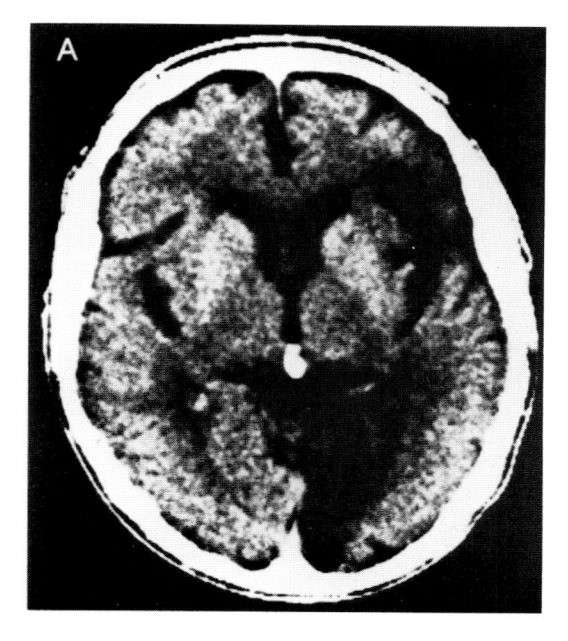

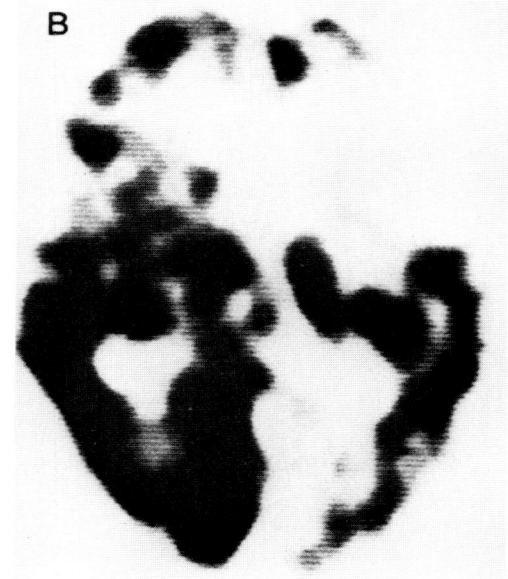

Figure 7–5. **A:** CT scan obtained 11 days after onset of right hemiparesis shows focal area of low attenuation in the left frontal lobe just anterior to the Sylvian fissure. The larger region of abnormality seen in the left occipital parietal lobe is secondary to a stroke that occurred 15 months earlier. **B:** I-123 IMP tomography shows decreased activity in left frontal area that is more extensive than the edema shown on the CT scan. Also note decreased activity in the left occiptal region that is related to the previous stroke.

brain function over the course of the disease, 2) it may be useful in documenting improvements in perfusion and vascular reserve and assessing complications after surgery, and 3) it may be used to determine prognosis after cerebral ischemic attacks as a guide to further management.

References

1. Baldwin RM, Wu JL, Lin TH, Salazar NE, Ma JM, Look S, VU CD, Boreinstein JS, Reele S, Hain D, Felix MJ (1986) Pharmacokinetics of I 123 N isopropyl p iodoamphetamine (IMP) in humans. In Billinghurst MW (ed): Current Concepts in Radiopharmacology. Proceedings of the 4th International Symposium on Radiopharmacology. Toronto: Pergamon Press, pp 35–41.
2. Brott TG, Gelfand MJ, Williams CC, Spilker JA, Hertberg VS (1986) Frequency and patterns of abnormality detected by iodine 123 amine emission CT after cerebral infarction. Radiology 158:729–734.
3. Buell U, Sceid KF, Lanksh W, Kleinhauss E, Ulbert V, Reger U, Rath M, Moser EA (1981) Sensitivity of computed assisted radionuclide angiography in TIA and PRIND. Stroke 12:829–834.
4. Cesaro P, Moretti JL, Defer G, Sergent A, Gaston A, Keravel Y, Degos JD (1987) Comparison of SPECT with isopropyl p (I-123) iodoamphetamine and CT scanner in reversible ischemia. Eur J Nucl Med. (in press).
5. Chang LT (1978) A method for attenuation correction in radionuclide computed tomography. IEEE Trans Nucl Sci 25:638–643.
6. de Bruine JF, van Royen EA, Vyth A, de Jong JMBV, van der Schoot JB (1985) Thallium-201 diethyldithiocarbamate: An alternative to iodine-123 N-isopropyl-p-iodoamphetamine. J Nucl Med 26: 925–930.
7. Defer G, Moretti JL, Cesaro P, Sergent A, Raynaud C, Degos JD (1987) Early and delayed SPECT using N-isopropyl–p– iodoamphetamine iodine 123 in cerebral ischemia: A prognostic index for clinical recovery. Arch Neurol, 44:715–718.
8. The EC-IC Bypass Study Group (1985) Failure of extracranial-intracranial arterial bypass to reduce the risk of ischemic stroke. N Engl J Med 313:1191–1200.
9. Ell PJ, Lui D, Cullum I, Jarritt PH, Donaghy M, Harrison MJG (1983) Cerebral blood flow studies with 123 iodine-labelled amines. Lancet 1:1348–1352.
10. Ell PJ, Hocknell JML, Jarritt PH (1985) A Tc-99m-labelled radiotracer for the investigation of cerebrovascular disease. Nucl Med Commun 6:437–441.

11. Fazio F, Lenzi GL, Gerundini P, Collice M, Gilardi MC, Colombo R, Taddei G, Del Maschio A, Piacentini M, Kung HF, Blau M (1984) Tomographic assessment of regional cerebral perfusion using intravenous I-123 HIPDM and a rotating gamma-camera. J Comput Assist Tomogr 9:911–921.

12. Halsey JH, Morawetz RB, Blaunstein UW (1982) The hemodynamic effect of STA-MCA bypass. Stroke 12:163–167.

13. Hartmann A (1985) Prolonged disturbances of regional cerebral blood flow in transient ischemic attacks. Stroke 6:932–939.

14. Hill TC, Holman BL, Lovett R, O'Leary DH, Front D, Magistretti P, Zimmerman RE, Moore SC, Clouse ME, Wu JL, Lin TH, Baldwin RM (1982) Initial experience with SPECT (single-photon computerized tomography) of the brain using N-isopropyl I-123 p-iodoamphetamine. J Nucl Med 23:1911–1195.

15. Hill TC, Magistretti PL, Holman BL, Lee RGL, O'Leary DH, Uren RF, Royal HD, Mayman CI, Kolodny GM, Clouse ME (1984) Assessment of regional cerebral blood flow (rCBF) in stroke using SPECT and N-isopropyl-(I-123)-p-iodoamphetamine (IMP). Stroke 15:40–45.

16. Holm S, Anderson AR, Vorstrup S, Lassen NA, Paulson OB, Holamn LA (1985) Dynamic SPECT of the brain using a lipophilic technetium-99m complex, PnAO. J Nucl Med 26:1129–1134.

17. Holman BL, Zimmerman RE, Schapiro JR, Kaplan ML, Jones AG, Hill TC (1983) Biodistribution and dosimetry of N-isopropyl I-123 p-iodoamphetamine in the primate. J Nucl Med 24:922–931.

18. Holman BL, Lee RGL, Hill TC, et al. (1984) A comparison of two cerebral perfusion tracers N-isopropyl I-123 p-iodoamphetamine and I-123 HIPDM in the human. J Nucl Med 25:25–30.

19. Holman BL, Wick MM, Kaplan ML, Hill TC, Lee RGL, Wu J-L, Lin T-H (1984) The relationship of the eye uptake of N-isopropyl p-I-123-iodoamphetamine to melanin production. J Nucl Med 25:315–319.

20. Jagust WJ, Budinger TF, Reed BR (1987) The diagnosis of dementia with single photon emission computed tomography. Arch Neurol 44:258–262.

21. Johnson KA, Mueller ST, Walshe TM, English RJ, Holman BL (1987) Cerebral perfusion imaging in Alzheimer's disease. Arch Neurol 44:165–168.

22. Kempinsky WH (1958) Experimental study of distant effects of acute focal brain injury: A study of diaschisis. Arch Neurol Psychiatry 79:376–389.

23. Kjallquist A, Nardini M, Siesjo BK (1969) The effect of acetazolamide upon tissue concentrations of bicarbonate, lactate, and pyruvate in the cat brain. Acta Physiol Scand 77:241–251.

24. Knapp W, Von Kummer R, Kubler W (1986) Imaging of cerebral blood flow to volume distribution using SPECT. J Nucl Med 27:455–470.

25. Kobayashi H, Hayashi M, Kawano H, Handa Y, Nozaki J, Yamamoto S, Matsuda H (1985) Cerebral blood flow studies using N-isopropyl I-123 p iodoamphetamine. Stroke 16:293–296.

26. Kuhl DE, Barrio JR, Huang S-C, Selin C, Ackermann RF, Lear JL, Wu JL, Lin TH, Phelps M (1982) Quantifying local cerebral blood flow by N-isopropyl-p-123-I-iodoamphetamine (IMP) tomography. J Nucl Med 23:196–203.

27. Kung HF, Blau M (1982) Regional intracellular pH shift: A proposed new mechanism for radiopharmaceutical uptake in brain and other tissues. J Nucl Med 21:147–152.

28. Kung HF, Tramposch KM, Blau M (1983) A new brain perfusion imaging agent: I-123 HIPDM: N.N.N' - trimethyl - N' - 2 - hydroxy - 3 - methyl - 5 - iodobenzyl-1.3-propanediamine. J Nucl Med 24:66–72.

29. Kung HF, Billings J, Farrell E, Blau M (1985) The effect of anaesthetics on the uptake of brain imaging agents in rats. Nucl Med Commun 6:75–81.

30. Lassen NA, Ingvar DH (1961) The blood flow of the cerebral cortex determined by radioactive krypton-85. Experientia 17:42–45.

31. Lassen NA, Hoedt-Rasmussen K, Sorensen S (1963) Regional cerebral blood flow in man determined by krypton[85]. Neurology 13:719–727.

32. Lassen NA (1966) The luxury perfusion syndrome and its possible relation to acute metabolic acidosis localized within the brain. Lancet 2:1113–1115.

33. Lassen NA (1982) Incomplete cerebral infarction-focal incomplete ischemic tissue necrosis not leading to emollition. Stroke 13:522–523.

34. Lassen NA, Henriksen L, Holm S, Paulson DI, Paulson OB, Vorstrup S, Rapin J, le Poncin-Lafitte M, Moretti JL, Askienazy S, Raynaud C (1983) Cerebral blood-flow tomography: Xenon-133 compared with isopropyl-amphetamine-iodine-123. N Nucl Med 24: 17–21.

35. Larsson SA, Bergstrand G, Bergstedt H, Berg J, Flygare O, Schnell P, Andersson N, Lagergren C (1984) A special cutoff gamma camera for high resolution SPECT of the head. J Nucl Med 24:1023–1031.

36. Laux BE, Raichle ME (1978) The effect of acetazolamide on cerebral blood flow and oxygen utilization in the rhesus monkey. J Clin Invest 62:585–592.

37. Lee RG, Hill TC, Holman BL, Clouse ME (1982) N-isopropyl-(I-123)p-iodoamphetamine brain scans with single-photon emission tomography: Discordance with transmission computed tomography. Radiology 145:795–799.

38. Lenzi GL, Frackowiack RSJ, Jones T (1982) Cerebral oxygen metabolism and blood flow in human cerebral ischemic infarction. J Cereb Blood Flow Metab 2:321–335.

39. Lever SZ, Burns HD, Kervitsky A, Goldfarb HW, Woo DV, Wong DF, Epps LA, Kramer AV, Wagner HN (1985) The design, preparation and biodistribution of a technetium-99m triaminodithiol complex to assess regional cerebral blood flow. J Nucl Med 26: 1287–1294.

40. Leonard J-P, Nowotnik DP, Nerinckx RD (1986) Technetium-99m-d,l-Hm-PAO: A new radiopharmaceutical for imaging regional brain perfusion using SPECT: A comparison with iodine-123 HIPDM. J Nucl Med 27:1919–1823.

41. Lucignani G, Nehlig A, Blasberg R, Patlak CS, Anderson L, Fieschi C, Fazio F, Sokoloff L (1985) The

use of [^{125}I]HIPDM for quantitative measurement of regional cerebral blood flow. *J Cereb Blood Flow Metab* 5:86–96.

42. Marcoux FW, Morawetz RB, Crowell RM, DeGirolami U, Halsey JH (1982) Differential regional vulnerability in transient focal cerebral ischemia. *Stroke* 13:339–346.

43. Mies G, Auer LM, Ebhardt G, Traupe H, Heiss WD (1983) Flow and neuronal density in tissue surrounding chronic infarction. *Stroke* 14:22–27.

44. Von Monakow C (1914) *Die localization LM Grosshirn and der Abbau der Funktion durch Korlihale Herde*. Wiesbaden: JF Bergmann.

45. Moore SC, Doherty MD, Zimmerman RE, Holman BL (1984) Improved performance from modifications to the Harvard multi-detector SPECT brain scanner. *J Nucl Med* 25:688–691.

46. Moretti J-L, Askienazy S, Raynaud C, Lassen N, Sanabria E, Soussaline F, Bardy A, Le Poncin-Lafitte M, Caron J-P, Chodkiewick J-P (1983) N-isopropyl p-iodoamphetamine I-123: An agent for brain imaging with SPECT. In Magistretti PL (ed.) *Functional Radionuclide Imaging of the Brain*. New York: Raven Press, pp 231–246.

47. Moretti JL, Cesaro P, Louarn F, Askienazy S, Sanabria E, Raynaud C, Rapin JR, Coornaert S, Iachetti D, Degos JD (1984) N isopropyl amphetamine I-123 et tomoscintigraphie monophotonique dans les affections ischemiques cerebrales. *Cir et Metab du Cerveau* 2:63–75.

48. Moretti JL, Askienazy S, Raynaud C, Sergent A, Cesaro P, Tardy M (1986) I-123 p iodo isopropyl amphetamine (IAMP) for brain tumor diagnosis. In Biersack HJ (ed): *Amphetamines and ph-Shift Agents for Brain Imaging: Basic Research and Clinical Results*. Berlin, New York: Walter de Gruyter Company, pp 125–128.

49. Moretti JL, Cesaro P, Cinotti L, Defer G, Raynaud C, Ducassou D (1987) Tomoscintigraphy and subacute strokes: Comparative application with HMPAO Tc-99m and IMP I-123. *J Nucl Med* 28:623.

50. Moretti JL, Defer G, Cesaro P, Sergent A, Raynaud C, Holman BL (1987) Early and delayed IMP I-123 SPECT as a prognostic index for clinical recovery in cerebral ischemia. *J Nucl Med* 28:623.

51. Moretti JL, Cinotti L, Cesaro P, Defer G, Joulin Y, Sergent A, Vigneron N, Rapin JR, Raynaud C (1987) Amines for brain tomoscintigraphy. *Nucl Med Commun*, 8:581–595.

52. Moretti JL, Kung HF, Cesaro P, Blau M, Defer G, Holman BL, Vigneron N, Rapin J (1987) Temporal evoluation of brain distribution of IMP and HIPDM. *Nucl Med Commun*, in press.

53. Mueller SP, Polak JF, Kijewski MF, Holman BL (1986) Collimator selection for SPECT brain imaging: The advantages of high resolution. *J Nucl Med* 27:1729–1738.

54. Neirinckx RD, Canning LA, Piper JM, Nowotnik DP, Pickett Rd, Holmes RA, Volkert WA, Forster AM, Weisner PS, Marriott JA, Chaplin SB (1987) Technetium 99m d.1 HMPAO: A new radiopharmaceutical for SPECT imaging of regional cerebral blood perfusion. *J Nucl Med* 28:191–202.

55. Norrving B, Nilsson B, Risberg J (1982) rCBF in pa-

tients with carotid occlusion: Resting and hypercapnic flow related to collateral pattern. *Stroke* 13:155–162.

56. Oldendorf W, Braun L, Cornford E (1979) pH dependence of blood brain barrier permeability to lactate and nicotine. *Stroke* 10:577–521.

57. Olsen TS, Larsen B, Kriver EE, Herning M, Enevoldsen E, Lassen NA (1981) Focal cerebral hyperemia in acute stroke: Evidence, pathophysiology, and clinical significance. *Stroke* 2:598–606.

58. Pantano P, Baron JC, Samson Y, Bousser MG, Derouesne C, Comar D (1986): Crossed cerebellar diaschisis. *Brain* 109:677–694.

59. Pardridge WM, Connor JD (1973) Saturable transport of amphetamine across the blood-brain barrier. *Experientia* 29:302–304.

60. Pardridge WM, Sakiyama R, Fierer G (1984) Blood-brain barrier transport and brain sequestration of propranolol and lidocaine. *Am J Physiol* 247:R582–588.

61. Polak JF, Holman BL, Moretti JL, Eisner RL, Lister-James J, English RJ, (1984) I-123 HIPDM brain imaging with a rotating gamma camera and slant-hole collimator. *J Nucl Med* 25:495–498.

62. Rapin JR, Dutertre D, Le Poncin-Lafitte M, Lageron A, Monmaur P, Rips R, Lassen NA (1983) Iodoamphetamine derivative as tracers for cerebral blood flow or not? Autoradiography and authohistoradiographie studies. *J Cereb Blood Flow Metab* 3(suppl):105–106.

63. Rapin JR, Le Poncin-Lafitte M, Duterte D, Rips R, Morier E, Lassen N (1984) Iodoamphetamine as a new tracer for local cerebral blood flow in the rat: Comparison with isopropyliodoamphetamine. *J Cereb Blood Flow Metabol* 4:270–274.

64. Raynaud C, Rancurel G, Samson Y, Baron JL, Soucy JP, Kieffer E, Cabanis E, Majdalani A, Ricard S, Bardy A, Bourguignon M, Syrota A, Lassen N (1987) Pathophysiologic study of chronic infarcts with I-123 isopropyl iodoamphetamine (IMP). The importance of periinfarct area. *Stroke* 18:21–29.

65. Sakai F, Nakazawa K, Tazaki Y, Ishii K, Hino H, Igarashi H, Kanda T (1985) Regional cerebral blood volume and hematocrit measured in normal human volunteers by SPECT. *J Cereb Blood Flow Metab* 5:207–213.

66. Sapirstein LA (1958) Regional blood flow by fractional distribution of indicators. *Am J Physiol* 193 (I):161–168.

67. Schneck DW, Pritchard JF, Hayes AH Jr (1977) Studies on the uptake and binding of propranolol by rat tissues. *J Pharmacol Exp Ther* 203:621–629.

68. Sharp PF, Smith FW, Gemmell HG, Lyall D, Evans NT, Gvozdanovic D, Davidson J, Tyrell DA, Pickett RD, Neirinckx RD (1986) Technetium-99m- HMPAO stereoisomers as potential agents for imaging regional cerebral blood flow. *J Nucl Med* 27:171–177.

69. Spreafico G, Cammelli F, Gadola G, Freschi R, Zancaner F (1987) Luxury perfusion syndrome in cerebral vascular disease evaluated with technetium-99m HM-PAQ. *Clin Nucl Med* 12:217–218.

70. Stokely EM, Sveinsdottir E, Lassen NA, Rommer P

(1980) A single-photon dynamic computer assisted tomograph (DCAT) for imaging brain function in multiple cross-sections. *J Comput Assist Tomogr* 4:230–240.

71. Sugiyama M, Christensen J, Olsen TS, Lassen NA (1986) Monitoring CBF in clinical routine by dynamic single photon emission tomography (SPECT) of inhaled Xenon-133. *Stroke* 17:1179–1182.

72. Szasz IJ, Lyster D, Morrison RT (1985) Iodine 123 IMP uptake in brain metastases from lung cancer. *J Nucl Med* 26:1342–1343.

73. Touya JJ, Rahimian J, Grubbs DE, Corbus HF, Bennett LR (1985) A noninvasive procedure for in vivo assay of lung amine endothelial receptor. *J Nucl Med* 26:1302–1307.

74. Trauble H (1971) The movement of molecules across lipid membranes a molecular theory. *J Membr Biol* 4:193–208.

75. Troutner De, Volkert WA, Hoffman TJ (1984) A neutral lipophilic complex of Tc-99m with a multidentate amine oxime. Int J Appl Radiat Isotop 35:467–470.

76. Tsui BMW, Gullberg GT, Ederton ER, Gilland DR, Perry JR, McCartney WH (1986) Design and clinical utility of a fan beam collimator for SPECT imaging of the head. *J Nucl Med* 27:810–819.

77. Van Royen EA, DeBruine JF, Hill TC, Vyth A, Limburg M, Byse BL, O'Leary DH, DeJong JM, Hijdra A, Van Der Schoot JB (1987) Cerebral blood flow imaging with Tl-201 diethydithiocarbamate SPECT. *J Nucl Med* 28:178–183.

78. Von Schulthess GK, Ketz E, Schubiger PA, Bekier A (1985) Regional quantitative non-invasive assessment of cerebral perfusion and function with N-isopropyl I-123 p iodoamphetamine. *J Nucl Med* 26:9–16.

79. Volkert WA, Hoffman TJ, Seger RM (1984) Tc-99m propyleneamine oxime (Tc-99m-PnAO): A potential brain radiopharmaceutical. *Eur J Nucl Med* 9:511–516.

80. Vorstrup S, Hemmingsen R, Henriksen L, Lindewald H, Engell HC, Lassen NA (1983) Regional cerebral blood flow in patients with transient ischemic attacks studied by xenon-133 inhalation and emission tomography. *Stroke* 14:903–910.

81. Vorstrup S, Henriksen L, Paulson OB (1984) Effect of acetazolamide on cerebral blood flow and cerebral metabolic rate for oxygen. *J Clin Invest* 74:1634–1639.

82. Vorstrup S, Lassen NA, Henriksen L, Haase J, Lindewald H, Boysen G, Paulson OB (1985) CBF before and after extracranial-intracranial bypass surgery in patients with ischemic cerebrovascular disease studied with xenon-133 inhalation tomography. *Stroke* 16:616–626.

83. Vorstrup S, Brun B, Lassen NA (1986) Evaluation of the cerebral vasodilatory capacity by the acetazolomide test before EC-IC bypass surgery in patients with occlusion of the internal carotid artery. *Stroke* 17:1291–1298.

84. Waltz AG, Sundt TM (1967) The microvasculature and microcirculation of the cerebral cortex after arterial occlusion. *Brain* 90:681–696.

85. Winchell HS, Baldwin RM, Lin TH (1980) Development of I-123-labeled amines for brain studies: Localization of I-123 iodophenylalkyl amines in rat brain. *J Nucl Med* 21:940–946.

86. Winchell HS, Horst WA, Braum L, Oldendorf WH, Hattner R, Parker H (1980) N-isopropyl (I123) p-iodoamphetamine: Single-pass brain uptake and washout, binding to brain synaptosomes and localization in dog and monkey brain. *J Nucl Med* 21:947–952.

8

Functional Imaging of Brain Ischemia

Michael Kushner, MD and Martin Reivich, MD

Cerebrovascular Research Center, Department of Neurology, University of Pennsylvania School of Medicine, Philadelphia, Pennsylvania 19104-6063.

INTRODUCTION

Historically the investigation of cerebrovascular disease in man has relied upon correlations between pathology, neurologic function, and vascular anatomy. Research dealing with the pathophysiology of brain ischemia was limited to global or 2-dimensional estimates of cerebral blood flow and global cerebral oxygen consumption derived from clearance techniques such as the Kety-Schmidt method [27] and the xenon-133 technique [36,45]. Over the last decade computed tomography using x-rays and magnetic waves more recently has permitted structural investigations to be performed during life [24].

In contrast, studies of cerebral ischemia in animals have enjoyed the benefits of laboratory methods that permit studies of high spatial resolution and multiple physiologic parameters [14,61]. Work from animal models has demonstrated that the physiologic consequences of hypoperfusion leading to eventual tissue damage are complex and manifest themselves both in gross alterations of tissue hemodynamics and cellular biochemistry [23,60].

For several years the technique of positron emission tomography (PET) has enabled quantitative 3-dimensional imaging of cerebral hemodynamics and metabolism [2,50]. During this time, work from a number of laboratories has begun to describe the pathophysiology of cerebral ischemia and infarction in quantitative physiologic terms [1,6,7,11,28,40,53,58]. Further, the correlation of ischemic brain damage with subsequent neurologic function and outcome has provided a new means with which to establish the clinical correlates of brain ischemia [31]. The insights gained from these studies have detailed the balance between cerebral blood flow, cerebral hemodynamics, and cerebral metabolism over a continuum ranging from early asymptomatic disturbances in cerebral hemodynamics to ischemia and infarction [16,38,67]. This review is intended to summarize the current understanding of the pathophysiology of brain ischemia gained from PET studies in man.

CEREBRAL HEMODYNAMICS

The process of cerebral infarction is a complicated one arising from alterations in local cerebral hemodynamics as well as cellular biochemical processes [60]. Within the ischemic cell, disruption of the plasma membrane and internal cytoarchitecture can lead to multiple and complex alterations in cellular biochemistry including ionic shifts, activation of prostaglandins, disruption in superoxide catabolism, and other potentially damaging events [51,56,60]. As yet these cellular processes have not lent themselves to 3-dimensional cerebral imaging in man. Current PET technology allows measurement of cerebral blood flow (LCBF), oxygen and glucose consumption (LCMRC$_2$ and LCMRglu), cerebral blood volume (CBV) and pH [3,12,52,64].

In mammalian brain the majority of the energy demand required for primary cellular activities and electrochemical transmission is

---

This work was supported in part by Program Project Grant NS-14867-08 from the United States Public Health Service. Dr. Kushner is the recipient of Clinical Investigator Development Award 1 KO8 NS 00999-03.

Noninvasive Imaging of Cerebrovascular Disease, pages 163–174
© 1989 Alan R. Liss, Inc.

met by the process of oxidative glycolysis [56]. Early studies employing the Kety-Schmidt method have demonstrated that the rate of substrate delivery far exceeds normal cerebral metabolic demand [27]. Studies in animal and man have also demonstrated that homeostatic mechanisms exist whereby the level of CBF is maintained at a relatively constant level over a wide range of perfusion pressures [19]. For practical purposes the mean cerebral perfusion pressure can be approximated by the difference between mean systemic arterial blood pressure and intracranial pressure, this being the pressure gradient over the arterial-venous circuit. This phenomenon has been termed autoregulation since early times and is dependent upon the interrelationships between perfusion pressure, cerebrovascular resistance, and cerebral blood flow (Ohm's law for fluids). A progressive decline in perfusion pressure must be met by a compensatory decline in resistance in the cerebrovascular bed for the CBF to be maintained. Below mean cerebral perfusion pressures of 70–80 torr, the relation between cerebral blood becomes linear and nonautoregulatory (Fig. 8–1). In this range, cerebral blood flow declines and varies directly with declining perfusion pressure. Here the reduction in cerebral vascular resistance is near maximal, and compensatory vasoreaction is no longer significant.

Beyond normal autoregulation other compensatory mechanisms are available whereby cerebral metabolism is maintained despite a declining cerebral blood flow (Fig. 8–1) [16]. This state of preserved metabolism in the face of declining levels of cerebral perfusion has been dubbed the "critical perfusion" state by Frackowiak [13] and the "misery-perfusion" state by Baron [5]. Normal levels of oxidative metabolism are maintained by increased efficiency with which oxygen is extracted from residual cerebral blood flow. This increase in oxygen extraction fraction (OEF) is likely the result of local tissue alterations arising from oligemia, decreased blood transit time, and the accumulation of local metabolic by-products that may serve to enhance the dissociation of oxyhemoglobin by the Bohr effect. In theory it is conceivable that oxygen extraction may rise from the normal rate of about 40% up to a near maximum rate of 100% before oxidative metabolism is placed in jeopardy. At maximal OEF values, oxygen delivery to tissue cannot increase, and $CMRO_2$ is jeopardized. It is in the range where $CMRO_2$ and CBF vary directly that true ischemia may be defined. Ischemia may be thought of as the state where all the compensatory hemodynamic mechanisms have been exhausted and cerebral tissue faces an increasing potential energy deficit as the actual rate of substrate delivery (e.g., CBF) progressively declines [26]. In theory, anaerobic glycolysis or the consumption of noncarbohydrate moieties may serve to fill this energy gap, but these processes would signal a shift away from normal cerebral oxidative metabolism [51,60].

With ischemia, and energy failure, the tissue is at risk for membrane ion-pumping failure, failure of electrochemical transmissions, and actual cytotoxic damage, or infarction. Energy consumption in infarcted regions may become vanishingly small, and residual cerebral metabolism is no longer limited by absolute levels of cerebral blood flow [56,60]. In infarction, residual substrate delivery far outstrips metabolic demand producing "luxury perfusion" or nonnutritive flow [7,12].

Ischemia and Infarction

Available evidence from clinical studies suggests that ischemia leading to eventual tissue destruction, or infarction, is resolved relatively quickly in a matter of hours or at least a few days [18,68]. To date PET studies of human cerebral ischemia have been limited by the vagaries of performing these studies within this time frame. Despite these limitations a characteristic disruption of the normal coupling between cerebral blood flow and metabolism has been demonstrated within areas of cerebral infarction [6,67]. Serial studies in a limited number of patients have demonstrated a uniformly low OEF in infarction indicating a failure of normal oxidative metabolism despite residual CBF in excessive metabolic demand [68]. Studies of LCMRglu using 18F-FDG also have demonstrated near uniform hypometabolism in infarcted regions [6,31]. The features of absolutely depressed levels of $CMRO_2$, LCMRglu and uncoupling of the normal flow-metabolism relationship, as evidenced by abnormally low OEF, comprise the characteristic

Functional Imaging of Brain Ischemia 165

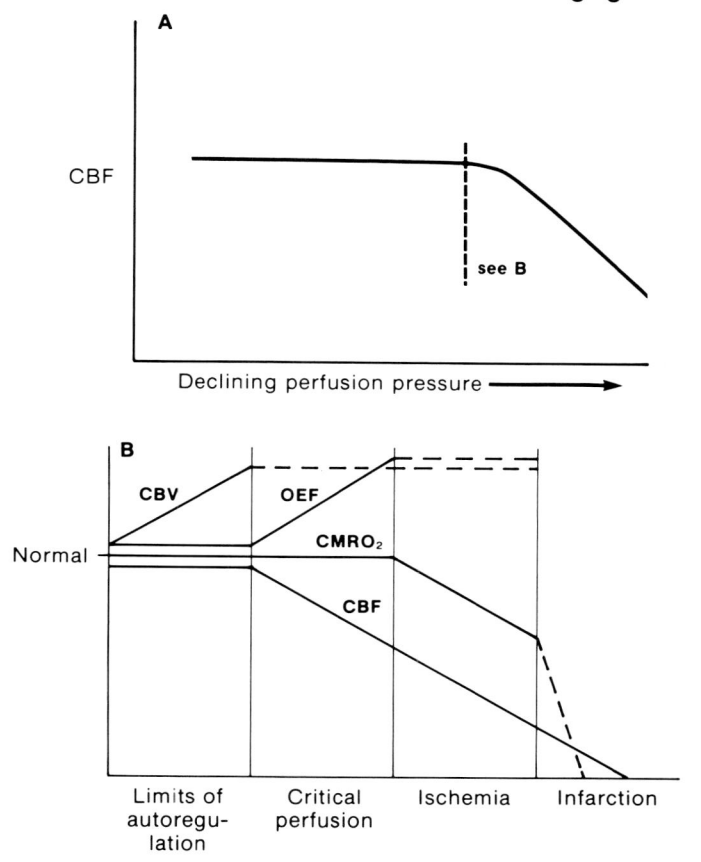

Figure 8–1. **A:** Autoregulation. CBF remains stable over a wide range of perfusion pressures. **B:** Compensatory mechanisms. At the limits of autoregulation, CBF may remain stable due to compensatory vasodilation, resulting in decreased cerebrovascular resistance. This can be accompanied by a measurable increase in CBV. With maximal vasodilation (critical perfusion) CBF declines linearly with further decrements in perfusion pressure, but CMRO$_2$ may remain stable due to an increasing OEF. With further declines in perfusion pressure, OEF becomes maximal and CMRO$_2$ is linked linearly with flow (ischemia). When CMRO$_2$ is strictly flow-dependent, the cell faces an energy deficit that may be manifested by disturbances in electrochemical transmission and other cytochemical processes. If the energy deficit is severe, then membrane disruption or other serious cellular defects may lead to irreversible damage (infarction). After infarction has occurred, then residual CBF may be in excess of residual cell energy requirement, e.g., luxury perfusion.

metabolic profile of tissue infarction beyond 72 hours after the ischemic ictus (Fig. 8–2).

Nearer to the time of the ischemic ictus the pattern of cerebral metabolism may be more variable. Several authors have noted the expected decrease in CBF coincident with an elevation of the OEF [6,67]. Acutely the imbalance between CMRO$_2$ and CBF is manifested by an abnormally elevated OEF, and this may be a more common finding within several hours of the ischemic ictus (Fig. 8–3). This phenomenon likely represents the transition from the state of the late critical perfusion phase and early ischemic phase to true infarction (Fig. 8–1B). As mentioned previously, a depressed oxygen extraction faction indicates the tissue metabolic demand is no longer limited by substrate delivery. However these ob-

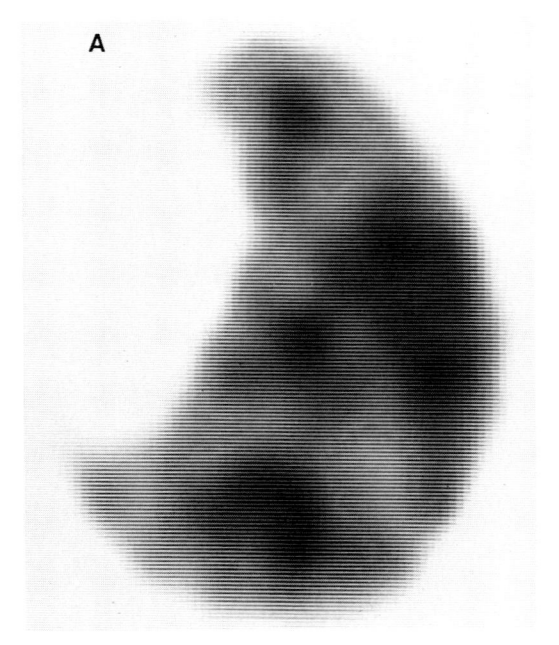

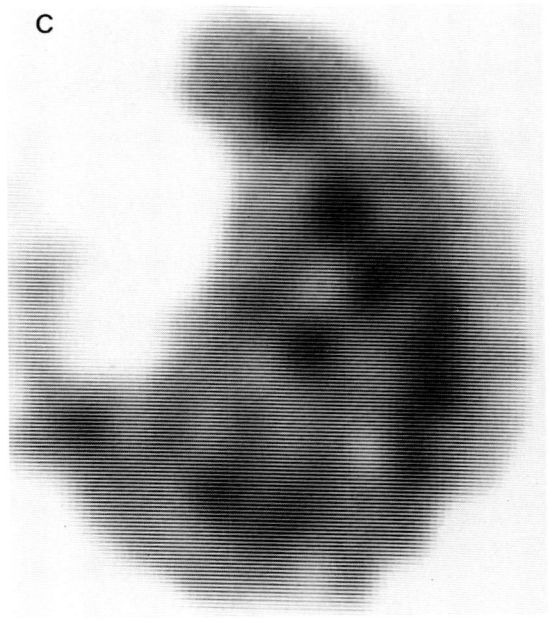

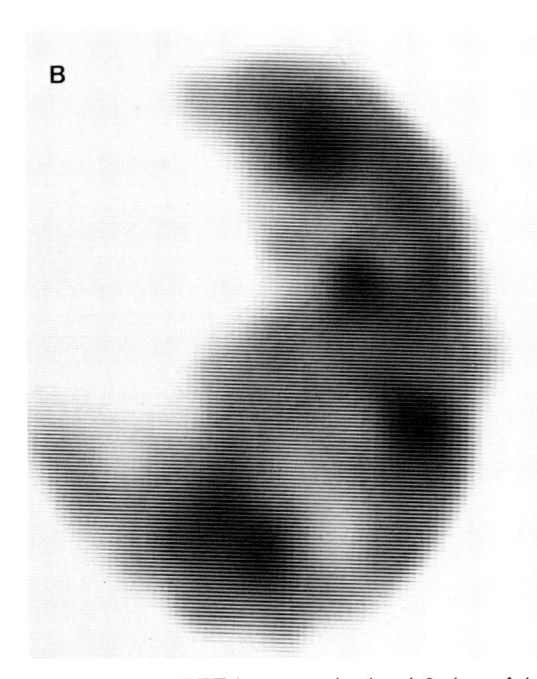

Figure 8–2. PET images obtained 3 days following right internal carotid artery occlusion in a 67-year-old man. There is a uniform reduction in LCBF (**A**), CMRO$_2$ (**B**), and LCMRglu (**C**).

servations have not been uniform. Baron et al. [6], Ackerman et al. [1], and Hakim et al. [18] have demonstrated that the CBF is variously depressed, normal, or even increased in areas of ischemic infarction. This may reflect the clinical heterogeneity of the primary vascular insult leading to ischemia. Persistently reduced levels of cerebral blood flow may accompany vascular occlusion, while normal levels of CBF or reactive hyperemia could follow embolic occlusion with secondary clot lysis and reperfusion, or shock-related cerebral ischemia.

It is likely that the change in the direction of the OEF is a reliable indicator of the transition from local tissue ischemia to true infarction [53]. An increased OEF may be regarded as a compensatory mechanism to derive maximal use of residual CBF substrate delivery capacity while a depressed OEF indicates that normal metabolic processes have been sorely, and probably irreversibly, disrupted. It is conceivable that measures designed to restore perfusion could have significant clinical impact if they could be initiated before the terminal decline of OEF [54,55]. Unfortunately the data of Wise et al. [67] have suggested that the transition of OEF from abnormally high to abnor-

Functional Imaging of Brain Ischemia 167

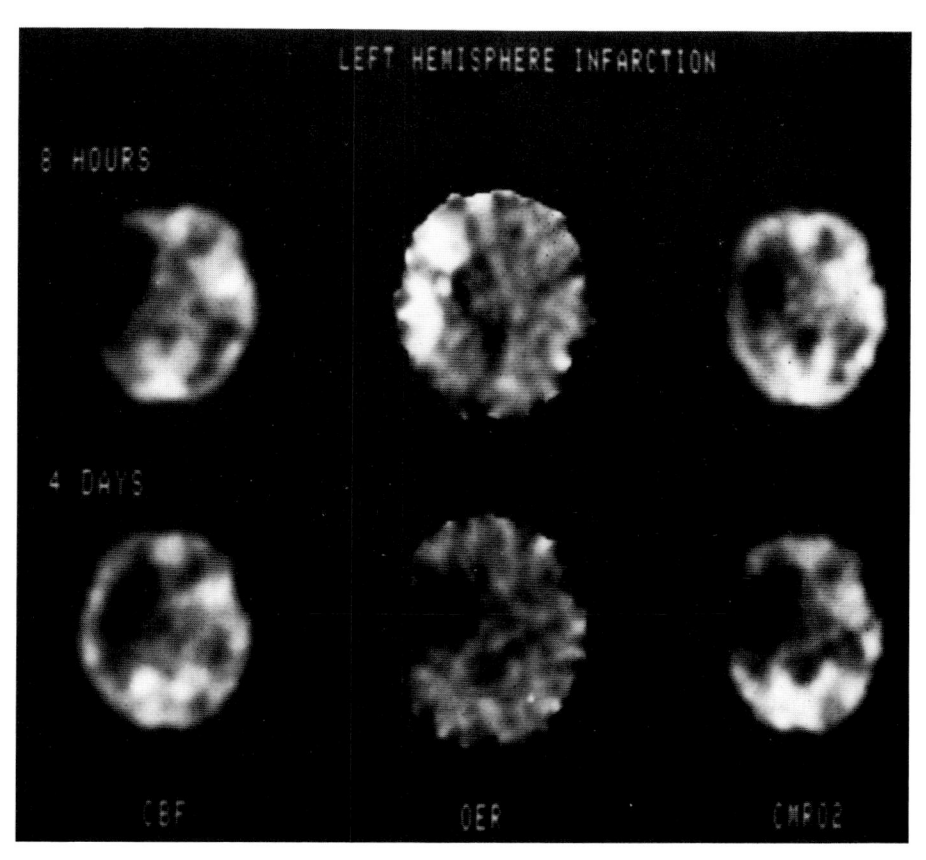

Figure 8–3. Serial studies of LCBF and LCMRO$_2$ following middle cerebral artery branch infarction. Eight hours after the ictus, there is a focal increase in our OEF (OER) in the area of hypoperfusion/hypometabolism. At 4 days, infarction is complete, and focally the OEF is subnormal. This indicates that residual CBF is in excess for residual tissue energy requirements in the infarction, e.g., redundant flow or luxury perfusion. The earlier study illustrates tissue hemodynamics in the ischemia range (see Fig. 8–1B) because an increase in OEF was accompanied by a decrease in LCMRO$_2$. (Photo courtesy of Dr. Richard Frackowiak).

mally low levels is established within only a few hours of the ischemic ictus. Regrettably standard clinical intervention generally cannot be expected to be accomplished within that period of time except under specialized circumstances.

Some uncertainties in current methodologies are raised by local metabolic conditions and ischemic brain. Firstly, tissue activity from unextracted O15-labeled molecular oxygen could lead to over estimates of CMRO$_2$ and OEF if the local cerebral blood volume is greater than normal [25,35]. Such a situation could arise in areas of ischemic brain evidencing reactive hyperemia or in areas subject to critical perfusion with a maximal dilation of the cerebral resistance vessels. Many centers now obtain measurements of cerebral blood volume in order to correct for this potential source of error [35]. Also ischemic conditions have been shown to alter the rate constants, and possibly the lumped constant, needed for estimation of LCMRglu by the Sokoloff model [17,20,21,57,62]. Wise et al. [68] observed that absolute levels of LCMRglu were significantly reduced in areas of infarction and that this residual glucose consumption was not wholly oxidative in nature. They suggested that some residual LCMRglu in areas of infarction actually reflect local metabolism by nonneural components such as macrophages and glial elements. The precise impact of these perturbations upon determinations of LCMRglu using the Sokoloff model are as yet uncertain. Recent work by Hakim et al. [18] has suggested that actual ischemic conditions may be prevalent only during the first few hours of infarction.

Syrota et al. [64] has noted an absolute alkalosis in areas of infarction using C11-DMO in studies of intracellular pH. These results do not support the notion of significant primary biochemical lactacidosis arising from hypoperfusion. The finding of a nonacidic pH coupled with other observations of physiologic early reflow in areas of infarction suggest that actual ischemia, or a depressed CBF, is often transient in symptomatic cerebral ischemia.

The absence of acidic pH in human infarcts is as yet unaccounted for. Numerous animal models of stroke employing autoradiographic techniques have demonstrated glycolysis in excess of oxygen consumption that has been thought to be due to anaerobic conditions arising in an acidic tissue milieu [14,51]. Despite this animal work, most human studies have indicated relatively coupled glucose and oxygen consumption in infarcted tissue [18,68].

States of Critical Perfusion

The relationship between cerebral arterial stenosis and tissue ischemia has long been recognized. Only recently has PET provided a pathophysiologic mechanism for the relationship between arterial stenosis and tissue hypoperfusion. A state of critical hemodynamics may be identified in cerebral tissue "downstream" from hemodynamically significant stenotic lesions [16,55,59]. Gibbs et al. [16] first noted an increase in CBV with normal CBF and $CMRO_2$ in the hemisphere ispllsilateral to carotid artery occlusion. This finding suggested that normal autoregulatory mechanisms permitted compensatory vasodilation and thus a reduction in cerebrovascular resistance. This reduction in resistance is produced by an increase in the caliber of the cerebral resistance vessels (Fig. 8–1).

Serial studies of the effects of extra-intracranial bypass surgery have demonstrated that CBV is reduced following surgery with either no change or increased in CBF [54,59]. Powers et al. [55] found a consistent decrease in CBV following bypass surgery for major vessel stenosis/occlusion with a variable change in CBF and $CMRO_2$. Patients with transient ischemia and no CT evidence of tissue damage tended to exhibit increased CBF and $CMRO_2$ following extra-intracranial bypass surgery. This was not the case in patients with fixed ischemic lesions in whom CBF and $CMRO_2$ did not change significantly despite a post-bypass increase in CBF. It was postulated that fixed tissue damage superimposed upon critical cerebral hemodynamics was responsible for this lack of metabolic response. Baron et al. [3] postulated that long-standing marginal perfusion may contribute to neural deactivation that manifests itself as persistently borderline or modestly depressed, CBF and $CMRO_2$ in the tissue area perfused following bypass surgery. It has been suggested that true increases in CBF can be produced following bypass surgery in the "borderzone" areas of anastomosis between the territories of the anterior and middle cerebral arteries and the carotid-vertebral basilar circulation [37].

The concept of a state of critical perfusion leading to the exhaustion of autoregulation capacity and subsequent hypoperfusion and ischemia is an attractive one. These states can be inferred by the observation of 1) increased CBV, 2) increased OEF, and 3) decreasing $CMRO_2$. Despite this formulation in the disappointing results of the cooperative EC-IC bypass trial dampens enthusiasm for general applications of this procedure [66]. Further studies employing PET might eventually identify an appropriate subpopulation where bypass surgery could be justified.

Remote Metabolic Effects of Cerebral Ischemia

Among the most surprising developments arising from functional imaging in cerebral ischemia and infarction has been the observation that metabolism in remote and intact neural tissue may be altered by focal ischemia [9, 22,29,30,41–43]. It is not surprising to find widespread metabolic disturbances following CT visualization of focal cortical infarction. Also PET images may reveal profoundly disturbed cerebral metabolism in the absence of structural change identified by CT or MRI [31]. As yet, precise mechanisms underlying these remote metabolic perturbations are not fully understood. Transneuronal inactivation, the release of neurotoxic substances or false neurotransmitters, and diaschisis have all been offered as mechanisms for this phenomenon [4,43,44,46,63]. Increasingly, however, new data suggest that there exists a close link between the functional neurologic state and the pattern of cerebral metabolism [31]. The evidence supporting this view will be outlined in the following section and the commonly observed patterns of remote cerebral dysmetabolism will be reviewed.

IPSILATERAL THALAMIC HYPOMETABOLISM

Numerous authors have described metabolic disturbance of the intact thalamus following cortical infarction following the original description by Kuhl et al. [28]. Thalamic hypometabolism has been noted with cortical infarction involving widespread regions of both right and left hemispheres [3,28,31]. Thalamic hypometabolism has also been seen with subcortical lacunar infarction (Fig. 8–4). Most reports have cited remote dysmetabolism in the structurally intact thalamus as being transient, generally clearing over subsequent weeks. Our results suggested that thalamic hypometabolism following left hemispheric infarction is closely related to the presence or absence of aphasia [32]. These data will be summarized below (Functional Correlates of Acute Ischemic Infarction). Several observers have described a halo effect where a surrounding zone of less-intense hypometabolism is observed about the ischemic core [6,28]. This is demonstrated by branch cortical artery occlusion where partial volume effects cannot be expected to generate this surrounding area of hypometabolism in adjacent neural tissue.

In addition to a halo of hypometabolism surrounding focal cortical infarction there is occasionally seen characteristic disturbances of metabolism in the cortical mantle overlying subcortical infarction [3,31]. This phenomenon (Fig. 8–4) appears to be transient, with restoration of more normal cortical metabolism over time. Again the mechanism for this phenomenon remains uncertain, but undercutting

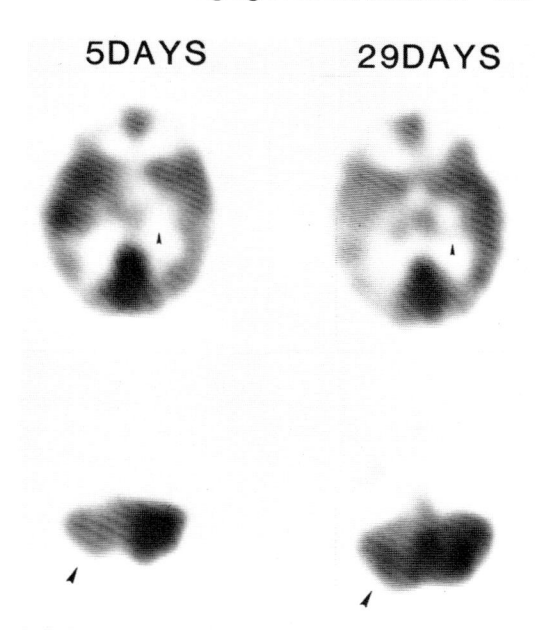

SUBCORTICAL LESION– REMOTE DEPRESSION

Figure 8–4. Remote depression of metabolism following subcortical infarction. At 5 days after the ictus, a focus of hypometabolism is present in the posterior limb of the right internal capsule. There is remote metabolic depression in the overlying cortical mantle, ipsilateral thalamus, and contralateral cerebellum. At 29 days, metabolism has normalized in these areas remote from the infarction, leaving a small area of subcortical hypometabolism (Reference 31).

of the cortex with interruption of afferent and efferent projections seems a popular explanation.

The mechanism of deafferentation clearly seems responsible for the characteristic visual cortical hypometabolism observed with lesions of the anterior optic pathways [9,28]. Striking depressions in striate metabolism are seen ipsilateral to lesions in the optic radiations, and these have been found to correspond specifically with the pattern of homonomous visual field loss [9].

CEREBELLAR HYPOMETABOLISM

Among the first regions to be recognized as being subject to remote hypometabolism was the cerebellar hemisphere contralateral to a supratentorial lesion (Fig. 8–4). Beginning with earliest report of Baron et al. [4], crossed cerebellar hypometabolism and hypoperfusion has been observed in the setting of cerebral infarction, transient ischemic attack, brain tumor, head trauma, and rarely in Alzheimer's disease [29,34,39,49]. With chronic disorders such as brain tumor, crossed cerebellar hypometabolism is generally chronic [29,48]. With ischemia, the phenomenon has been seen to resolve during the subacute phase, but persists in the majority of cases [39,47]. The determinants of resolution (or persistence) of remote cerebellar hypometabolism are not understood. Neither are the clinical correlates of this phenomenon clear-cut. Several observers have found a striking association between parietal hypometabolism and contralateral cerebellar hypometabolism [29,39]. Others have maintained that large lesions involving portions of both the parietal and the frontal lobes are needed [4,41,47]. In contrast to these observations we have found that small subcortical lesions, often nonresolvable by CT scan, may be associated with striking crossed cerebellar hypometabolism [31]. In our experience the presence of clear-cut clinical signs of ataxia have been seen in only one case with cerebellar hypometabolism and frontal brain tumor with falsely localizing ataxia [15]. The actual correlation of neurologic abnormalities with cerebellar hypometabolism remain unresolved.

Functional Correlates of Acute Ischemic Infarction

Most work to date dealing with emission computed tomography in cerebral infarction has focused on the local interrelationship between cerebral blood flow and metabolism in ischemic and infarcted tissue [3,31]. In part, these human studies have been influenced by the vast animal literature dealing with experimental stroke models [14]. Beyond these considerations, noninvasive studies of cerebral blood flow and metabolism in man have begun to suggest that the clinical state may influence, and in turn be influenced, by patterns of cerebral metabolism [8,31]. Certainly the clinician has a keen interest in prognosis, degree of recovery, and integrating the patterns of anatomic metabolic disruptions with the overall clinical picture. Current PET results suggest that useful information concerning degree of functional impairment and recovery can be gained from studies of cerebral blood flow and metabolism. In addition, these techniques hold forth the promise of providing a powerful new means for the clinicoanatomic localization of cerebral function.

Studies by Kuhl et al. [28] and Metter et al. [42] suggested that the area of metabolic disturbance could exceed the extent of anatomic damage. Results from our laboratory have suggested that widespread metabolic disruption in the left cerebral hemisphere is the rule in patients with acute ischemic asphasia (Fig. 8–5). In 15 asphasic patients, we have found ispilateral depression of thalamic metabolism in 11 of 13 cases; in nine of these 11 cases the thalamus was uninvolved by edema, mass effect, or possible ischemia [32]. Quantitative analysis of regional cerebral metabolism and patient performance on standized asphasia testing has indicated a high degree of correlation between residual language ability and regional LCMRglu. This finding is independent of the presence of anatomic disturbance seen on CT or MR. Of the recognized language-associated areas of the left hemisphere (including Wernicke's area, Broca's area, basal ganglia, thalamus, and opercular cortex), it is metabolism in the temporoparietal junction, or Wernicke's area, that is most highly correlated with language performance (Fig. 8–6). These results reinforce the notion that the left cerebral hemisphere is specialized for language function [65]. Further these observations suggest that language, and possibly other higher cortical functions, are affected by anatomically disparate, but functionally interconnected brain regions. It is conceivable that a lesion anywhere within this functionally interconnected network may lead to aphasia. Rather than the exact location of the lesion, it is possible that the specific disruption of the integrative processes of language may underly the clinical "phenotype" of aphasia. Such speculations as these will benefit from further study in lesioned patients and by studies of cerebral language processing by the normal brain [33].

We have found that ictal studies of cerebral metabolism may have been useful in establishing prognosis following acute ischemic infarction [31]. These results suggest that the spatial extent of metabolic disruption, rather than fo-

Functional Imaging of Brain Ischemia 171

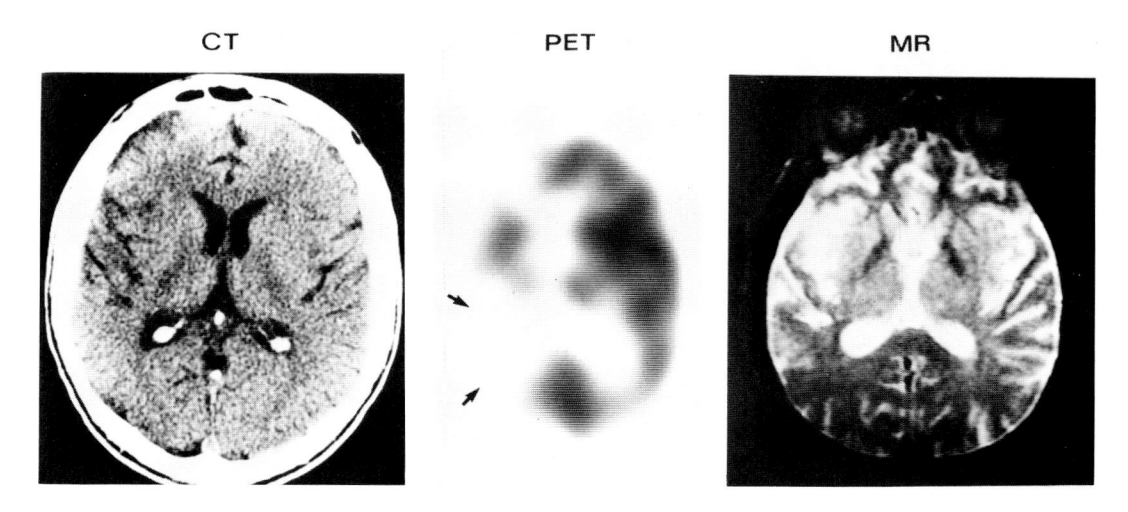

CT   PET   MR

Figure 8–5. Metabolic derangement in the absence of anatomic abnormality. This patient had left parietal cortical branch occlusion documented by cerebral arteriography. The clinical syndrome included dense Wernicke's aphasia and minimal motor weakness. Profound hypometabolism is noted at the temporoparietal junction. There is also hypometabolism of the ipsilateral thalamus, basal ganglia, and posteroinferior frontal region. Acute and chronic CT showed no abnormality. Also, MRI using multiple pulse sequences was normal (Reference 31).

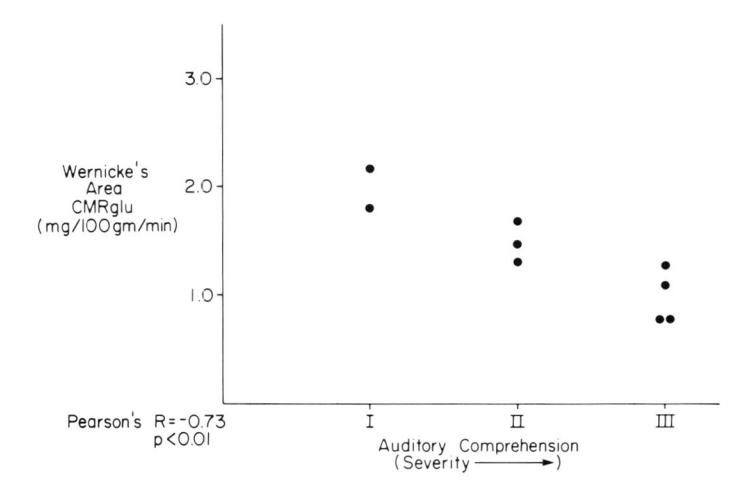

Figure 8–6. Correlation of language performance with LCMRglu. Metabolism in Wernicke's area was compared with the severity of auditory comprehension deficits. I = paragraph level errors, II = sentence level errors, and III = word level errors. The comprehension deficit correlated directly with Wernicke's area LCMRglu.

cal intensity of metabolic disruption in the area of infarction, is more closely related to degree of recovery (Fig. 8–7). In general, our results have indicated the ictal and subacute CT and MR do not correlate with degree of eventual recovery. Metabolic disturbances in multiple lobes predict polysymptomatic neurologic dysfunction and are associated with a

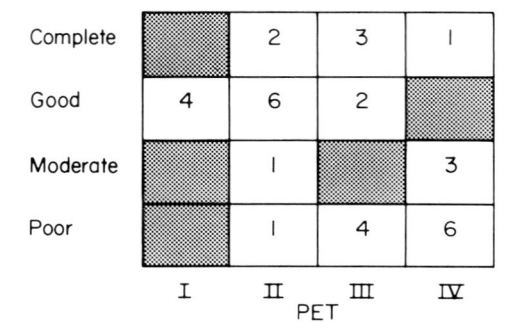

Figure 8–7. Comparison of PET with recovery. The degree of recovery following stroke was compared with the extent of the metabolic abnormality. PET grade I = normal scan, II = lesion less than 2 cm, III = subpolar lesion, IV = lobar or multilobar. The greater the PET abnormality, the greater the likelihood of a poor outcome (Reference 31).

worse prognosis. A retrospective analysis has shown that patients destined for a complete recovery or only mildly persisting deficits, regardless of the initial degree of functional impairment, have an overwhelming tendency for normal patterns of cerebral metabolism or only mild metabolic derangement. This approach may become more widespread in the future [8].

As mentioned previously, the presence of local increase of OEF in the area is consider indicative of retained, although tenuous, tissue viability. Recent developments using SPECT imaging and perfusion agents such as IMP have suggested that a retained, although delayed, uptake of IMP is suggestive of some retention of neural tissue viability [10]. Future studies examining remote metabolic function and clinical parameters may clarify the balance between local and remote tissue function and clinical outcome.

References

1. Ackerman RH, Correia JA, Alpert NM, Baron JC, Gouliamos A, Grotta JC (1981) Positron imaging in ischemic stroke disease using compound labeled with oxygen 15. *Arch Neurol* 38:537–543.
2. Alavi A, Reivich M, Jones SC, Greenberg JH, Wolf AP (1982) Functional imaging of the brain with positron emission tomography. In *Nuclear Medicine Annual* pp 319–372.
3. Baron JC (1985) Positron tomography in cerebral ischemia. *Neuroradiology* 27:509–516.
4. Baron JC, Bousser MG, Comar D, et al. (1981) Crossed cerebellar diaschisis: A remote functional depression secondary to supratentorial infarction in man. *J Cereb Blood Flow Metab* 1(Suppl 1):S500–S501.
5. Baron JC, Bousser MG, Guillard A, Comar D, Castaigne R (1981) Reversal of focal "misery-perfusion syndrome" by extra-intracranial arterial bypass in hemodynamic cerebral ischemia. *Stroke* 12:454–459.
6. Baron JC, Rougemont D, Bousser MG, Lebrun-Grandie P, Iba-Zizen TM (1983) Local CBF, oxygen extraction fraction (OEF), and $CMRO_2$: Prognostic value in recent supratentorial infarction in humans. *J Cereb Flood Flow Metab* 3(Suppl):S1–S2.
7. Baron MD, Rougemont D, Soussaline F, Bustany P, Crouzel C, Bousser MG, Comar D (1984) Local interrelationships of cerebral oxygen consumption and glucose utilization in normal subjects and in ischemic stroke patients: A positron tomography study. *J Cereb Blood Flow Metab* 4:140–149.
8. Beil C, Hebold I, Pawlik G, et al. (1987) Correlative clinco-metabolic short term follow-up in ischemic stroke by positron emission tomography of 2(18F)-fluorodeoxyglucose and standardized clinical ratings. *J Cereb Blood Flow Metab* 7(Suppl 1):S20.
9. Bosley TM, Dann R, Silver F, Alavi A, Kushner M, Sussman NM, Savino PJ, Sergott RR, Schatz WJ, Reivich M (1987) Recovery of vision after ischemic lesions: Positron emission tomography. *Ann Neurol* 21:444–450.
10. Defer G, Moretti JL, Cesaro P, et al. (1987) Early and delayed SPECT using N-isopropyl p-todoamphetamine iodine 123 in cerebral ischemia. *Arch Neurol* 44:715–718.
11. Frackowiak RSJ (1985) Pathophysiology of human cerebral ischemia: Studies with positron tomography and ^{15}oxygen. In Sokoloff L (ed): *Brain Imaging and Brain Function*. New York: Raven Press, 139–161.
12. Frackowiak RSJ (1985) The pathophysiology of human cerebral ischemia: A new perspective obtained with positron tomography. *Q J Med* 223:713–727.
13. Frackowiak RSJ, Wise RJS (1983) Positron tomography in ischemic cerebrovascular disease. *Neurol Clin* 1:183–200.
14. Garcia JH (1984) Experimental ischemic stroke: A review. *Stroke* 15:5–14.
15. Gassel MM (1964) False localizing signs. *Arch Neurol* 4:70–98.
16. Gibbs JM, Leenders KL, Wise RJS, Jones T (1984) Evaluation of cerebral perfusion reserve in patients with carotid-artery occlusion. *Lancet* 1:310–314.
17. Gjedde A, Wienhard K, Heiss W-D, Kloster G, Diemer NH, Herholz K, Pawlik G (1985) Comparative regional analysis of 2-fluorodeoxyglucose and methylglucose uptake in brain of four stroke patients. With special reference to the regional estimation of the lumped constant. *J Cereb Blood Flow Metab* 5:163–178.
18. Hakim AM, Pokrupa RP, Villanueva J, et al. (1987)

The effect of spontaneous reperfusion on metabolic function in early human cerebral infarcts. Ann Neurol 21:279–289.
19. Harper AM, Glass HI (1965) The effect of alterations in the arterial carbon dioxide tension on the blood flow through the cerebral cortex at normal and low arterial blood pressures. J Neurol Neurosurg Psychiatry 28:449–452.
20. Hawkins RA, Phelps ME, Huang S-C, Kuhl DE (1981) Effect of ischemia on quantification of local cerebral glucose metabolic rate in man. J Cereb Blood Flow Metab 1:37–51.
21. Heiss W-D, Pawlik G, Herholz K, Wagner R, Goldner H, Wienhard K (1984) Regional kinetic constants and cerebral metabolic rate for glucose in normal human volunteers determined by dynamic positron emission tomography of [^{18}F]-2-fluoro-2-deoxy-D-glucose. J Cereb Blood Flow Metab 4:212–223.
22. Heiss W-D, Pawlik G, Wagner R, Ilsen HW, Herholz K, Wienhard K (1983) Functional hypometabolism of noninfarcted brain regions in ischemic stroke. J Cereb Blood Flow Metab 3(Suppl 1):S582–S583.
23. Hossmann K-A (1982) Treatment of experimental cerebral ischemia. J Cereb Blood Flow Metab 2:275–297.
24. Hounsfield G (1980) Computed medical imaging. Science 210:22–28.
25. Jones T, Chesler DA, Tar-Pugussian MM (1976) The continuous inhalation of oxygen-15 for assessing regional oxygen extraction in the brain of men. Br J Radiol 49:339–343.
26. Jones TH, Morawetz RB, Crowell RM, Marcoux FW, FitzGibbon SJ, DeGirolami U, Ojemann RG (1981) Thresholds of focal cerebral ischemia in awake monkeys. J Neurosurg 54:773–782.
27. Kety SS, Schmidt CG (1945) Determination of cerebral blood flow in man by use of nitrous oxide in low concentrations. Am J Physiol 143:53.
28. Kuhl DE, Phelps ME, Kowell AP, Metter EJ, Selin C, Winter J (1980) Effects of stroke on local cerebral metabolism and perfusion: Mapping by emission computed tomography of ^{18}FDG and ^{13}NH$_3$. Ann Neurol 8:47–60.
29. Kushner MJ, Alavi A, Reivich M, et al. (1984) Contralateral cerebral hypometabolism following cerebral insult. A PET study. Ann Neurol 15:425–434.
30. Kushner MJ, Fazekas F, McElhany K, Rosen M, Alavi A, Chawluk J, Reivich M (1987) Patterns of cerebral metabolism in ischemic aphasia. J Cereb Blood Flow Metab 7(Suppl 1):S47.
31. Kushner MJ, Fieschi C, Silver F, Chawluk J, Rosen M, Greenberg J, Burke A, Alavi A (1987) Metabolic and clinical correlates of acute ischemic infarction. Neurology 37:1103–1110.
32. Kushner MJ, Reivich M, Fazekas F, et al. (1987) Studies of cerebral metabolism and language dysfunction after acute ischemic aphasia. Ann Neurol 22:135.
33. Kushner MJ, Schwartz R, Alavi A, et al. (1987) Cerebral glucose consumption following normal auditory stimulation. Brain Res 409:79–87.
34. Kushner MJ, Tobin M, Alavi A, et al. (1987) Cerebellar glucose consumption in normal and pathological states. J Nucl Med 28:1667–1670.

35. Lammertsma AA, Jones T, Frackowiak RSJ, Lenzi GL (1981) A theoretical study of the steady-state model for measuring regional cerebral blood flow and oxygen utilization using oxygen-15. J Comput Assist Tomogr 5:544–550.
36. Lassen NA, Ingvar DH (1963) Regional cerebral blood flow measurement in man. Arch Neurol 9:615–622.
37. Leblanc R, Tyler J, Mohr G, Meyer E, Diksic M, Yamamoto L, Taylor L, Gauthier S, Hakim A (1987) Hemodynamic and metabolic effects of cerebral revascularization. J Neurosurg Sci 66:529–535.
38. Lebrun-Grandie P, Baron J, Soussaline F, et al. (1983) Coupling between regional blood flow and oxygen utilization in the normal human brain: A study with positron emission tomography and oxygen. Arch Neurol 40:230–236.
39. Lenzi GL, Frackowiak RSJ, Jones T (1982) Cerebral oxygen metabolism and blood flow in human cerebral ischemic infarction. J Cereb Blood Flow Metab 2:321–335.
40. Lenzi GL, Frackowiak RSJ, Jones T (1981) Regional cerebral blood flow (CBF), oxygen utilization (CMRO$_2$) and oxygen extraction ratio (OER) in acute hemispheric stroke. J Cereb Blood Flow Metab (Supp) 1:S504–505.
41. Martin WRW, Raichle ME (1983) Cerebellar blood flow and metabolism in cerebral hemisphere infarction. Ann Neurol 14:168–176.
42. Metter EJ, Mazziotta JC, Itabashi HH, Mankovich NJ, Phelps ME, Kuhl DE (1985) Comparison of glucose metabolism, x-ray CT, and postmortem data in a patient with multiple cerebral infarcts. Neurology 34:1695–1701.
43. Metter EJ, Wasterlain CG, Kuhl DE, Hanson WR, Phelps ME (1981) ^{18}FDG positron emission computed tomography in a study of aphasia. Ann Neurol 10:173–183.
44. Mies G, Auer LM, Ebhardt G, Traupe H, Heiss W-D (1983) Flow and neuronal density in tissue surrounding chronic infarction. Stroke 14:22–27.
45. Obrist WD, Thompson HK, Wang HS, Wilkinson WE (1967) Determination of regional cerebral blood flow by inhalation of 133-xenon. Circ Res 22:124–135.
46. Olsen TS, Larsen B, Herning M, Skriver EB, Lassen NA (1983) Blood flow and vascular reactivity in collaterally perfused brain tissue: Evidence of an ischemic penumbra in patients with acute stroke. Stroke 14:332–341.
47. Pantano P, Baron JC, Samson Y, et al. (1986) Crossed cerebellar diaschisis. Brain 109:677–694.
48. Patronas NJ, DiChiro G, Smith BH, et al. (1984) Depressed cerebellar glucose metabolism in supratentorial tumors. Brain Res 291:93–101.
49. Paragni D, Gerandini P, Lenzi GL (1987) Cerebral hemispheric and contralateral cerebellar hypoperfusion during a transient ischemic attack. J Cereb Blood Flow Metab 7:507–509.
50. Phelps ME, Mazziotta JC, Huang SC (1982) Study of cerebral function with positron computed tomography. J Cereb Blood Flow Metab 2:113–162.
51. Plum F (1983) What causes infarction in ischemic

brain? The Robert Wartenberg lecture. *Neurology* 33:222–233.

52. Powers WJ, Raichle ME (1985) Positron emission tomography and its application to the study of cerebrovascular disease in man. *Stroke* 16:361–376.

53. Powers WJ, Grubb RL, Raichele ME (1984) Physiological responses to focal cerebral ischemia in humans. *Ann Neurol* 16:546–552.

54. Powers WJ, Martin WRW, Herscovitch P, Raichle M, Grubb RL (1984) Extracranial-intracranial bypass surgery: Hemodynamic and metabolic effects. *Neurology* 34:1168–1174.

55. Powers WJ, Press GA, Grubb RL, Gado M, Raichle ME (1987) The effect of hemodynamically significant carotid artery disease on the hemodynamic status of the cerebral circulation. *Ann Intern Med* 106:27–35.

56. Raichle ME (1983) The pathophysiology of brain ischemia. *Ann Neurol* 13:2–10.

57. Reivich M, Alavi A, Wolf A, Gowler J, Russel J, Arnett C, MacGregor RR, Shiue CY, Atkins H, Anand A, Dann R, Greenberg JH (1985) Glucose metabolic rate kinetic model parameter determination in man: The lumped constants and rate constants for 18F-fluorodeoxyglucose and 11C-deoxyglucose. *J Cereb Blood Flow Metab* 5:179–192.

58. Reivich M, Greenberg JH, Kushner MJ, Alavi A (1985) Measurement of local cerebral glucose metabolism: Application to the study of stroke. In Heiss WD, Phelps ME et al. (eds): *Positron Emission Tomography of the Brain*. New York: Springer-Verlag, 153–161.

59. Samson Y, Baron JC, Bousser MG, Rey A, Deilon JM, Daniel P, Comay J (1985) Effect of extra-intracranial arterial bypass on cerebral blood flow and oxygen metabolism in humans. *Stroke* 16:609–614.

60. Siesjo BJ (1981) Cell damage in the brain: A speculative synthesis. *J Cereb Blood Flow Metab* 1:155–185.

61. Sokoloff L (1982) Localization of functional activity in the central nervous system by measurement of glucose utilization with radioactive deoxyglucose. *J Cereb Blood Flow Metab* 1:7–36.

62. Sokoloff L, Reivich M, Kennedy C, Des Rosiers MH, Patlak CS, Pettigrew KD, Sakurada O, Shinohara M (1977) The [14C]-deoxyglucose method for the measurement of local cerebral glucose utilization: Theory, procedure, and normal values in the conscious and anesthetized albino rat. *J Neurochem* 28:897–916.

63. Strong AJ, Venables GS, Gibson G (1983) The cortical ischemic penumbra associated with occlusion of the middle cerebral artery in the cat. 1. Topography of changes in blood flow, potassium ion activity, and EEG. *J Cereb Blood Flow Metab* 3:86–96.

64. Syrota A, Castaing M, Rougemont D, Berridge M, Baron JC, Bousser MG, Pocidalo JJ (1983) Tissue acid-base balance and oxygen metabolism in human cerebral infarction studies with positron emission tomography. *Ann Neurol* 14:419–428.

65. Tallal P, Schartz J (1981) Hemispheric specialization for language processes. *Science* 211:961.

66. The EC/IC Bypass Study Group (1986) Failure of extracranial-intracranial arterial bypass to reduce the risk of ischemic stroke: Results of an international randomized trial. *N Engl J Med* 313:1191–1200.

67. Wise RJS, Bernardi S, Frackowiak RSJ, Legg NJ, Jones T (1983) Serial observations on the pathophysiology of acute stroke. *Brain* 106:197–222.

68. Wise RJS, Rhodes CG, Gibbs JM, Hatazawa J, Palmer T, Frackowiak RSJ, Jones T (1983) Disturbance of oxidative metabolism of glucose in recent human cerebral infarcts. *Ann Neurol* 14:627–637.

Cerebral Blood Flow Measurements During Carotid Endarterectomy

Thoralf M. Sundt, Jr., MD

Department of Neurosurgery, Mayo Clinic, Rochester, Minnesota 55904

INTRODUCTION

Approximately 14 years ago, we adopted routine intracerebral blood flow measurements and continuous electroencephalography as a method for monitoring patients undergoing carotid endarterectomy at the Mayo Clinic. Our interest in monitoring patients undergoing this surgery was related to the high risk category of individuals coming to us for endarterectomy and to our dissatisfaction in terms of results for patients with major risk factors. At that time, our overall morbidity-mortality (not synonymous with complications, as many complications do not result in morbidity if addressed promptly) was less than 5% [28], but the high risk patient had a much higher complication rate than did the low risk patient. Parenthetically, this should be kept in mind when one analyzes surgical results from one institution to another. There is a vast difference in the surgical material from one institution compared to another, with asymptomatic patients comprising the bulk of individuals undergoing surgery in some centers. This subject is beyond the scope of the present chapter, but it is necessary to keep these facts in mind in order to place in perspective the role of monitoring for the patient undergoing carotid endarterectomy. In our judgment, monitoring is especially indicated in the high risk patient and patients with frequent symptoms of ischemia. We have little doubt that the asymptomatic patient may undergo surgery without a major increase in risk associated with the lack of monitoring techniques.

In spite of the fact that we seldom took more than 15 to 20 minutes for the arterial procedure itself in our early experience, a number of patients awoke from surgery with either a major or a minor neurologic deficit; some were transient, others were permanent. Although ever-cognizant of the risk of intraoperative embolization, we did not feel that these deficits were attributable to that cause in all instances. In fact, it was our conclusion that most of these deficits were related to inadequate cross flow from the opposite hemisphere and to our failure to shunt these cases at that point. Balanced against shunting in the average case is the fact that shunting undeniably complicates the operative procedure and places the distal internal carotid artery at some risk and introduces the small but definable risk of intraoperative embolization through the shunt [1].

Our agonizing reappraisal at that time led us to the decision to perform a more meticulous endarterectomy and to use routinely a saphenous vein patch graft. Coupled with this approach was the need to provide better cerebral protection by indwelling shunts either routinely or selectively during the period of carotid occlusion, as the period of occlusion and reconstruction obviously would be greater. Subsequently we have discovered the extreme importance of meticulous reconstruction of the external carotid artery as well, which of course adds even more time to the operative procedure.

In modern neurovascular surgery there is no place for the rapid carotid endarterectomy.

176 Sundt et al.

The surgery must be carefully performed with adequate time devoted to the multiple technical aspects of the operation, which can result in major postoperative complications if not performed precisely. The only way to do this type of surgery in our judgment is with knowledge about cerebral blood flow and cerebral metabolic function during the operation, and these can only be revealed with adequate monitoring techniques.

METHOD OF MEASURING CEREBRAL BLOOD FLOW

Cerebral blood flow is measured by the rapid injection of 300 μCi of xenon-133 in 0.4 ml of isotonic saline through a 27-gauge needle into the common carotid artery with the external carotid artery occluded [2]. A single scintillation detector is used with a sodium iodide (NaI) crystal $1\frac{1}{4}''$ in diameter and $\frac{1}{4}''$ thick. The crystal is recessed 1" behind a tapered lead collimator with a $\frac{7}{8}''$ opening, widening to $1\frac{1}{8}''$ at the surface of the crystal. The detector is mounted on a Zeiss operating microscope stand and placed adjacent and perpendicular to the scalp overlying the hand and face area of the motor strip.

It is possible (after the operation) to compute CBF values by the kinetic (H/A) method or by exponential analysis [3,4]. Early in our series, this was done for correlation with the measurements obtained at surgery calculated by the initial slope technique. Our confidence in the initial slope technique is now so great that we seldom employ the other methods of measurement.

CBF values are calculated using the initial slope technique of Waltz [5]. The formula's derivation is available in his work comparing analytical methods for the derivation of CBF. The use of the following formula is illustrated in Figure 9–1: CBF (ml/100g/min) = $3600/T_{\frac{1}{2}}$ (sec), where $T_{\frac{1}{2}}$ is the time required in seconds for the curve to reach a value one-half its original maximum or peak. Flows are calculated from a number or with a slide rule and are available to the surgeon within several minutes after injection. Examples of typical clearance curves before, during, and following carotid occlusion are depicted in Figure 9–2.

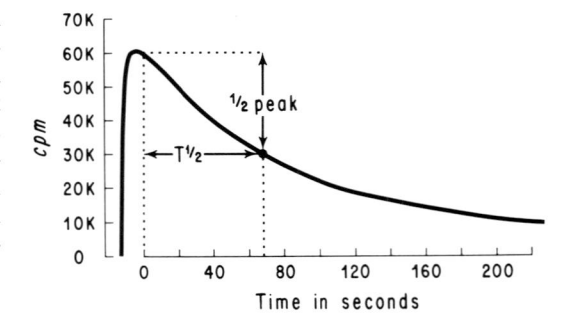

Figure 9–1. Typical cerebral blood flow (CBF) curve following intraarterial injection of xenon-133 (^{133}Xe) into the internal carotid artery (ICA). CBF is determined by dividing 3,600 by the time in seconds for curve to fall to one-half its peak value. CBF here equals 3,600 ÷ 65 = 55.5 ml/100 g/min. K = kilocounts (1,000 counts); cpm = counts per minute.

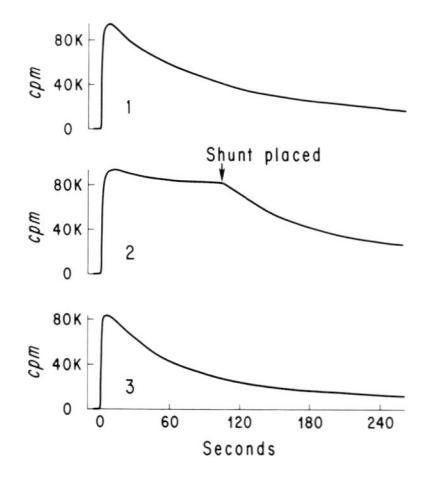

Figure 9–2. Sequential CBF curves in a patient during endarterectomy. CBF values (ml/100 g/min) were 46, baseline; < 5, with occlusion (washout slope too flat to measure accurately and rapidly); 44, with placement of a shunt; and 67, following restoration of flow.

METHOD OF ELECTROENCEPHALOGRAPHIC MONITORING

Technique

Forty-five minutes before the patient is taken to the operating room, two ear and 21 scalp electrodes are applied with collodion [6]. The

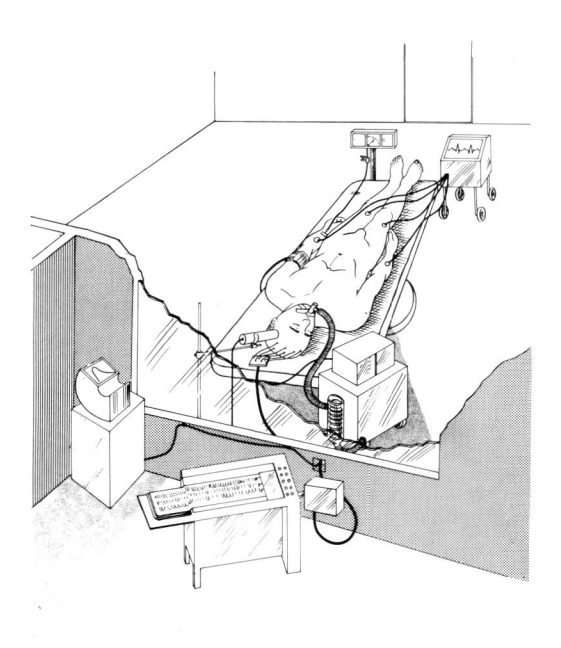

Figure 9–3. Equipment arrangement for simultaneous cerebral blood flow measurements and electroencephalograms during the operative procedure. All cumbersome equipment and paraphernalia are housed in an adjacent monitoring room so that it does not encroach upon the working space of the surgical or anesthesia teams.

10 and 20 international system of electrode placement is employed. A 16-channel EEG recording is obtained with a Grass model 6 machine. A baseline trace is obtained prior to induction. The EEG is then recorded continuously, beginning with induction and ending with extubation. Both routine (30 mm/second) and slow (5 mm/second) paper speeds are employed. The EEG and CBF recording equipment are positioned in a monitoring room adjacent to the operating room or in a corner of the operating room well away from the surgical field (Fig. 9–3).

Results
BACKGROUND EEG PATTERN UNDER ANESTHESIA

There are two basic patterns seen during a surgical level of anesthesia: a symmetric pattern and a grossly asymmetric pattern with a persistent delta focus [6].

The symmetric pattern is noted in most cases in which the patients are free of significant preoperative neurologic deficits and persistent focal findings in their waking EEG. The records are usually dominated by symmetric, sustained, rhythmic activity of 10 to 14 Hz that range between 25 and 100 uV. Some records show faster activity, of 15 to 24 Hz, but the activity is usually of lesser amplitude and persistence. In addition, especially with deeper levels of anesthesia, slower activity in the delta frequency range, with amplitudes ranging between 50 and 150 uV, becomes more apparent. All of these patterns tend to show a midline maximum in either the frontal or the central regions. In Figure 9–4 these normal anesthetic patterns are demonstrated in the first eight channels, all of which record activity from a normal hemisphere.

A persistent delta focus and asymmetry of the background patterns throughout anesthesia are noted in most patients, with a persistent delta focus in their waking EEG taken prior to surgery. In addition, some cases show a persistent delta focus during anesthesia in spite of the fact that their waking trace was free of such a delta focus. Figure 9–4 illustrates the baseline anesthetic EEG in a patient with previous right cerebral hemodynamic TIAs and a residual right-sided EEG abnormality that consists of reduction in the normal faster-background activity associated with increased, persistent, long-wave length irregular delta slowing (last eight channels).

MAJOR FOCAL EEG CHANGES OCCURRING WITH CAROTID CLAMPING

Approximately 24% of our cases have had a major focal EEG change with carotid clamping. The severity of these changes has closely paralleled the relative reduction of blood flow. In general, the onset of change is less rapid and less severe, with reductions of CBF to levels between 10 ml and 18 ml/100 g/min than it is when flow falls below 10 ml/100 g/min. It is rare for CBF to fall to levels below 10 ml/100 g/min without EEG evidence of ischemia (this varies somewhat with the anesthetic agent). In some cases in which the opposite ICA is occluded, the EEG changes are bilateral, but only

EEG UNDER FORANE ANESTHESIA

♂ Age: 66 yrs (2-23-83)

Hemodynamic right cerebral TIA

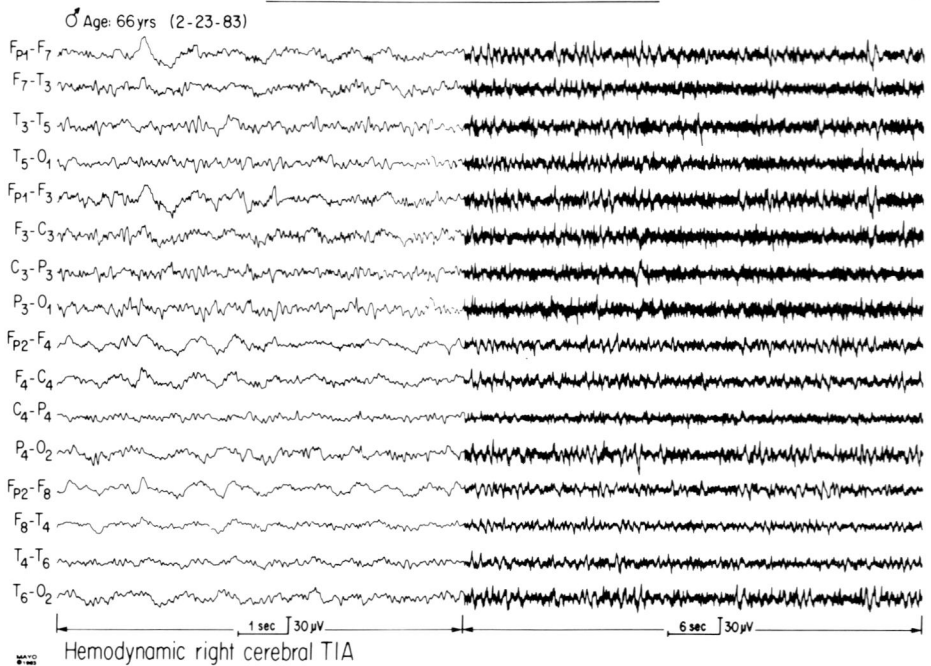

Figure 9–4. Anesthetic EEG recorded at regular (30/mm/sec) (**left**) and slow (5/mm/sec) (**right**) paper speeds. The first eight channels record the usual anesthetic pattern from a normal left hemisphere demonstrating the sustained rhythmic anesthetic pattern in the 10–14-Hz frequency range. In addition, there are triangular slow waves of briefer duration, maximal in the anterior head region, and lower voltage, more widespread, irregular slow, generally maximum more posterior. The lower eight channels record the right hemisphere with the residual EEG changes related to previous right hemodynamic TIAs. In these channels, the rhythmic anesthetic pattern is reduced (compare the lower four channels to the upper four channels), and there is an increased amount of irregular slowing. This effect can be appreciated both at the regular and slow paper speeds.

rarely are they more severe on the contralateral side.

The changes with clamping are usually stereotyped with attenuation of faster background frequencies. With less severe ischemia, this is associated with higher amplitude, longer wavelength slow waves; but with more severe ischemia, even the slow waves attenuated (Fig. 9–5). In most cases, the EEG returns to normal within 1 to 2 minutes after the shunt is in place, but with more severe changes and prolonged clamps, it takes longer. We have had no cases in which the EEG did not return to normal with placement of a shunt.

In all cases following placement of a shunt, the focal EEG changes resolved within 2 to 7 minutes after shunting. However, four patients have sustained an EEG change with the shunt in place that was proven angiographically to be related to small emboli arising from the functioning shunt.

MAJOR FOCAL EEG CHANGES NOT IMMEDIATELY ASSOCIATED WITH CAROTID CLAMPING.

A number of patients have had major transient focal or generalized slowing not immediately associated with or due to carotid clamping. These changes usually persist for a few minutes and in most cases appear in both hemispheres. Early in our experience, it was our impression that when these changes were

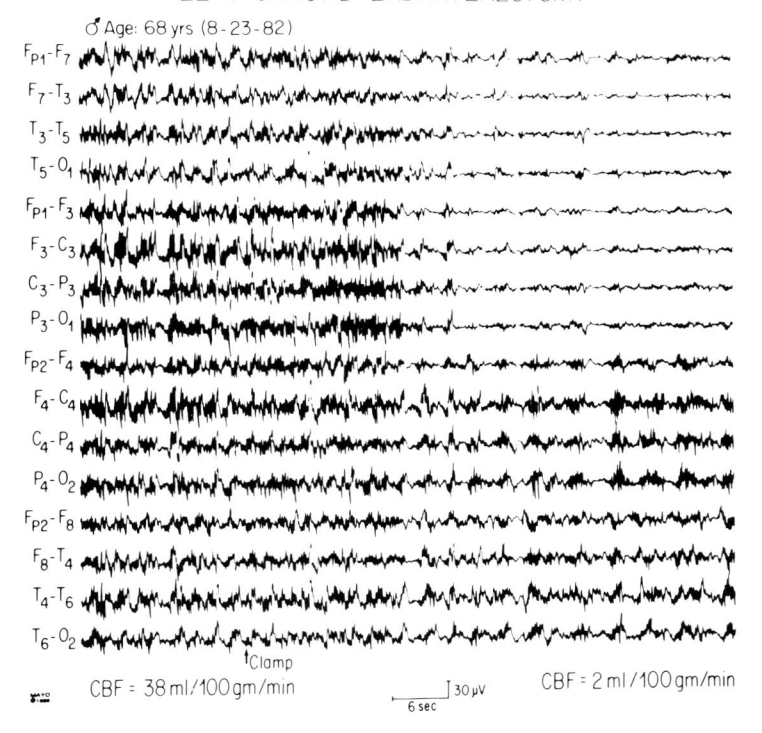

Figure 9–5. EEG recorded at slow paper speed (5 mm/sec) and demonstrating the dramatic attenuation of both the faster as well as the slower components that occurred with carotid clamping, which reduced cerebral blood flow from 38 to 2 ml/100 g/min.

seen predominantly on the side of surgery they were in fact related to small emboli. This indeed can be the case, but fortunately this is much less common than changes related to subtle alteration in the level of anesthesia. When the changes come on more slowly and are seen in both hemispheres, invariably they are related to an increase in the depth of anesthesia, and quite often this can be attributed to nitrous oxide rather than the primary anesthetic agent. Lightening the level of anesthesia usually results in a prompt improvement in the EEG.

In patients with a preexisting neurologic deficit and a baseline asymmetrical EEG, a change in the level of anesthesia can be preferentially reflected in the hemisphere with the abnormal EEG. Thus, a lateralized EEG change in these patients is not necessarily attributable to intraoperative embolization.

Intraoperative embolization can usually be identified on the EEG by its focality, as well as failure to respond to altering the anesthetic level. However, the embolic changes usually are not as dramatic as those associated with total hemispheric ischemia following occlusion of the internal carotid artery in patients with inadequate collateral flow (Fig. 9–6).

CEREBRAL BLOOD FLOW VS. ANESTHETIC AGENT AND PATIENT CATEGORY

Cerebral blood flow measurements performed prior to occlusion, with shunting, and following endarterectomy are summarized in Table 9.1 for patients having the three major anesthetics used during the period of this report. Additional cases having a variety of anesthetic agents are not included in this table as the anesthetic agent has considerable bearing

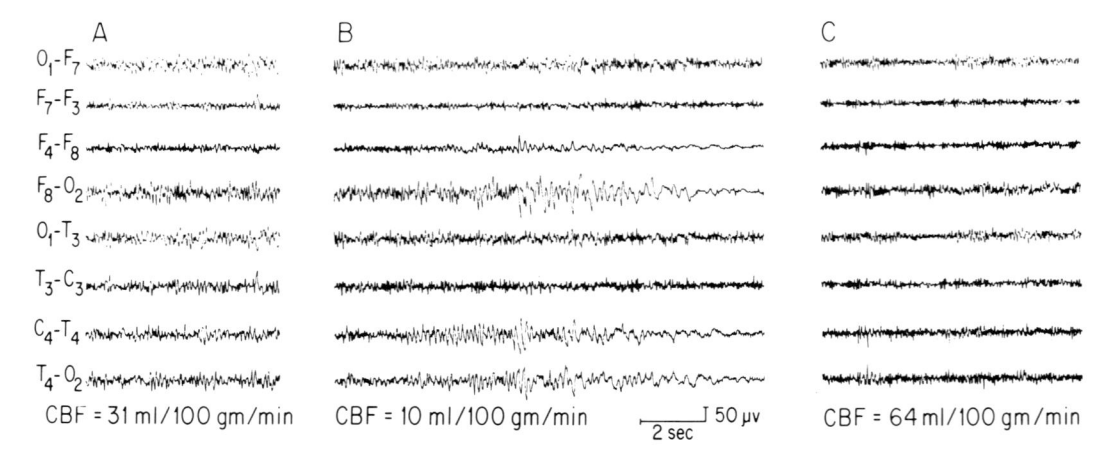

Figure 9–6. EEG in a 59-year-old man undergoing left carotid endarterectomy. **A:** EEG recording before left carotid clamping shows a symmetric pattern. **B:** EEG recording 40 seconds after clamping shows left-sided delta slowing and reduced background activity when the blood flow is reduced to 10 ml/100 g/min; **C:** EEG 4 minutes after internal shunting has returned to baseline levels.

Table 9.1
Cerebral Blood Flow According to Anesthetic Used and Grade of Risk, January 1, 1972–June 30, 1986*

Time of measurement	Grade 1 N	Grade 1 CBF ± SD	Grade 2 N	Grade 2 CBF ± SD	Grade 3 N	Grade 3 CBF ± SD	Grade 4 N	Grade 4 CBF ± SD
Halothane (470 cases)								
Baseline	150	62 ± 26	89	59 ± 27	143	51 ± 21	81	48 ± 21
Occlusion	148	35 ± 18	88	31 ± 18	145	26 ± 16	77	24 ± 13
Shunt	41	44 ± 16	42	53 ± 17	66	43 ± 17	48	42 ± 12
Postocclusion	151	69 ± 27	90	70 ± 25	145	61 ± 23	84	61 ± 22
Ethrane (854 cases)								
Baseline	290	50 ± 19	197	44 ± 18	198	42 ± 18	143	37 ± 21
Occlusion	287	28 ± 13	195	23 ± 13	194	21 ± 11	140	18 ± 11
Shunt	91	39 ± 15	102	35 ± 11	105	36 ± 13	89	35 ± 14
Postocclusion	297	51 ± 18	200	50 ± 19	205	48 ± 19	152	51 ± 21
Forane (789 cases)								
Baseline	213	36 ± 15	179	34 ± 19	242	31 ± 13	117	27 ± 13
Occlusion	211	23 ± 11	177	18 ± 11	239	18 ± 10	116	16 ± 9
Shunt	52	26 ± 9	70	29 ± 9	103	26 ± 9	72	29 ± 11
Postocclusion	216	41 ± 17	181	42 ± 17	256	36 ± 14	136	46 ± 43

*N = number of cases, CBF = cerebral blood flow, SD = standard deviation.

on cerebral blood flow measurements. There is a statistically significant difference in blood flow among comparable grades of patients operated on under these three anesthetic agents. There is also a significant difference between the baseline and occlusion flows in the grade IV group of patients when they are compared to the better-risk (grades I and II) patients operated on under that same anesthetic agent ($P < 0.05$). Thus, the high risk group had both

Table 9.2
Percentage of Cases Shunted by Grade, January 1, 1972–June 30, 1986

Grade	Percentage
1	27
2	45
3	44
4	54

Table 9.3
Occlusion Flows in Endarterectomies, January 1, 1972–June 30, 1986

Occlusion flow (ml/100 g/min)	Percentage total
0–4	4
5–9	9
10–14	15
15–20	21

marginal baseline perfusion and inadequate collateral flow.

The frequency of shunt use according to the anesthetic agent employed and the grade of the patient can be determined by comparing the number of patients in whom shunt measurements were obtained to the number of patients in whom baseline measurements were obtained. The discrepancy between the number of patients having a postocclusion flow and the number of patients having a baseline flow relates to technical problems in delivering the indicator to the brain in patients with a very high grade stenosis (99.9%) or a physiologic occlusion. The data from all three anesthetic agents are compiled in Table 9.2. One finds that shunts were used in 27% of grade I, 45% of grade II, 44% of grade III, and 54% of grade IV patients. Forty-one percent of all patients were shunted.

Table 9.3 summarizes the cerebral blood flow data from all three anesthetic agents during the period of carotid occlusion. During occlusion, cerebral blood flow fell to 0–4 ml/100 g/min in 4% of the cases, 5–9 ml/100 g/min in 9% of the cases. Virtually all of these patients were shunted. In addition to these cases with flows clearly below what has been determined to be minimal perfusion requirements, 21% of patients had flows between 15 and 20 ml/100 g/min. A large number of these cases were also shunted, as many of these patients had preoperative alterations in the electroencephalogram, indicating areas of marginal neuronal function.

CORRELATION OF EEG AND CBF MEASUREMENTS

The severity of EEG changes observed with varying degrees of ischemia under halothane anesthesia is illustrated in Figure 9–7. Table 9.4 summarizes the frequency of changes seen in the EEG with carotid occlusion according to the anesthetic agent used. It should be noted that patients with a low CBF often were shunted prior to the development of an EEG change.

CEREBRAL BLOOD FLOW AND STUMP PRESSURES

Stump pressures were measured consecutively in 100 patients in order to correlate these measurements with the occlusion of CBF. These data have been previously reported [7] and are summarized in Figure 9–8. On the basis of that experience, we have not used stump pressure measurements as a monitoring technique. However, other experienced groups report excellent results using this technique [8–10].

EMBOLIC COMPLICATIONS

Embolic complications during the operation are identified by a focal change in the EEG. There were a total of 15 embolic complications in patients undergoing surgery for primary stenosis during the surgery that led to a major or minor neurologic deficit. This gives an incidence of about 1%. Embolic complications were more common in patients with recurrent stenosis.

There were four cases of emboli through a functioning shunt during the operation in this series. These were major events and related to proximal atherosclerosis and might possibly have been avoided, retrospectively, with more experience. There were additional cases in which the shunt became transiently occluded from a platelet thrombus or fragment of atherosclerosis. The occlusion was identified by an EEG change and actually visualized through

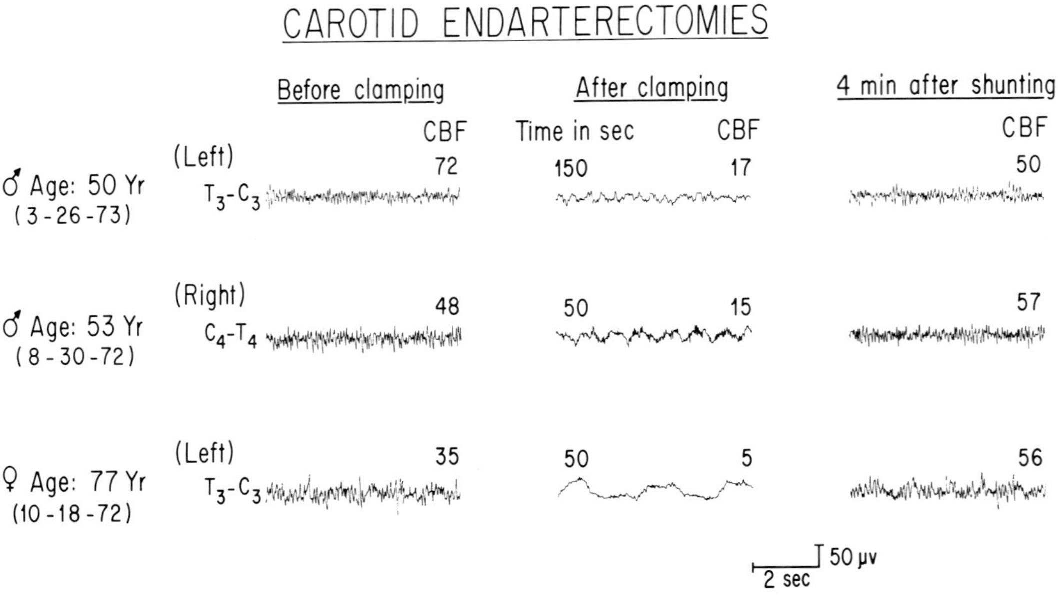

CAROTID ENDARTERECTOMIES

Figure 9–7. Correlation between the electroencephalograms and cerebral blood flow measurements under halothane anesthesia. The severity of the EEG change parallels the reduction in cerebral blood flow.

Table 9.4
Cerebral Blood Flow During Carotid Occlusion, January 1, 1972–June 30, 1986

Flow (ml/100 g/min)	No. of cases without change in EEG within 3 minutes of occlusion			No. of cases with change in EEG within 3 minutes of occlusion		
	Halothane	Ethrane	Forane	Halothane	Ethrane	Forane
0–4	0	1	8	12	23	33
5–9	1	2	44	20	76	47
10–14	8	52	107	42	74	34
15–19	25	91	128	41	46	16
20–24	48	122	131	0	0	3
25–29	56	104	84	0	0	0
30+	214	249	123	0	0	0
Total	352	621	625	115	219	133

the shunt wall. Removal of the shunt with clearance of the thrombus resulted in normalization of the EEG; both patients awoke from surgery with normal neurologic function.

There were 11 embolic complications not related to shunt usage. Nine of these occurred during the exposure of the vessel, one with induction of anesthesia and one as the patient was awakening from surgery.

VALUE OF MONITORING AND SHUNTING DURING ENDARTERECTOMY

From January 1972 through June 1986, we performed 2,183 endarterectomies for primary carotid stenosis and 59 procedures for recurrent stenosis using the intraoperative monitoring techniques described above. The correlation of CBF measurements with EEGs in these cases has been excellent, as indicated in Table

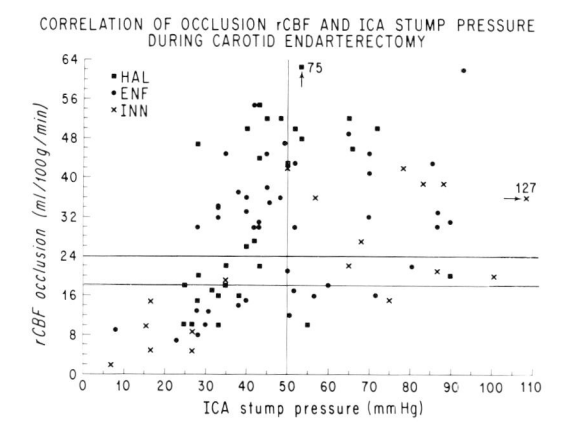

Figure 9-8. Scattergram of occlusion regional cerebral blood flows (rCBF) plotted against internal carotid artery (ICA) stump pressures. The vertical line represents a stump pressure of 50 torr (considered the critical level). The two horizontal lines represent the critical flow level (rCBF ≤ 18 ml/100 g/min) and the marginal zone (rCBF 18-24 ml/100 g/min). Regression lines for each anesthetic agent were calculated. Expressed for halothane, rCBF$_{occl}$ = 0.51 (stump pressure) ± 9.94, r = 0.43. Expressed for enflurane, rCBF$_{occl}$ = 0.26 (stump pressure ± 16.51, r = 0.39. Expressed for Innovar, rCBF$_{occl}$ = 0.27 (stump pressure) ± 0.93, r = 0.68.

9.4, which summarizes data from 2,065 cases operated on under halothane, ethrane, or forane. We have had 77 cases with occlusion flows between 0 and 4 ml/100 g/min, 190 with flows between 5 and 9 ml/100 g/min, and 317 with flows between 10 and 14 ml/100 g/min. Using the xenon washout technique, flows below 5 are difficult to quantitate and can be equated essentially to zero flow. Thus, we believe that 4% of the patients in our group would definitely have sustained a cerebral infarction without shunting because of inadequate collateral flow. Another 9%, that is patients with flows between 5 and 9 ml/100 g/min, probably would have sustained an infarction with any prolonged period of occlusion. Patients with flows between 10 and 14 ml/100 g/min, representing 15% of the group, may or may not have withstood the period of ischemia. Shunts were also used in a large number of patients with flows between 15 and 20 ml/100 g/min for fear that the EEG would fail to reveal regions of focal ischemia in the deep white matter of basal ganglia with these borderline flows or because of a preoperative region of infarction or ischemia. Occasionally patients with flows above 20 ml/100 g/min were also shunted if they had a preexisting EEG abnormality related to preoperative infarct, as we have found (as have others) that these patients are particularly vulnerable to marginal flow [11-17]. Shunts are usually not inserted until the plaque has been removed from the distal internal carotid artery except in cases in which flow is below 5 ml/100 g/min or in which there has been a dramatic and catastrophic change in EEG (usually these are simultaneous events and one does not occur without the other).

There was a statistically significant difference in blood flows among patients categorized according to the anesthetic agent employed. The highest flows were seen with halothane and the lowest flows were seen with forane (supplemented in many cases with fentanyl). A data analysis of Table 9.1 shows significant differences in baseline and postocclusion CBF in patients operated under the three agents studied ($P < 0.001$). Halothane had higher flows than ethrane, which in turn had higher flows than forane. Halothane occlusion and shunt flows were also significantly higher when compared to ethrane and forane, but there were less striking differences between the latter agents.

In comparing CBF according to the grade of the patient, there were statistically significant differences in the baseline and occlusion flows when grade 4 patients were compared to grade 1 patients, with values in the grade 4 patients being lower ($P < 0.001$). There were no differences in the postocclusion flow values.

Shunts were required in only 30% of grade 1 candidates for surgery, but were required in 56% of patients who were grade 4 candidates for surgery. Furthermore, both the baseline and occlusion flows were lower in the higher risk category of patients. This leads one to the conclusion that the microembolic and hemodynamic theories for transient ischemic attacks and infarctions are not mutually exclusive. Areas of brain functioning on a marginal flow of 40 to 50% of normal are particularly vulnerable to the effects of emboli [2,18,19].

Conversely, Whisnant found from a detailed multivariant analysis of a group of patients with transient ischemic attacks undergoing surgery in the period 1970–1974 that no patients with a high occlusion flow had an intraoperative or postoperative stroke [20]. Furthermore, this group had no stroke in 4.5 years of followup evaluation, indicating that individuals with high collateral flow have a good prognosis.

CRITICAL FLOW AND ISCHEMIC TOLERANCE

The reader is directed to other reports for a discussion concerning the concepts of critical cerebral blood flow and ischemic tolerance of neural tissue [21]. In general, there is good correlation between laboratory studies in primates and clinical studies in humans [3,4,22,23]. It appears that the critical flow required to maintain normal electrical activity in the brain varies somewhere between 15 and 20 ml/100 g/min and that the critical flow required to maintain basic cell metabolism is somewhere between 10 and 15 ml/100 g/min. There is now general agreement about the protective effects of barbiturate anesthesia for cerebral ischemia. However, there is less information concerning the possible beneficial effects of inhalation general anesthesia agents [24]. Our data suggest that there is a difference, however, in these critical flows related to the anesthetic agent. Thus, the critical flow is higher for halothane than it is for forane. The best available data to date suggest that flows below 10 ml/100 g/min result in ionic shifts that may be irreversible if allowed to persist. The true level of tolerance for ischemia in patients who have flows between 5 and 10 or between 10 and 15 ml/100 g/min is unknown. Furthermore, in areas of marginal flow, brain blood flow is nonhomogenous, and there may be considerable focal variability in regions of incomplete focal ischemia.

We prefer not to speculate how long a particular person can retain a physiologic paralysis without developing neuronal damage. Thus, we shunt the patient routinely whenever there is a doubt regarding the adequacy of cerebral blood flow and when placement of the shunt is safe and does not jeopardize the arterial repair. A number of other groups with considerable experience in this field have adopted intraoperative EEG monitoring as a means of increasing the safety of the procedure [11,13,15,16,25–27].

References

1. Sundt TM Jr, Ebersold MJ, Sharbrough FW, Piepgras DG, Marsh WR, Messick JM (1986) The risk-benefit ratio of intraoperative shunting during carotid endarterectomy. Ann Surg 203:196–204.
2. Sundt TM Jr, Sharbrough FW, Anderson RE, Michenfelder JD (1974) Cerebral blood flow measurements and electroencephalograms during carotid endarterectomy. J Neurosurg 41:310–320.
3. Boysen G (1971) Cerebral blood flow measurement as a safeguard during carotid endarterectomy. Stroke 2:1–10.
4. Boysen G, Ladegaard-Pedersen HJ, Henriksen H, Oleson J, Paulson OB, Engell HC (1971) The effects of $PaCO_2$ on regional cerebral blood flow and internal carotid arterial pressure during carotid clamping. Anesthesiology 35:286–300.
5. Waltz AG, Wanek AR, Anderson RE (1972) Comparison of analytic methods for calculation of cerebral flow after intracarotid injection of 133-Xe. J Nucl Med 13:66–72.
6. Sharbrough FW, Messick JM Jr, Sundt TM Jr (1973) Correlation of continuous electroencephalograms with cerebral blood flow measurements during carotid endarterectomy. Stroke 4:674–683.
7. McKay RD, Sundt TM Jr, Michenfelder JD, Gronert GA, Messick JR, Sharbrough FW, Piepgras DG (1976) Internal carotid artery stump pressure and cerebral blood flow during carotid endarterectomy: Modification by halothane, enflurane, and innovar. Anesthesiology 45:390–399.
8. Hays RF, Levinson SA, Wylie EJ (1972): Intraoperative measurement of carotid back pressure as a guide to operative management of carotid endarterectomy. Surgery 72:953–960.
9. Hunter GC, Sieffert G, Malone JM, Moore WS (1982) The accuracy of carotid back pressure as an index for shunt requirements. Stroke 13:319–326.
10. Moore WS, Hall AD (1969) Carotid artery back pressure. A test of cerebral tolerance to temporary carotid occlusion. Arch Surg 99:702–710.
11. Callow AD, Matsumoto G, Baker D, Cossman D, Watson W (1978) Protection of the high risk carotid endarterectomy patient by continuous electroencephalography. J Cardiovasc Surg 19:55–64.
12. Callow AD, O'Donnell TF (1983) Electroencephalogram monitoring in cerebrovascular surgery. In Bergan JJ, Yao JS (eds): Cerebral Vascular Insufficiency. New York: Grune & Stratton, pp 327–341.
13. Gianotta SL, Dicks RE, Kindt GW (1980) Carotid endarterectomy: Technical improvements. Neurosurgery 7:309–312.
14. Imparato AM, Ramirez A, Riles T, Mintzer R (1982) Cerebral protection in carotid surgery. Arch Surg 117:1073–1078.
15. Leech PJ, Miller JD, Fitch W, Barker J (1974) Cerebral blood flow, internal carotid artery pressure,

and the EEG as a guide to the safety of carotid ligation. J Neurol Neurosurg Psychiatry 37:854–862.
16. Ojemann RG, Crowell RM, Roberson GH, Fisher CM (1975) Surgical treatment of extracranial carotid occlusive disease. Clin Neurosurg 22:214–263.
17. Thompson JE (1979) Complications of carotid endarterectomy and their prevention. World J Surg 3:155–165.
18. Sundt TM Jr, Sharbrough FW, Piepgras DG, Kearns TP, Messick JM Jr, O'Fallon WM (1981) Correlation of cerebral blood flow and electroencephalographic changes during carotid endarterectomy. Mayo Clin Proc 56:533–543.
19. Wylie EJ, Ehrenfeld WK (1970) Extracranial Occlusive Cerebrovascular Disease: Diagnosis and Management. Philadelphia: W.B. Saunders.
20. Whisnant JP, Sandok BA, Sundt TM Jr (1983) Carotid endarterectomy for unilateral carotid system transient cerebral ischemia. Mayo Clin Proc 58:171–175.
21. Sundt TM Jr (1986) Occlusive Cerebrovascular Disease: Diagnosis and Surgical Management. Philadelphia: W.B. Saunders.
22. Astrup J, Symon L, Branston NM, Lassen NA (1977) Cortical evoked potential and extracellular K^+ and H^+ at critical levels of brain ischemia. Stroke 8:51–57.
23. Astrup J, Siesjo BK, Symon L (1981) Thresholds in cerebral ischemia: The ischemic penumbra. Stroke 12:723–725.
24. McDowall DG (1965) The effects of general anaesthetics on cerebral blood flow and cerebral metabolism. Br J Anaesth 37:236–245.
25. Matsumoto GH, Baker JD, Watson CW, Gleucklich B, Callow AD (1976) EEG surveillance as a means of extending operability in high risk carotid endarterectomy. Stroke 7:554–559.
26. Phillips MR, Johnson WC, Scott RM, Vollman RW, Levine H, Nabseth DC (1979) Carotid endarterectomy in the presence of contralateral carotid occlusion: The role of EEG and intraluminal shunting. Arch Surg 114:1232–1239.
27. Trojaborg W, Boysen G (1973) Relation between EEG, regional cerebral blood flow and internal carotid artery pressure during carotid endarterectomy. Electroencephalogr Clin Neurophysiol 34:61–69.
28. Sundt TM Jr, Sandok BA, Whisnant JP (1975) Carotid endarterectomy: Complications and preoperative assessment of risk. Mayo Clin Proc 50:301–306.

Index

Acetazolamide, 76, 155, 157
Acetylsalicylic acid, 44
Acidosis, 147, 152, 154, 155
Acquired immunodeficiency syndrome, 133
Aging process, 129, 136
Algorithms, 63, 150
Alzheimer's disease, 134–135, 151, 157, 170
Amine transport, 147
Anastomosis, 45, 168
Anastomotic pathways, 40
Anesthesia, 113, 148, 177–181
Aneurysms, 9, 94, 142–143
Angioendotheliomatosis, cerebral, 133
Angiography
    B-mode imaging and, 21
    carotid, 141–142
    cerebral, 94
    digital subtraction, 27, 99–100
    Doppler ultrasound and, 40, 43
    duplex scanning and, 51, 53–54, 58, 60, 63
    magnetic resonance imaging and, 136–142
    transcranial Doppler and, 99–100, 107
Angioma, 100, 102, 105, 142
Anterior
    cerebral artery (ACA)
        angioma in, 100
        CCA compression testing, 85, 87, 97
        extracranial occlusive disease in, 103–105
        identification of, 77–78, 81
        occlusion, 94
    communicating artery, 77
Aortic
    regurgitation, 57
    sclerosis, 7
    stenosis, 5, 7, 9, 11, 20
Aortocoronary bypass, 60
Aortographs, 27
Aphasia, 153
Arteriography
    cerebral, 27, 105
    digital subtraction, 96, 99
    ultrasonic, 49, 105
Arteriosclerosis, 36, 77, 181
Arteriosclerotic vascular disease, 128–136
Arteriovenous malformations, 76, 99–106, 115, 139–140, 142–143
Atheroma, 17, 58
Atherosclerosis, 17, 58
Atherosclerotic
    lesions, 22–23, 32, 34

    plaque, 18, 21–22, 58
Atrial myxomas, 7–10
Attenuation, 151–152
Autoregulation
    cerebral, 115, 117, 155, 165, 168
    defined, 164

Basilar artery, 77, 84–85, 91, 96
Blood flow, 107–108, 110–111
    magnetic resonance and, 135
    occlusion, 42, 107
    stenosis, 97
    thrombosis, 41–42, 102
Bifurcation, carotid. *See* Carotid bifurcation
Binswanger's disease, 128–129 132–133
Blind stump, 32, 34, 44, 94
Blood-brain barrier, 147, 149
Blood flow, cerebral. *See* Cerebral blood flow
Blood pressure, 115, 118
B-mode ultrasonography
    angiography and, 21
    of carotid bifurcation, 36, 47
    color-flow imaging and, 64
    duplex scanning and, 20, 49–65
    real-time, 18, 20, 21–22, 49, 64
Bohr effect, 155, 164
Brachial artery pressure, 18
Brachial claudication, 45–46
Broca's area, 170
Bulbar syndrome, 117
Bypass
    aortocoronary, 60
    carotidosubclavian, 45
    EC/IC, 107–108, 115, 157, 168

Calcarine artery, 85
Calcium, 21, 53, 105
Calvaria, 149
Camera, gamma, 150, 154, 158
Carbon dioxide, 107–108, 115
Carbon monoxide asphyxia, 133
Cardiac
    catheterization, 9
    gaiting, 139
    tamponade, 9
Cardiomyopathy, 6, 9, 11–12
Carotid angiography, 141–142
Carotid artery(ies)
    bifurcation, 17, 49
        atherosclerotic plaque, 18, 21–22

188 Index

B-mode imaging of, 36, 47
continuous-wave Doppler imaging of, 19–21, 30–31
contralateral disease of, 60
duplex scanning of, 60
embolization in, 17
and flow disturbances, 21
common. *See* Common carotid artery
disease, cervical, 17
external. *See* External carotid artery
internal. *See* Internal carotid artery
lesion, 17
magnetic resonance and, 135
occlusion, 20, 31–34, 140
stenosis, 20
   diagnosis, 31–34
   ophthalmic pressure and, 19
   recurrent, 60, 181
   signal intensity in, 141
velocity waveform analysis, 19–21
Carotid bulb, 58–59
Carotid endarterectomy
   CBF measurements during, 175–185
   continuous-wave Doppler screening for, 35
   postsurgical lesions, 58
   recurrent stenosis and, 60, 181
   SPECT screening for, 157
   transcranial Doppler monitoring during, 111–114
   for transient ischemic attack, 17, 177–178, 183–184
Carotidosubclavian anastomosis, 45
Carotid sinus, 18, 21, 23
CCA. *See* Common carotid artery
Cerebellar artery, 22
Cerebellar hypometabolism, 169–170
Cerebral angiography, 94
Cerebral arterial vasospasm, 75
Cerebral arteriography, 27, 105
Cerebral blood flow
   anesthesia and, 179–181
   direction of, 27–28, 30, 58, 137
   EEG's and, 176–185
   measurement of, 175–185
   monitoring by TCD, 109–114
   patterns, 58
   PET and, 163–168
   pressure, 115, 118
   regional. *See* Regional cerebral blood flow
   resistance index, 102
   separation, 59–61, 63
   SPECT and, 155–157
   stenosis and, 19–20, 27, 94
   stump pressure and, 181
   turbulence, 19–21
   velocity, 27, 30, 64, 75, 78–90
   waveform analysis, 50–53

Cerebral blood volume
   PET and, 163, 167–168
   SPECT and, 149–150, 155–157
Cerebrospinal fluid, 124–126, 133, 135
Cerebrotendinous xanthomatosis, 133
Circle of Willis, 17, 28–30, 76, 82, 87, 91, 100, 102, 107, 112
Clamping, intraoperative, 111–114, 177–182
Claudication, brachial, 45–46
$CMRO_2$, 163–168
Collateral blood flow
   carotid clamping and, 114
   ophthalmic pressure and, 27, 29
   pathways, 82–84, 88
Collimator design, 150
Collodion, 176
Color-flow Doppler imaging, 5–6, 15
   B-mode imaging and, 64
   duplex scannimg and, 63–64
   mitral regurgitation and, 7–8
   shunts and, 14
   stenosis and, 6
Common carotid artery(ies)
   CBF measurement and, 176
   compression testing, 82–90, 97–99, 106, 113, 119
   duplex scamning of, 50, 55, 57, 59
   identification of, 19, 36
   insonation, 30–33, 36
Computerized spectral waveform analysis, 61–62
Computerized tomography, 85–86, 123–146
Congestive heart failure, 9
Continuous-wave Doppler echocardiography, 5, 15
Continuous-wave Doppler ultrasound
   accuracy, 34–35
   applications, 91
   of carotid artery flow, 19–21
   of carotid bifurcation, 19–21, 30–31
   of carotid endarterectomy, 35
   compared to B-mode imaging, 35
   duplex scanning and, 49–65
   of extracranial cerebral arteries, 27–48
   insonation angle, 28
   limitations, 34–35
   in screening for TIA, 35
   stenosis, 5, 20
   transcranial Doppler and, 103
   in vertebrobasilar system, 36–47, 103
   zero crossing waveforms, 31–32, 34
Contralateral compression test, 83–84, 88
Contrast medium-enhanced (CME) CT, 85–86
Cortical infarction, 123–125
Coumarin, 44
Covibration phenomena, 94, 100
Creutzfeldt-Jakob disease, 133
"Critical perfusion" state, 164–165, 168

Index

Cross-clamping, 111–114
Cytomegalovirus encephalitis, 133

Deafferentation, 169
Dementia, 128, 132, 134–135, 143, 157
Dental prophylaxis, 7
Diabetes, 125
Diamine dithiol (DADT), 149
Diamox. *See* Acetazolamide
Diaschisis, 154, 169
Diethyldithiocarbamate (DDC), 149, 151, 154
Diffuse white matter hypodensities, 128, 133–136
Digital subtraction angiography, 27, 99–100
Digital subtraction arteriography, 96, 99
Diplopia, 46
Direct imaging, 18
Directional Doppler techniques, 18–21, 29, 31
Disturbances, flow, 2, 19, 20–21, 27–28, 94
Doppler
    angle and duplex scanning, 55–57
    echocardiography, 1–15
    effect, 19
    frequency analysis, 51–54, 56
    shift, 2, 64, 100, 105
Duplex scanning. *See* Ultrasonic duplex scanning
Dysmetabolism, 169

ECA. *See* External carotid artery
Echocardiography, 1–15, 36, 91
Electrocardiogram, 11
Electroencephalogram, 75, 105, 112, 176–184
Embolization, 11, 21
    in carotid bifurcation, 17
    in carotid endarterectomy, 111, 175
    intraoperative, 175, 179, 181–182
Encephalitis
    cytomegalovirus, 133
    subcorticalis chronica progressiva, 128
Encephalomalacia, macrocystic, 124–126
Encephalopathy
    acute necrotizing hemorrhagic, 133
    hypertensive, 133
    postoperative, 111
    subcortical arteriosclerotic, 47 128–136
Endarterectomy, carotid. *See* Carotid endarterectomy
Endocarditis, 6, 11
Epileptic seizures, 154
Epinephrine, 117
Ethrane, 180, 183
External carotid artery(ies)
    collateralization, 85
    identification of, 19
    insonation, 30–32
    spikes in, 58
    stenosis, 21
    velocity waveform of, 19–21, 50, 57
External occipital artery, 36

Extracranial carotid artery disease, 60, 105–109
Extracranial vertebral arteries, 36–47
Extraventricular obstructive hydrocephalus, 133–134

Fan beam collimator, 150
Fast Fourier transform, 31-32, 51
FDG, 164
Fentanyl, 183
Fibrosis, 6
Fistulas, 99–105
Fluorodeoxyglucose, 164
Focal neurologic dysfunction, 17
Foramen transversarum, 22, 24, 40
Forane, 180, 183–184

Gadolinium diethylenetriaminepentaacetic acid, 123
Galen's veins, 138
Gamma camera, 150, 154, 158
Gated blood pool scanning, 9
Gd-DTPA, 123
Gliosis, 124, 126
Glucose, 147, 163–164, 166–168, 170–171
Glycolysis, 164, 168
Gray matter, 127, 129, 148, 152

Halothane, 180–184
Hammocking, 8
Hemiparesis, 153, 159
Hemodynamic patency, 155–157
Hemorrhage, 94, 140
Heparin, 44, 47, 96, 99, 102
Hexamethyl propylene amine oxime. *See* HMPAO
HIPDM, 148–151
HMPAO, 149, 151, 152, 154
Hunt and Hess scale, 105
Hydrocephalus, 133
Hydrogen density, 123
Hypercapnia, 107–108, 114, 155
Hyperemia, 36, 108, 111, 166
Hyperperfusion, 112
Hyperplasia, 58
Hypertension, 125, 128
Hypocapnia, 100, 102, 107–108, 114
Hypoperfusion, 111, 114, 150, 155, 163, 168
Hypoplasia, 102, 107
Hypoxia, 114, 154

ICA. *See* Internal carotid artery
IMP, 147–162, 172
Indicator fractionation technique 150–151
Inferior petrosal sinus, 137
Initial slope technique, 176
Insonation angle, 28
Insonation depths, 78–85, 96–98, 100–102
Internal carotid artery(ies)

blind stump, 32, 34
CCA compression testing, 82–85, 87, 92, 97
continuous-wave Doppler and, 30–35
disease classification, 54, 60
identification of, 19, 82–85, 87, 103
insonation, 81, 92
lesions, 29
occlusion of, 20, 28, 30, 32, 35, 49, 96, 107–109, 115, 150, 166
recanalization, 96
stenosis, 20, 21, 24, 30, 33, 35, 49, 51, 64, 94, 150, 155
velocity waveform of, 19–21
Internal jugular vein, 50, 64
Interventricular septum, 3–5, 11–12
Intracardiac shunts, 11
Intracerebral neuronal diaschisis, 154
Intracranial
    artery identification, 82–90, 97, 103
    cerebrovascular disease, 96–99
    pressure, 112–113
    vertebrobasilar segment, 40–43
Intraluminal thrombus, 22, 51, 136
Intraoperative monitoring, 111–114
Intraosseous vertebral segment, 40
Intraplaque thrombus, 22
Intrathoracic anastomatic channels, 40
Intravenous angiography, 27
Intraventricular obstructive hydrocephalus, 133–134
Iodoamphetamines. *See* IMP
Ischemic brain infarction, 124, 152–155
N-Isopropyl-*p*-iodoamphetamine. *See* IMP

Jugular vein, 22, 50, 55, 64

Kappa statistic, 51, 53, 63
Karmann's eddy formation, 27
Kety-Schmidt method, 163, 164

Lactacidosis, 168
Lacunar infarction, 47, 94, 125–126
Language processing, 170–171
Leiomyosarcoma, 9
Leptomeningeal anastomosis, 90
Leukoaraiosis, 128
Leukoencephalopathy, 128–129, 131 133, 135
Leukomalacia, 128
Lipophilic sequestration system, 147
Long-bore collimator, 150
Lumbar tap, 99
Lupus vasculitis, 124
"Luxury perfusion" syndrome, 154, 164–165

Magnetic resonance imaging, 123–146, 169–171
Malformations, arteriovenous, 76, 99–106, 115, 139–140, 142–143

Mastoidal process, 36
Medullary infarction, 128
Meningitis, bacterial, 133
Methotrexate-induced leukoencephalopathy, 133
Microangiopathy, 36, 94
Middle cerebral artery (MCA)
    angioma in, 100
    blood flow velocity, 75
    CCA compression testing, 82–89
    extracranial occlusive disease in, 103–105, 107–119
    hyperemia in, 96
    identification of, 77–78
    infarction, 152
    occlusion, 94
Migraine, 114, 115
"Misery-perfusion" state, 164
Mitral regurgitation, 5, 6–8, 20
Mitral stenosis, 1, 6–7
Mitral valve
    leaflet, 3–4, 7, 13
    prolapse, 6–8, 11, 20
M-mode echocardiography, 1–8, 10
Mountain sickness, 76, 114, 115
Multidetector gamma camera, 150
Multiple sclerosis, 133, 142
Muscular dystrophy, 133
Myocardial function, 9–11
Myocardial infarction, 6, 9, 11
Myointimal hyperplasia, 58

"No reflow" phenomenon, 112
Nystagmus, 46

Oat cell tumors, 147
Occlusion
    basilar artery, 42
    carotid artery, 20, 31–34, 140
    common carotid artery, 58
    diagnosis, 31–35, 96
    internal carotid artery, 20, 28, 30, 32, 35, 49, 96, 107–109, 115, 150, 166
    segmental, 40
    "top-of-basilar," 97
    vascular, 138–141
    vertebral artery, 22
Oculoplethysmography, 18, 21
Oculopneumoplethysmography, 49
Ohm's law for fluids, 164
Ophthalmic artery
    insonation, 77, 81
    occlusion, 29
    as periorbital collateral channel, 27, 29
    pressure, 18–19, 20, 49
    reverse flow in, 28
    stenosis, 18
Ophthalmodynamometry, 18
Oscillatory shear stress, 58, 60
Osteodysplasia, polycystic, 133

Oxygen consumption, 163-168
Oxygen extraction fraction, 164-168

PAO, 149
Patency, hemodynamic, 155-157
Pendulum-like flow signal, 32, 34, 102, 105
Percutaneous transliminal angioplasty, 44, 108
Perfusion agents, 147-149
Perfusion pressure, 18-19, 29, 41, 43, 103, 105, 111, 114, 150, 155, 164-165
Pericardial diseases, 9
Periorbital Doppler flow studies, 28-30
Periventricular
    atherosclerotic leukoencephaly, 128
    hypodensity, 128-129, 131-132
    leukomalacia, 128
    translucencies, 94
Permanent regressive ischemic neurologic deficits, 155, 157
PET. *See* Positron emission tomography
Phonoangiography, quantitative, 49
N-Piperidinyl ethyl DADT, 149
Plasminogen activator, 102
Pneumooculoplethysmography, 18
Polycystic lipomembranous osteodysplasia, 133
Positron emission tomography, 123, 152, 154-155, 163-174
Post-endarterectomy stenosis, 59
Posterior cerebral artery (PCA)
    angioma, 100
    CCA compression testing, 82-87, 89
    extracranial occlusive disease in, 103-105, 117, 119
    identification of, 77, 79, 92
    occlusion, 94
Posterior collateral pathway, 82-84
Posterior communicating artery, 77, 82-84, 87, 97, 99, 109, 114
Posterior fossa infarction, 126-128
Posterior inferior cerebellar artery, 22, 96-97, 102, 153
Poststenotic disturbed flow, 27
PRIND, 155, 157
Propyleneamine oxime, 149
Prostaglandins, 163
Pulsatility index, 112
Pulsed Doppler echocardiography, 2-5
Pulsed Doppler ultrasound, 49-65

rCBF. *See* Regional cerebral blood flow
Real-time B-mode ultrasonography, 18, 20, 21-22, 49, 64
    see also Ultrasonic duplex scanning
Real-time Doppler imaging. *See* Color-flow Doppler imaging
Recanalization, 96, 107-108, 111, 113, 140
Regional cerebral blood flow
    with SPECT, 148, 149-151

    transcranial Doppler and, 75
Region of interest, 151
Reperfusion, 166
Rephasing phenomenon, 138
Resistance index, 102
Respiratory acidosis, 147
Restenosis, incidence of, 60
Reverberating flow signal, 32, 34, 41, 102, 105
Reversed flow, 28, 30, 36, 58
Reversible ischemic neurologic deficit, 129
Rheumatic disease, 6, 7
RIND, 129
Rotating gamma camera, 150, 154, 157

Sagittal sinus, 138
Saphenous vein patch graft, 175
SEP, 75
Shift, Doppler, 2, 64, 100, 105
Shunt(s)
    carotid endarterectomy and, 114, 175-176, 178-184
    flow, 14
    intracardiac, 11
    intracranial arteriovenous, 103
Shuttle flow, 30, 36, 41
Sigmoid sinus, 138-139
Single photon emission computerized tomography (SPECT)
    applications of, 152-157
    for carotid endarterectomy, 157
    cerebral blood volume and, 149-150
    instrumentation, 150
    perfusion agents in, 147-149
    regional CBF and, 148, 149-151
    techniques of, 151-152
    in TIA, 155-157
Slant-hole collimator, 150
Sokoloff model, 167-168
Somatosensory evoked potention (SEP), 75, 112
SPECT. *See* Single photon emission computerized tomography
Spectral waveform analysis
    computer-aided, 61-62
    duplex scanning with, 51-54, 56
    pattern recognition process, 63-64
Steal mechanism. *See* Subclavian steal mechanism
Stenosis
    aortic, 5, 7, 9, 20
    arterial, 31
    blood flow and, 27
    carotid artery
        external, 21
        internal, 20, 21, 24, 35, 49
        ophthalmic pressure and, 19
        recurrent, 60, 181
        signal intensity in, 141
    color-flow Doppler and, 6
    continuous-wave Doppler and, 5, 20

diagnosis, 27, 31–35, 96, 107
  duplex scanning and, 50–51, 54, 60
  mitral, 1, 6–7
  ophthalmic artery, 18
  post-endarterectomy, 59
  pulsed Doppler and, 5
  recurrent, 60, 181
  vertebral artery, 22–23
Sternocleidomastoidal muscle, 36
Stump pressure, 111–112, 114, 181
Subarachnoid hemorrhage, 75, 105, 112
Subclavian artery, 24, 36, 38, 40, 42
Subclavian steal mechanism, 36, 38–40, 42, 45–46, 76, 97, 100, 108–111
Subcortical
  arteriosclerotic encephalopathy, 47, 128–136
  incidental lesions, 128, 170
  lacunar infarction, 169
Submandibular TCD approach, 77, 85–87, 92, 94
Suboccipital TCD approach, 77, 79, 85–87, 91
Superficial temporal artery, 36, 58
Supraclinoidal carotid siphon, 77, 85
Supraorbital directional Doppler, 19, 21, 49
Supratrochlear artery, 29

Tapered lead collimator, 176
TCD. See Transcranial Doppler ultrasonography
Technetium-99m, 149, 151, 154, 155
Thalamic hypometabolism, 169
Thallium-201 diethyldithiocarbamate, 149, 151, 154
Three-dimensional imaging, 117, 163
Thromboembolism, 23–24
Thrombosis, basilar, 41–42
Thrombus
  atrial, 12
  diagnosis of, 138–140
  formation, 23–24, 40, 44
  intraluminal, 22, 51, 136
  intraplaque, 22
  ventricular, 13
TIA. See Transient ischemic attack
Transcranial Doppler ultrasonography (TCD), 40
  angiography and, 99–100, 107
  applications of, 76
  AV malformations and, 99–105
  CBF monitoring by, 109–114
  in cerebral vasospasm, 105
  cerebrovascular disease diagnosis, 90–96
  compression testing in, 86–90, 97–99
  continuous-wave Doppler and, 103
  errors in, 99
  extracranial occlusive disease, 105–109
  fistulas and, 99–105
  functional tests with, 114–117
  future of, 117–119
  intracranial blood flow velocity and, 105–109

  intracranial cerebrovascular disease and, 96–99
  in subarachnoid hemorrhage, 105
  techniques, 36, 76–85
  ultrasound windows, 77–85
Transient flow reversal, 58
Transient ischemic attack (TIA)
  carotid endarterectomy for, 17, 177–178, 183–184
  CW Doppler screening for, 35
  diagnosis, 17
  magnetic resonance in, 123, 129
  SPECT and, 155–157
  vasomotor reactivity in, 115
Transneuronal inactivation, 169
Transnuchal anastomotic channels, 40
Transorbital TCD approach, 77, 80–81, 87, 90, 94, 97, 105–106
Transtemporal TCD approach, 77–78, 87–89, 98, 119
Transverse foramina, 22, 24, 40
Transverse process, 24
Transverse sinus, 135–136, 138
N,N,N'-Trimethyl-N'-(2-hydroxy-3-methyl-5-iodobenzyl)-1,3-propanediamine. See HIPDM
Tuberous sclerosis, 133
Turbulence, 2, 19, 20–21, 27–28, 94
Two-dimensional echocardiography, 1, 6–13

Ultrasonic arteriography, 49, 105
Ultrasonic duplex scanning
  blood flow velocity and, 50–53
  B-mode imaging and, 20, 49–65
  of carotid bifurcation, 60
  compared with CW Doppler, 49–65
  and Doppler angle, 55–57
  errors in, 55–58
  as postoperative followup, 60
  technique, 53–60
  waveforms in, 51–53
Ultrasonoscope, 1
Ultrasound windows, 77–85, 92
Urokinase, 99

Valsalva's maneuver, 102
Valvular disease, 11
Vasculitis, 133
Vasomotor reactivity, 107–109, 114–115, 157
Vasospasm, 99, 105, 112
Ventricular aneurysms, 9
Vertebral artery(ies)
  compression testing, 96–97
  extracranial, 36–47
  extradural distal, 79, 85
  imaging, 22–24, 36
  insonation, 81
  intradural distal, 80, 85, 102

stenosis, 22–23
Vertebrobasilar system
   continuous-wave Doppler in, 36–47
   disease diagnosis in, 59
   TCD in, 91, 96–119
Vertigo, 22–23, 46

Waveform analysis, 51–54, 56, 61–64

Wernicke's area, 170–171
White matter, 126–129, 131, 133–136, 148, 152, 183

Xenon computerized tomography
   blood flow measurements and, 75, 163, 176
   rCBF and, 75, 149, 155, 157
Zero-crossing meter, 31–32, 34, 39

AES2909